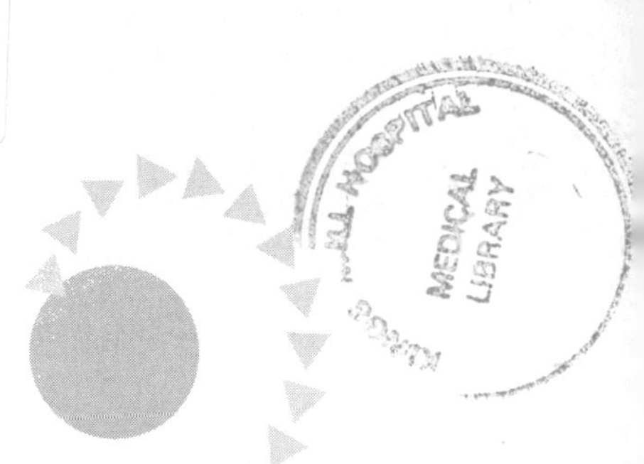

Recent Advances in

Surgery 28

Recent Advances in Surgery 27

Edited by C. D. Johnson & I. Taylor

ISBN 1–85315–571–3
ISSN 0143–8395

Recent Advances in

Surgery 28

Edited by

I. Taylor MD ChM FRCS FMedSci FRCPS(Glas)Hon

Vice-Dean and Director of Clinical Studies
David Patey Professor of Surgery, Royal Free and University College London Medical School, University College London, London, UK

C. D. Johnson MChir FRCS

Reader and Consultant Surgeon, University Surgical Unit, Southampton General Hospital, Southampton, UK

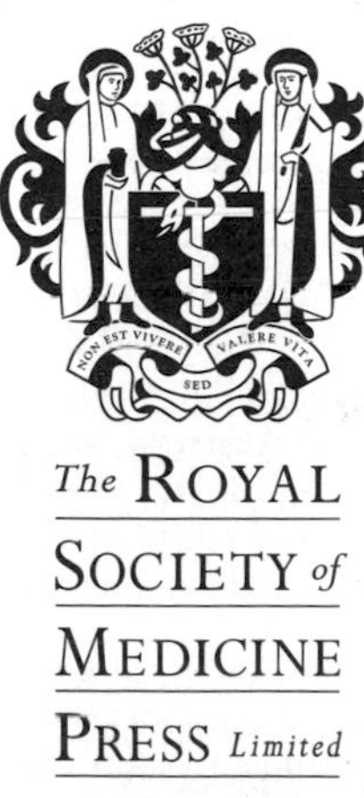

The ROYAL SOCIETY of MEDICINE PRESS Limited

Published by the Royal Society of Medicine Press Ltd
1 Wimpole Street, London W1G 0AE, UK
Tel: +44 (0) 20 7290 2921
Fax: +44 (0) 20 7290 2929
Email: publishing@rsm.ac.uk
Website: www.rsmpress.co.uk

The authors are responsible for the scientific content and for the views expressed, which are not necessarily those of the Royal Society of Medicine, or of the Royal Society of Medicine Press Ltd. Medical knowledge is constantly changing. As new information becomes available, changes in treatment, procedures, equipment and the use of drugs become necessary. The editors and the publishers have, as far as possible, taken care to ensure that the information given in this text is accurate and up to date. However, readers are strongly advised to confirm that the information, especially with regard to drug usage, complies with current legislation and standards of practice.

British Library Cataloguing in Publication Data
A catalogue record for this book is available from the British Library
ISBN 1-85315-610–8
ISSN 0143 8395

Distribution in Europe and Rest of World:
Marston Book Services Ltd
PO Box 269, Abingdon, Oxon OX14 4YN, UK
Tel: +44 ((0) 1235 465500
Fax: +44 (0) 1235 465555
Email: direct.order@marston.co.uk

Distribution in USA and Canada:
Royal Society of Medicine Press Ltd
c/o Jamco Distribution Inc., 1401 Lakeway Drive, Louisville, Texas 75057, USA
Tel: +1 800 538 1287
Fax: +1 972 353 1303
Email: jamco@majors.com

Distribution in Australia and New Zealand:
Elsevier Australia, 30–52 Smidmore Strreet, Marrickville NSW 2204, Australia
Tel: +61 2 9517 8999
Fax: +61 2 9517 2249
Email: service@elsevier.com.au

Commissioning editor - Peter Richardson
Editorial assistant - Shirley Mukisa
Production by BA & GM Haddock, Midlothian, UK
Printed in Great Britain by Bell & Bain, Glasgow, UK

Contents

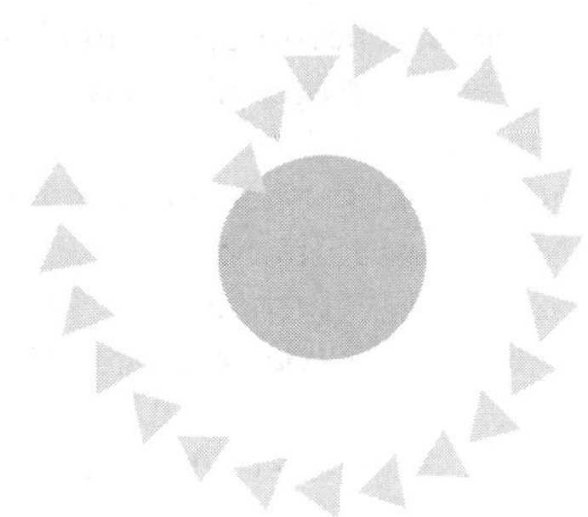

Contributors

Sayed Aly PhD FRCS
Consultant Vascular & Endovascular Surgeon, Mater University Hospital, Dublin, Ireland

Stephen G.E. Barker MS FRCS
Senior Lecturer/Consultant, The Academic Vascular Surgery Unit, Middlesex Hospital, London, UK

Fernando Bello PhD BSc MIEEE
Lecturer in Surgical Graphics and Computing, Department of Surgical Oncology & Technology, Imperial College, London, UK

Willem A. Bemelman MD
Academic Medical Center, Department of Surgery, Amsterdam, The Netherlands

Owen Boyd FRCA FRCP MD
Lead Consultant in Intensive Care Unit, Royal Sussex County Hospital, Brighton, UK

Nicholas R. Brook BSc MSc BM MRCS(Ed)
Specialist Registrar in Urology, Transplant Surgery Group, Department of Cardiovascular Sciences, University Hospitals of Leicester NHS Trust, Leicester, UK

Orf R.C. Busch MD
Academic Medical Center, Department of Surgery, Amsterdam, The Netherlands

David Chao BMBCh MRCP DPhil
Consultant Medical Oncologist, Department of Clinical Oncology, Royal Free Hospital, London, UK

Marcel Gatt MD, MRCSEd
Surgical Research Registrar, Combined Gastroenterology Unit, Scarborough Hospital, Scarborough, North Yorkshire, UK

Talvinder Singh Gill MBBS MS FRCS(Glas)
Specialist Registrar, Department of Surgery, Queen's Medical Centre, University Hospital NHS Trust, Nottingham, UK

Dirk J. Gouma MD
Professor, Academic Medical Center, Department of Surgery, Amsterdam, The Netherlands

Alison Halliday MS FRCS
Consultant Vascular Surgeon and Reader in Cardiovascular Sciences, St George's Hospital, London, UK

Majid Hashemi FRCS
Senior Lecturer/Consultant in Upper Gastrointestinal and Bariatric Surgery, Royal Free and University College Medical School, Whittington Campus, London, UK

Colin D. Johnson MChir FRCS
Reader in Surgery, University Surgical Unit, Southampton General Hospital, UK

Allan E. Kark FRCS FACS
Surgeon, British Hernia Centre, London, UK

Mohammed R.S. Keshtgar FRCSI FRCS(Gen) PhD
Senior Lecturer and Consultant Surgical Oncologist, Department of Surgery, University College London, London, UK

Roger L. Kneebone PhD FRCS FRCSEd MRCGP
Senior Lecturer in Surgical Education, Department of Surgical Oncology & Technology, Imperial College, London, UK

Sunil Kumar MS DNB FRCS(Ed), FRCS(Eng)
Senior Consultant, Department of Surgery, Tata Main Hospital, Jamshedpur, India

Martin Kurzer MBBS FRCS
Surgeon, British Hernia Centre, London, UK

Richard Leigh BSc MChS
Chief Podiatrist, Department of Podiatry, UCLH Trust, Middlesex Hospital, London, UK

John MacFie MB ChB MD FRCS
Consultant Surgeon, Combined Gastroenterology Unit, Scarborough Hospital, Scarborough, North Yorkshire, UK

Ursula B. McGovern BSc MBCh MRCP
SpR Medical Oncology, Department of Oncology, North Middlesex Hospital, London, UK

Michael L. Nicholson MD FRCS
Professor of Transplant Surgery, Transplant Surgery Group, Department of Cardiovascular Sciences, University Hospitals of Leicester NHS Trust, Leicester, UK

Hari I. Pandey MS MCh
Consultant Surgeon, Tata Main Hospital, Jamshedpur, India

Prabhjot Saggu MBBS DNB(Std)
Resident Surgeon, Tata Main Hospital, Jamshedpur, India

John H. Scholefield MB ChB FRCS ChM
Professor of Surgery, Queen's Medical Centre, University Hospital NHS Trust, Nottingham, UK

Nigel Scott FRCS
Consultant Surgeon, Hope Hospital, Salford, Manchester, UK

Dinesh Singhal MS, DNB
Consultant, Department of Surgical Gastroenterology, Max Healthcare Group of Hospitals, Patarganj and Saket, New Delhi, India

Dominic Slade MBChB FRCS
Specialist Registrar in General Surgery, Hope Hospital, Manchester, UK

Irving Taylor MD ChM FRCS FMedSci FRCPS(Glas)Hon
David Patey Professor of Surgery, Vice-Dean and Director of Clinical Studies, Royal Free and University College Medical School, London, UK

Jane Turner BSc
Research Assistant, Academic Vascular Surgery Unit, Middlesex Hospital, London, UK

Stella Vig MCh FRCS
Consultant Vascular Surgeon, St George's Hospital, London, UK

Jonathan Winehouse MSc FRCS
Lecturer and Honorary Registrar in Surgery, Royal Free and University College Medical School, London, UK

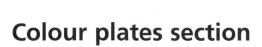

Colour plates section

All the colour figures are printed in order of appearance. The chapter reference is given for each figure.

CHAPTER 1

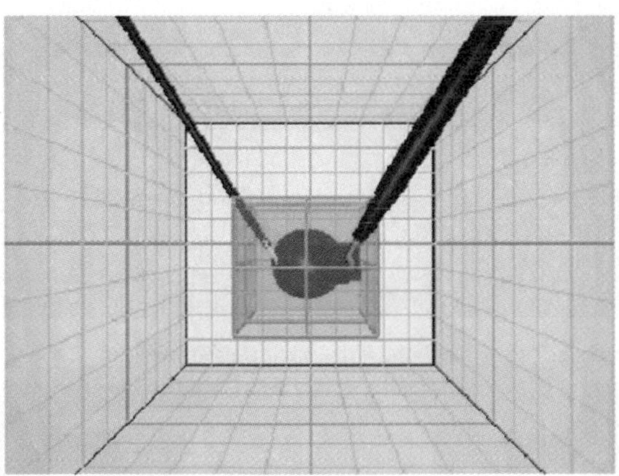

Plate I Basic skills simulator using abstract scenes.

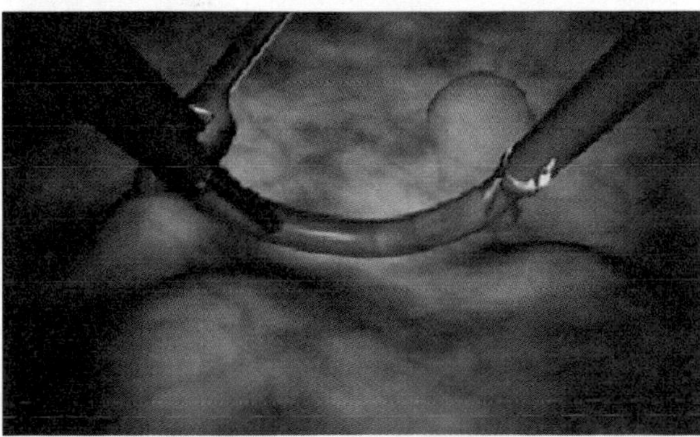

Plate II Basic skills simulator using procedure-related tasks.

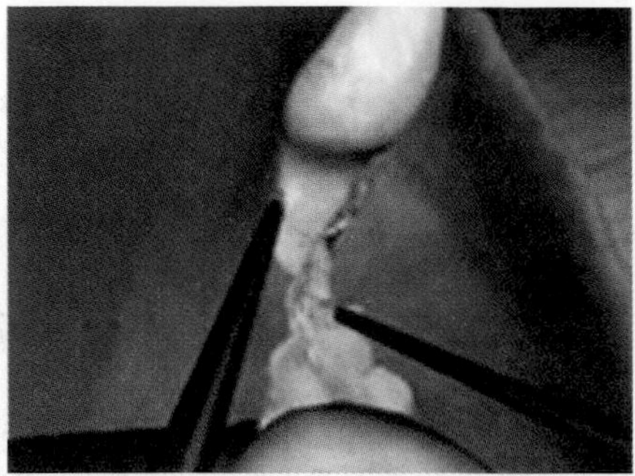

Plate III Simulation of laparoscopic cholecystectomy.

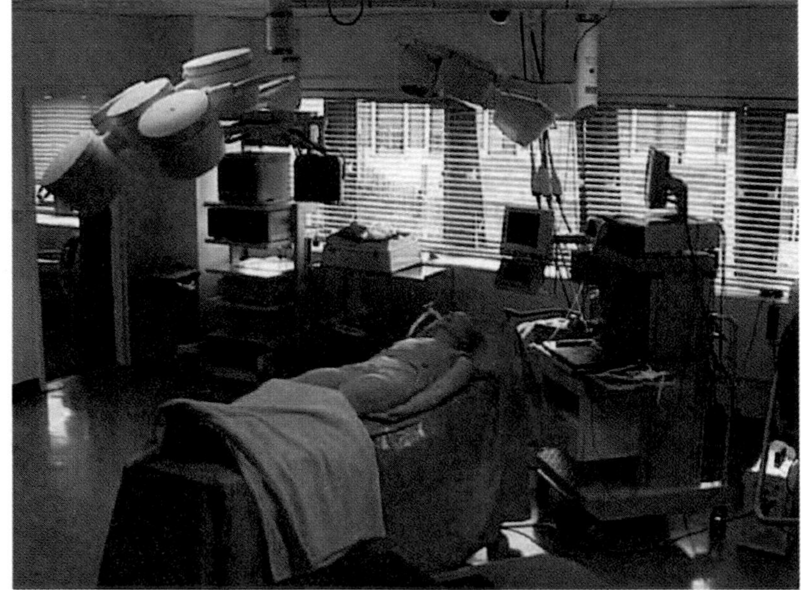

Plate IV Simulated operating theatre with patient mannequin.

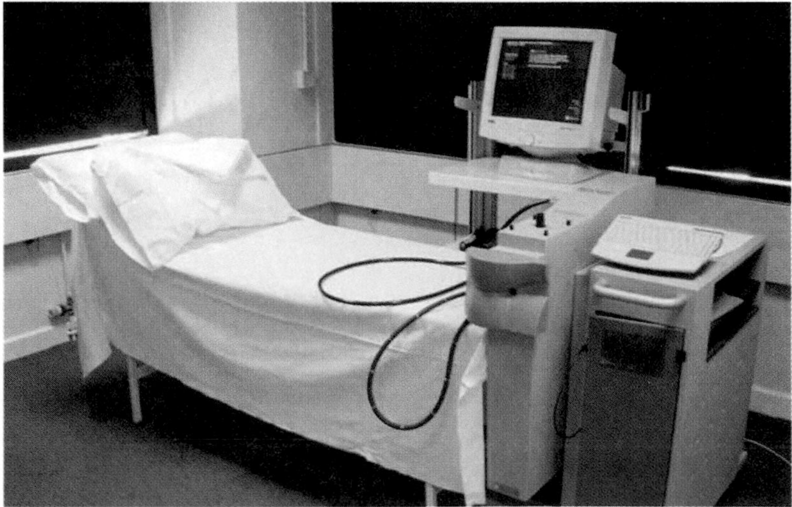

Plate V Endoscopy simulator in patient–practitioner setting.

CHAPTER 4

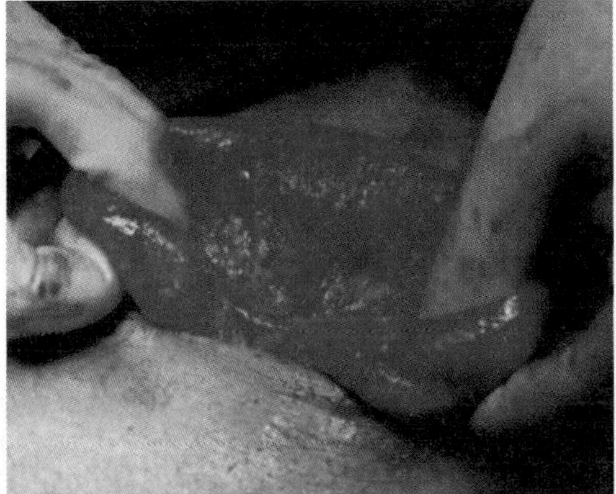

Plate VI Miliary tubercles.

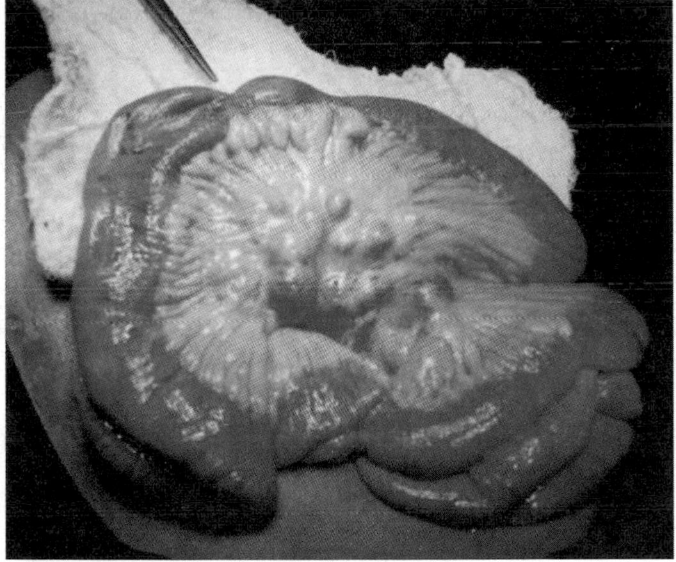

Plate VII Tuberculous stricture and nodes.

CHAPTER 5

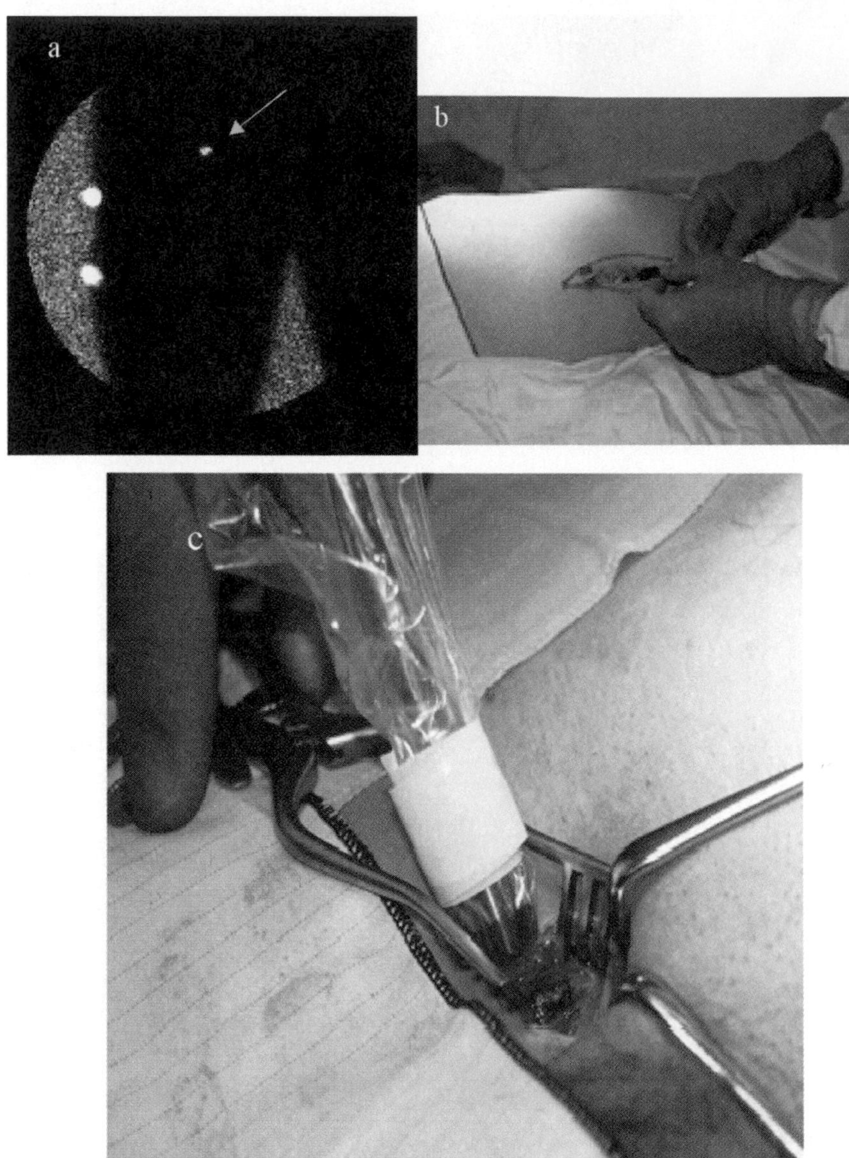

Plate VIII (a) A lymphoscintigram showing the injection site of radiocolloid at the site of excision scar right thigh. (b) Injection of patent blue dye. (c) Intra-operative detection of SLN using combined technique.

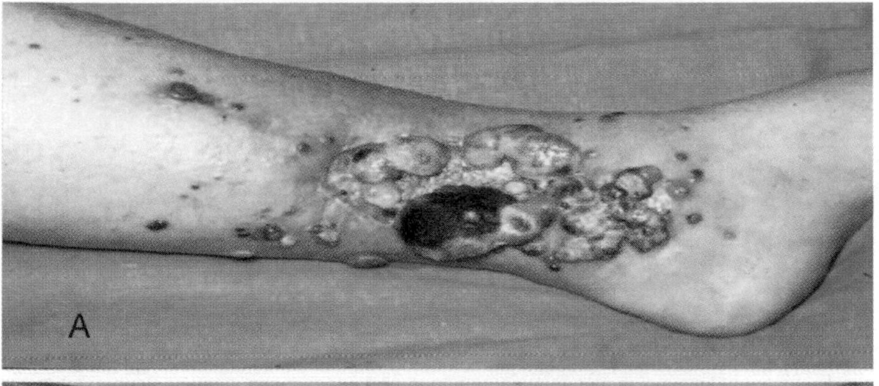

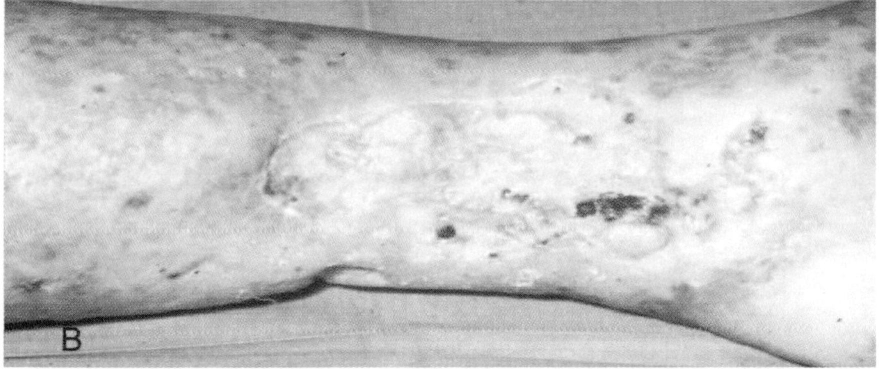

Plate IX Inoperable satellite metastases: (a) before regional chemotherapy; (b) after regional chemotherapy.

CHAPTER 8

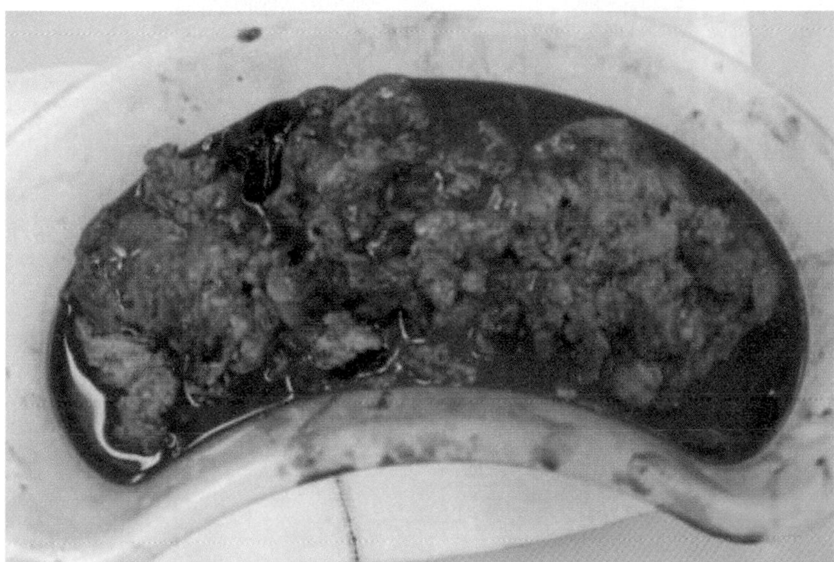

Plate X Solid material removed at necrosectomy. Radiological descriptions of necrosis often use terms such as 'fluid infiltrate' or 'fluid collections'. Percutaneous drainage of necrotic areas may release some pus, but the resolution of the infective process usually requires removal of solid material by a surgical approach.

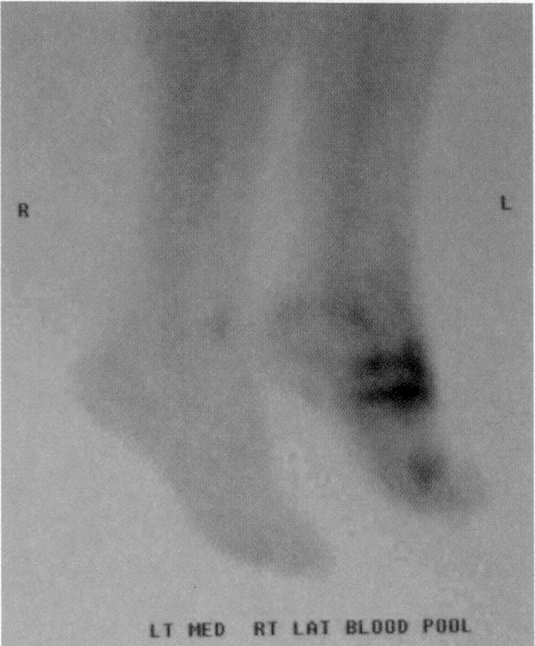

CHAPTER 13

Plate XI Bone scan showing unilateral increased radiolabel uptake in mid-tarsal Charcot's arthropathy.

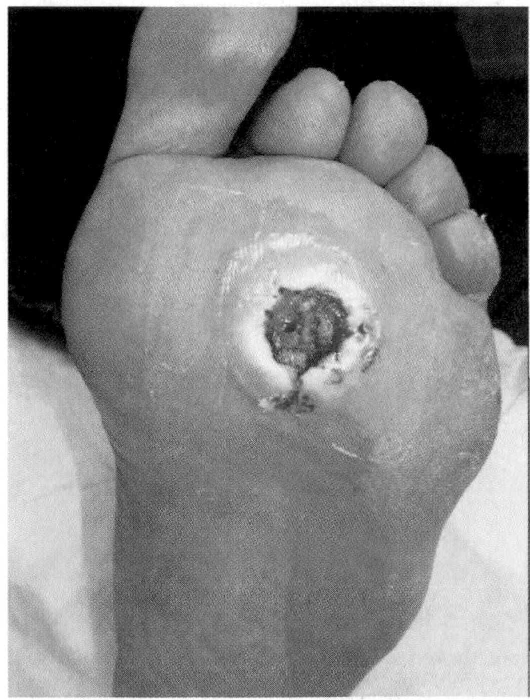

Plate XII Diabetic neuropathic ulceration.

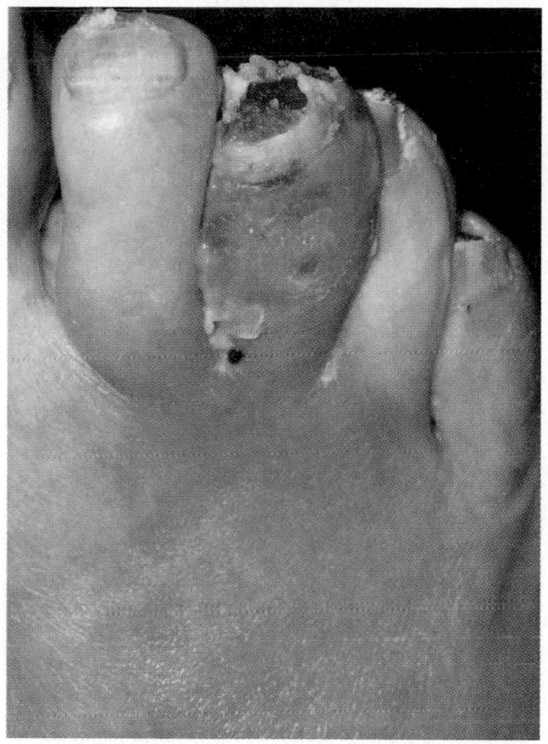

Plate XIII Cellulitis, gangrene and osteomyelitis in an infected 'sausage' toe.

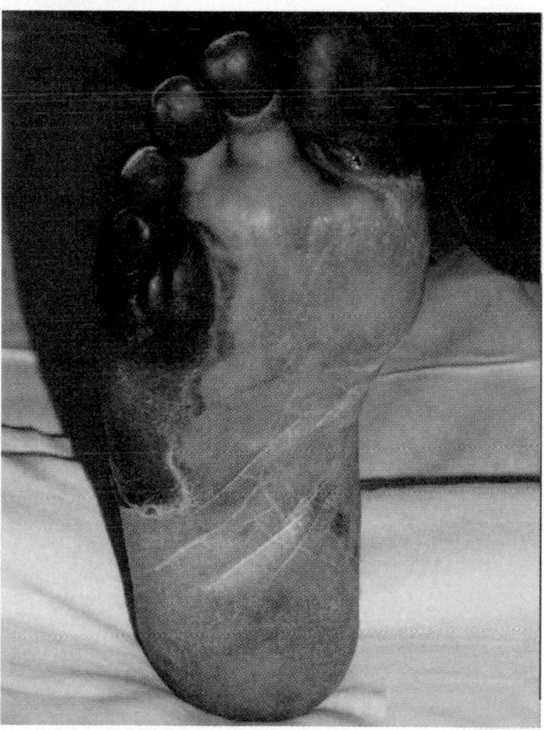

Plate XIV Dry gangrene associated with microvascular disease.

Chapter 14

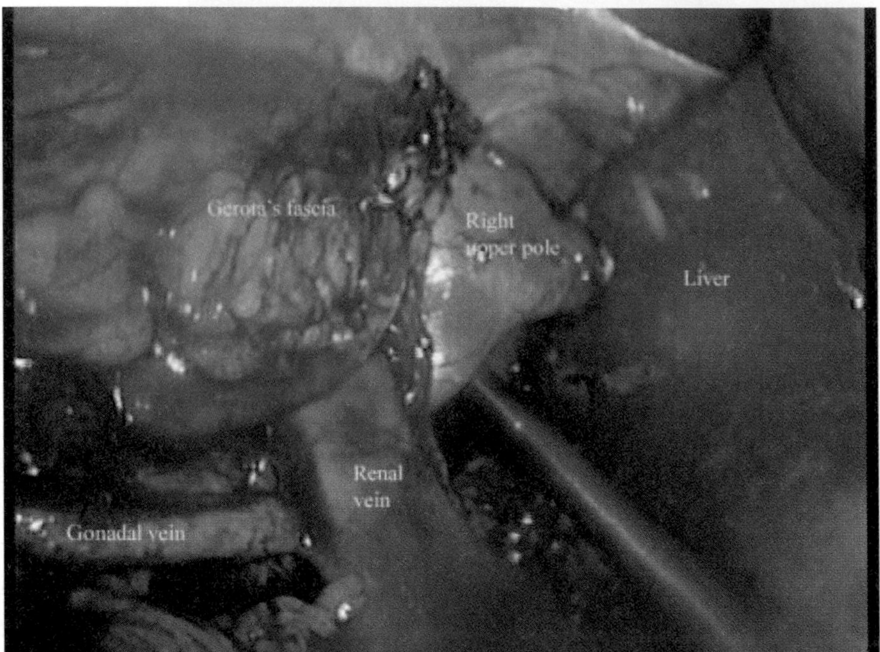

Plate XV Laparoscopic view at right donor nephrectomy.

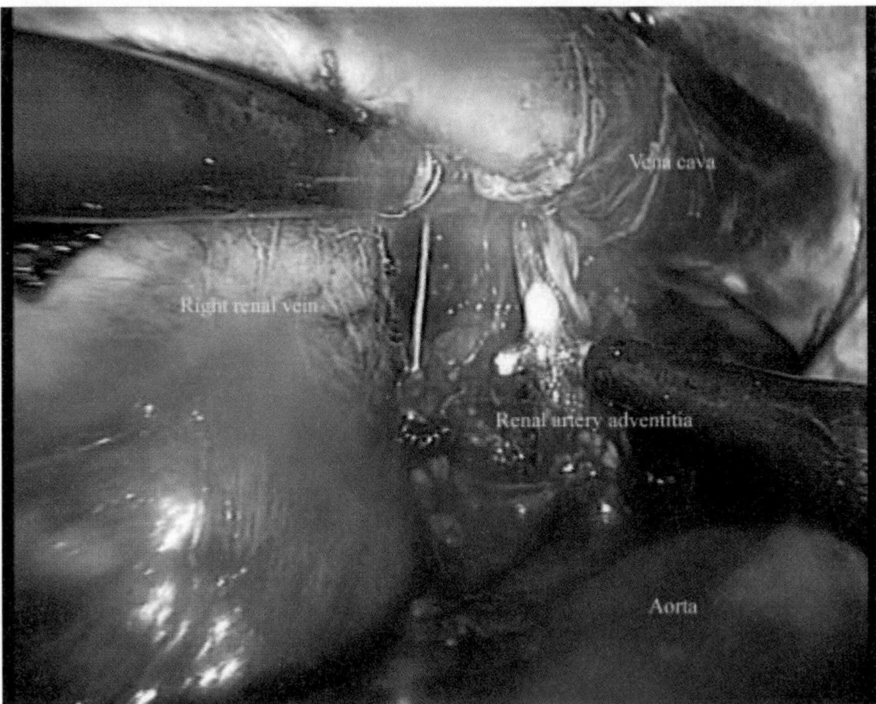

Plate XVI Laparoscopic view of the inter-aortocaval dissection, demonstrating the right renal artery. The vena cava is displaced anteriorly. Adventitia is being dissected from the artery with hook diathermy.

Roger L. Kneebone Fernando Bello

1

Technology in surgical education

This chapter considers the place of technology a time of far-reaching change for surgical training. A summary of relevant educational theory will be followed by a critical discussion of current technologies. The chapter ends with speculation about likely directions for future development.

BACKGROUND

In the past, surgeons learned their craft through a prolonged apprenticeship. Operating on patients within a service-driven system was a mainstay of training. At its best, this system offered excellent preparation for independent consultant practice. However, levels of supervision varied greatly, there was no generally accepted strategy for training, and learning objectives were often unclear.

Surgery is becoming increasingly specialised, new techniques are proliferating, and the wide-spread adoption of minimal access surgery places demands upon surgeons to acquire, maintain and develop a widening range of operative skills during the course of their careers. Such demands must be met within an increasingly cost-dominated NHS. The duration of training, moreover, has been dramatically reduced, and the Calman reforms have had far-reaching effects throughout the UK NHS.

These pressures have been compounded by the Working Time Directive, which will have a profound impact on patterns of surgical learning. The

*Colour figures (plates) referred to in this chapter are to be found in the 'Colour plates section' at the front of this volume (p1–8).

Roger L. Kneebone PhD FRCS FRCSEd MRCGP
Senior Lecturer in Surgical Education, Department of Surgical Oncology & Technology, Imperial College, London, UK. (E-mail: r.kneebone@imperial.ac.uk)

Fernando Bello PhD BSc MIEEE
Lecturer in Surgical Graphics and Computing, Department of Surgical Oncology & Technology, Imperial College, London, UK. (E-mail: f.bello@imperial.ac.uk)

introduction of the Foundation Programme, although aimed primarily at doctors in their first two years of practice, will also have repercussions at higher levels of surgical training. These changes are taking place against a background of rising public expectations and a growing sensitivity to ethical issues around the involvement of patients for training, especially in the early stages.

Since the traditional apprenticeship approach is undergoing such radical change, it can no longer be taken for granted that trainees will become competent simply by participating in surgical care. A much more structured approach is required, designed to achieve specified learning outcomes. Such training must address the needs of all learners, from novices to experienced consultants. It is here that technology has much to offer.

Educational technologies, including simulation, provide obvious benefits and will undoubtedly play an expanding role in the future. However, such technologies are driven by the commercial interests of developers as well as by the needs of trainees and educational providers, and pitfalls surround the uncritical adoption of new technology.[1] A familiarity with educational theory provides an essential framework.

Key point 1

- Surgical practice is changing dramatically and preservation of the status quo is not an option. Innovative approaches to training are essential if high standards are to be maintained.

EDUCATIONAL THEORY

Of the many factors which contribute to surgical expertise, operative skill often steals the limelight. In fact, of course, knowledge, professional judgement, decision-making skills, communication, team-working and a range of other attributes are also essential. Effective surgical education must address all of these. The following section summarises key educational theories and outlines how these relate to developments in technology.

Key point 2

- Surgical practice demands a complex mixture of knowledge, judgement, technical skill and effective team-working. Technology can improve learning in all these areas.

Creating conditions for learning

Effective learning needs a structure where learners and teachers share common aims. Although a curriculum is clearly essential, current training is often fragmented, with skills being learned in isolation as opportunities arise.

It is also clear that the conditions in which learning occurs exert a strong influence on learning outcomes. For example, a powerful though underestimated affective component to learning can exert positive or negative effects.[2–4] A supportive environment is essential if learning is to be maximised.[5]

This aim of giving priority to the learner's needs often conflicts with the pressures of real-world clinical practice, where opportunities for learning are circumscribed by the clinical needs of the patient. Simulation allows learners' needs to take centre stage, avoiding danger to real patients. Such technology can help learners to 'experience' aspects of practice, including those which might be profoundly distressing in real life, within a safe milieu specifically designed to support learning.[6]

Gaining expertise

In order to develop a secure knowledge base, learners require information. This should be relevant, immediately accessible and available when and where needed. Web-based learning environments, hand-held computers and the introduction of wireless 'information grids' have much to offer (see later).

Technical skills are crucial for every surgeon. The acquisition of psychomotor skill in any domain requires sustained deliberate practice over many years, underpinned by focused feedback.[7,8] Although much of the literature on expertise relates to sport and the performing arts, similar principles can be seen within surgery. Moreover, it is clear that simple repetition of tasks is not enough to ensure progress – each practitioner must be motivated to improve.[9] Expert tuition should be available when required, but should 'fade' when no longer needed in order to allow learners to become self-reliant.[10] The concept of 'scaffolding' describes expert support which remains sensitive to individuals' learning needs as they evolve.[11–13]

There is evidence, too, that any gains in psychomotor skill must be regularly reinforced, and that skills evaporate rapidly if such reinforcement does not occur.[14] It follows that effective training programmes should combine factual information with opportunities for repeated practice, underpinned by clear learning aims.

Simulation technology offers the opportunity to practise key tasks repeatedly, without jeopardising the safety of real patients. Task-based skills' workshops embody some of these principles, but isolated courses often fail to provide opportunities for extended practice.

Key point 3

- Training should allow regular context-based practice, providing expert feedback within a supportive, learner-centred *milieu*.

The importance of clinical context

Competence in performing specific tasks is only part of a wider picture. Safe surgical practice is a complex amalgam of knowledge, judgement, psychomotor skill and effective team-working. Technical skill is necessary, but not sufficient, for expert practice, and training must address wider issues of clinical context. Unless this happens, there is a risk that training will be confined to a parallel universe which fails to connect with real-world practice.

A contemporary view of apprenticeship highlights the importance of 'communities of practice', where newcomers learn by joining a group of professionals who share a common aim.[15,16] Although at first peripheral within the group, each newcomer's role becomes increasingly central as their experience and skills develop.[17] It follows that effective communication with other members of the surgical team (both within and beyond the operating theatre) is a key skill.

High fidelity situational simulations with debriefing allow members of surgical and anaesthetic teams to work together in conditions which reflect real-life practice. Such approaches allow teams to explore safely the consequences of potentially harmful actions and develop strategies for avoiding them. The successful integration of technical and team-working skills within an educational framework is a major challenge.[18]

Key point 4

- The context of learning is inseparable from the skills which are learned. Each surgical learning experience is unique and must be related to the specific needs of the learner.

Current practice

It is salutary to examine current surgical training in the light of the above summary. Relevant information may be difficult to access efficiently. Few training programmes provide opportunities for clinical reinforcement of newly acquired psychomotor skills. Sustained deliberate practice is often difficult to arrange, and expert tutors are in short supply. Team-working and communication are seldom addressed explicitly, and learning environments may or may not be perceived as supportive and learner centred.

The following sections will address specific areas where technology can assist in achieving these educational goals.

ACCESSING INFORMATION

The wide-spread use of the Worldwide Web, advances in mobile devices (PDAs, palmtop computers, tablet PCs) and the increased availability of broadband connections and wireless networks have resulted in vast improvements to the delivery and efficiency of information. Multimedia training packages[19] and collaborative web-based courseware materials incorporating advanced three-dimensional graphics, video footage and interactive simulation modules[20] are already having an impact in surgical education.[21–23]

Further efficiency in data integration, data processing and data exchange will be achieved through a new paradigm for distributed computing where information is stored, pre-processed and managed on a diverse collection of interconnected servers which together form an information Grid.[24] By combining Grid computing with wireless technology it will be possible to provide on-demand, mobile exchange of integrated patient information (*e.g.*

from medical records, laboratory results, clinical imaging) and trainee information (*e.g.* activity logs, video streams, personal notes, reference material) throughout a hospital or medical school.

> **Key point 5**
>
> - Technology is only one component of effective learning. A theory-grounded curriculum should underpin surgical training and ensure a connection between clinical and simulator-based experienced.

TRAINING BY SIMULATION

Simulation is already well established within surgical education and is used for teaching a wide variety of surgical skills, ranging from simple devices for knotting and suturing to elaborate recreations of actual operative procedures.

Simulators can be divided broadly into three categories – physical models, virtual reality (VR) computing, and hybrid simulators (Table 1). The next section will summarise current technology in this rapidly changing field, then offer a critique of its place in education.

PHYSICAL MODELS

Benchtop models are widely used within surgical training, especially at undergraduate and early postgraduate levels. Such models address a range of clinical procedures (*e.g.* venous cannulation, urinary catheterisation, basic suturing) as well as bowel and vascular anastomosis, hernia repair and other commonly performed surgical tasks. Advances in materials' technology have improved the realism of such models, which allow novices to practise tasks repeatedly, although divorced from their clinical context.

Recently, imaginative combinations of inanimate models with simulated patients (professional actors who take the part of patients) allow learners to practise and perform within realistic scenarios which reproduce the rich clues of an authentic clinical encounter.[25]

VIRTUAL REALITY COMPUTING

A rapidly expanding range of computer-generated simulations can now recreate many surgical procedures with a high degree of realism, allowing learners to interact with a convincing computer-based environment. Minimal access (MAS) procedures lend themselves especially to such simulations, as manipulating objects with surgical instruments on a 2-D screen reflects the reality of minimal access surgery. Learners choose procedures from a menu of varying levels of difficulty, and performance metrics (*e.g.* time taken, bleeding encountered, errors made) are recorded automatically.

The first generation of VR simulators focused on training basic skills by performing isolated tasks (*e.g.* pick and place, navigation) using abstract scenes (Plate I, p1). The second generation attempted to teach such skills using

Table 1 Summary of existing commercial surgical simulator systems

Type	Simulator	Comments
PHYSICAL		
	Pulsatile Heart Model[27]	Physical model of a beating heart including rib cage and pump
	Suture Tutor[27]	Skin pad and multimedia instruction CD ROM for practising basic wound closure
	Bowel and vascular trainers[27]	Benchtop models for anastomosis practice
VIRTUAL REALITY		
	MIST-VR[28]	Low fidelity key laparoscopic surgical techniques and high fidelity suturing
	LapSim[29]	High fidelity basic laparoscopic skills plus suturing and dissection. Gynaecology module available
HYBRID		
	VIST-VR[28]	Vascular interventional procedures, such as coronary, carotid and renal stenting, plus pacemaker lead placement. Incorporates force feedback
	SEP[30]	Basic laparoscopic skills and procedure-related tasks
	RLT[31]	Laparoscopic cholecystectomy simulator with force feedback
	LS500[32]	Laparoscopic cholecystectomy simulator with force feedback
	Angio Mentor[33]	Interventional endovascular basic skills and complete procedures
	LAP Mentor[33]	Basic laparoscopic skills and those required for cholecystectomy. Incorporates force feedback and high fidelity graphics
	PERC Mentor[33]	Percutaneous access procedures using fluoroscopy
	URO Mentor[33]	Cystoscopy and ureteroscopy procedures with real-time fluoroscopy. Flexible and rigid scopes
	GI Mentor[33]	Endoscopy simulator for colonoscopy and gastroscopy. Includes modules for ERCP practice
	Accutouch/ Cathsim[34]	Endoscopy and cardiac catheterisation simulators
	ProMIS[35]	Basic skills and techniques of minimally invasive surgery
	Metiman,[36] Simman,[37] Medsim[38]	Intelligent anaesthetic, ultrasound and emergency scenario dummies already employed in some universities

more realistic procedural tasks, such as clipping blood vessels or intracorporeal knotting (Plate II, p1). The current generation allows entire procedures (*e.g.* laparoscopic cholecystectomy) to be simulated (Plate III, p2).

The more complex a simulation and the more variables it offers, the greater the computing power it requires. There is, therefore, a trade-off between high visual fidelity on the one hand and the program's ability to respond in real time on the other. In addition, some simulators combine high-quality graphics with miniature servo motors that generate haptic feedback (the sensation of interacting with tissue while operating) to increase fidelity. This increases the demand for computing power even further, and most existing haptic feedback devices are not yet robust and reliable enough to be used routinely.

HYBRID SIMULATORS

These are perhaps the most interesting development, as they offer great potential for recreating the clinical context of practice. Hybrid simulators combine a physical model (replicating the instruments or interface) with a computer program (which creates interactive settings within which learning can take place). A key advantage of such technology is its potential for team training.

Sophisticated patient mannekins

Sophisticated patient mannekins (SimMan, METI) already offer a range of pathophysiological variables and can respond to the administration of drugs. They are well established within anaesthetic training, for example, and are becoming increasingly common within other domains. Such simulators may be used within a dedicated educational facility, such as a training centre or simulated operating theatre (Plate IV, p2), but also in the field. Portable mannekins allow realistic disaster scenarios to be mounted in a range of authentic settings.

Hybrid endoscopy simulators

Hybrid endoscopy simulators combine an authentic interface (the endoscope) with realistic VR displays of the endoluminal view seen by the operator (Plate V, p2). Different levels of difficulty allow novice and intermediate learners to gain the basics of manipulative skill through repeated practice. Recent work combining simulated patients with hybrid simulators introduces the additional dimension of patient–practitioner interaction during the procedure.[26]

ASSESSMENT AND VALIDATION

Simulation offers obvious benefits as a formative tool for training and is extensively used for this purpose already. A well-designed simulation can fulfil many of the educational desiderata outlined above, allowing repeated practice with expert feedback in a learner-centred environment which recreates the context of clinical practice without jeopardising patient safety.

> **Key point 6**
>
> - Simulation offers the opportunity to practise within a learner-centred environment which meets criteria for educational effectiveness yet avoids risk to patients.

As a tool for summative assessment, however, the place of simulation has yet to be confirmed. The need for objective assessment of skill in surgery is widely acknowledged,[39] and various tools for assessing psychomotor skills in open and laparoscopic surgery are now available. These include observational and video-based qualitative assessment systems (*e.g.* OSATS[40]) and quantitative motion analysis systems (*e.g.* ICSAD[41] and ADEPT[42]). The use of such assessment tools within simulator-based practice is increasing, but many simulators are introduced without robust validation.

Key point 7

- There is compelling evidence that simulation is an effective formative tool. Evidence of its effectiveness for assessment is much less robust.

The problem here is not obtaining data (VR and hybrid simulators can provide a multitude of quantitative performance metrics, including markers of technical error) but in validating simulators as proxies for surgical performance. Rigorous validation is, therefore, key to the acceptance of simulation within surgical practice. Clearly, the reliability of any validation, both across evaluators (inter-rater reliability) and between repeated tests (test-retest reliability), must also be established.

In the validation process, objective studies are used to demonstrate resemblance to a real world task (face validity) and to measure an identified and specific situation (content validity). Simple tests, such as construct validation, may show that an expert performs better than a novice in the model under test, while more complex, randomised controlled studies (concurrent validation) correlate the new method with a gold standard, such as apprenticeship.[43] Simulator-based competence should improve over time and with increasing operative experience, and it should be possible to discriminate between surgically naive and more experienced subjects.

If simulators are to be valid measures of operative ability, a surgeon's competence in a simulator should correlate with actual performance in the operating theatre. Although several studies have demonstrated the feasibility, reliability and validity of simulators as training aids in laparoscopic surgery,[44,45] very limited work has been done in studying the transfer of simulator training into operative performance.[46] Ultimately, predictive validity evaluates the impact on performance in a real procedure.

Key point 8

- Any new technology needs to be validated. The acid test for simulation is whether it maps onto clinical performance and leads to improved outcomes. Rigorous evaluation of educational technology is essential.

EVALUATING SIMULATIONS

Simulator-based training systems allow trainees to practice repeatedly, with permission to fail and to experience the consequences of error without endangering patients. Such an environment has clear educational, economic and efficiency advantages, particularly when learning technically complex procedures such as MAS – procedures whose very limitations make them especially suitable for computer-based simulations. Conditions which typically lead to erroneous behaviour can be recreated, and will support error-prevention strategies.

Educational resources are limited, however, and not all simulations are equally effective. When allocating resources, an informed yet critical detachment is essential. Successful simulation demands a symbiotic relationship between users and developers. For end-users (surgical trainers and trainees), simulators must meet educational needs and improve clinical practice. For simulator developers, however, technical development and profitability are key drivers. This tension can lead to unhelpful confusion about who is leading and who is following. This may divert attention from the key tasks of identifying training needs and working collaboratively towards reliable and valid systems which satisfy them.

The issue of simulator fidelity (realism) illustrates this point. At first sight, the highest achievable degree of realism might seem desirable for any simulation, and many developers go to great lengths to achieve this. However, the necessary degree of fidelity for any given set of skills is still open for discussion. Seen from this wider perspective, a lower level of fidelity may sometimes be preferable, as it can reduce technological limitations and cost while still ensuring educational effectiveness. No single level of realism will meet all needs, and effective decisions will require a closer collaboration between users and designers/manufacturers.

Key point 9

- The relationship between fidelity of a simulation and its effectiveness is not a simple one. Levels of realism should be tailored to meet educational goals within practical constraints of cost and technical feasibility.

Before adopting simulation within a training programme, it is important to ask key questions, including the following:

Which specific skills does the system address?

What level of fidelity is required to learn these skills?

To what extent do these skills transfer to the operating room?

Does the simulation system work reliably?

Does the system create conditions conducive to learning?

How does an hour of simulator time compare to an hour of traditional training methods?

Is this simulator cost effective? If not, when will it become so?

How can this simulator be integrated with existing training curricula? KP9

WHERE NEXT?

Surgical technology moves fast, and predicting the future is notoriously difficult. Based on current trends, likely areas for development in the immediate and medium-term include the following:

1. An increased availability of technology for learning needs prompted by clinical triggers ('just in time' learning), rather than reinforcing an artificial division between learning and clinical practice.
2. Cheaper and more widely available simulators, supported by increased access to wireless 'information grids' within clinical settings. This will allow clinical data to be accessed alongside learner-centred training programmes.
3. Patient-specific simulations of specific operative procedures which will allow surgeons to practise pre-operatively, combining scanned images of a patient's anatomy and pathology with computerised simulations of the procedure itself (augmented reality).
4. An increasing awareness of the importance of context will be strengthened by a move away from task-based training to a more team-based approach, recreating the pressures and realities of everyday practice.
5. Hybrid simulations will continue to expand, providing clinical challenges within a realistic, yet safe, environment. Such simulators will allow individuals and teams to explore the consequences of their actions or decisions, and test alternative pathways of care 'to destruction' without putting patients at risk.

CONCLUSIONS

Until recently, educational technology has been a blunt instrument, offering generic skills but not addressing each learner's needs unique needs. However, any 'one size fits all' approach is doomed to failure. A novice grappling with the basics of minimal access surgery has entirely different requirements from an experienced consultant acquiring a new technique in their own speciality. While a generic approach may be appropriate for entrants into surgical training, established specialists will require opportunities of a different kind. Emerging technology offers the potential to customise training, ensuring that it is tailored to fit individuals' requirements.

Traditionally, discussions of technology within surgical education have focused on the isolated acquisition of technical surgical skills. Such a view risks oversimplification. Technology must be seen as a component of curriculum development, not as an end in itself. To realise its potential, technology must form a part of integrated learning packages which are aimed at the needs of specific groups, underpinned by clear objectives and supported by validated assessment.

There seems little doubt that technology will play an increasing role in surgical education in the future. The challenge is to ensure that learners' educational needs occupy centre stage, that developments take place within a rigorous scientific framework, and that training both reflects and supports the care of surgical patients in the real world.

Key points for clinical practice

- Surgical practice is changing dramatically and preservation of the status quo is not an option. Innovative approaches to training are essential if high standards are to be maintained.
- Surgical practice demands a complex mixture of knowledge, judgement, technical skill and effective team-working. Technology can improve learning in all these areas.
- Training should allow regular context-based practice, providing expert feedback within a supportive, learner-centred milieu.
- The context of learning is inseparable from the skills which are learned. Each surgical learning experience is unique and must be related to the specific needs of the learner.
- Technology is only one component of effective learning. A theory-grounded curriculum should underpin surgical training and ensure a connection between clinical and simulator-based experienced.
- Simulation offers the opportunity to practise within a learner-centred environment which meets criteria for educational effectiveness yet avoids risk to patients.
- There is compelling evidence that simulation is an effective formative tool. Evidence of its effectiveness for assessment is much less robust.
- Any new technology needs to be validated. The acid test for simulation is whether it maps onto clinical performance and leads to improved outcomes. Rigorous evaluation of educational technology is essential.
- The relationship between fidelity of a simulation and its effectiveness is not a simple one. Levels of realism should be tailored to meet educational goals within practical constraints of cost and technical feasibility.

References

1. Kneebone R. Simulation in surgical training: educational issues and practical implications. *Med Ed* 2003; **37**: 267–277.

2. Boud D, Miller N. Synthesizing traditions and identifying themes in learning from experience. In: Boud D, Miller N. (eds) *Working with Experience: Animating Learning*. New York: Routledge, 1996.
3. Boud D, Keogh R, Walker D. Promoting reflection in learning: a model. In: Edwards R, Hanson A, Raggatt P. (eds) *Boundaries of Adult Learning*. New York: Routledge, 1996; 32–56.
4. Ferro TR. The influence of affective processing in education and training. In: Flannery DD. (ed) *Applying Cognitive Learning Theory to Adult Learning*. San Francisco, CA: Josey-Bass, 1993; 25–33.
5. Cassar K. Development of an instrument to measure the surgical operating theatre learning environment as perceived by basic surgical trainees. *Med Teach* 2004; **26**: 260–264.
6. Gordon JA, Oriol NE, Cooper JB. Bringing good teaching cases 'to life': a simulator-based medical education service. *Acad Med* 2004; **79**: 23–27.
7. Ericsson KA, Krampe RT, Tesch-Römer C. The role of deliberate practice in the acquisition of expert performance. *Psychol Rev* 1993; **100**: 363–406.
8. Ericsson KA, Charness N. Expert performance. Its structure and acquisition. *Am Psychol* 1994; **49**: 725–747.
9. Guest CB, Regehr G, Tiberius RG. The life long challenge of expertise. *Med Educ* 2001; **35**: 78–81.
10. Tharp R, Gallimore R. Theories of teaching as assisted performance. In: Light P, Sheldon P, Woodhead M. (eds) *Learning to Think*. New York: Routledge, 1991; 42–59.
11. Bruner JS. *The Process of Education*. Cambridge, MA: Harvard University Press, 1960.
12. Bruner JS. *Toward a Theory of Instruction*. Cambridge, MA: Harvard University Press, 1967.
13. Wood D. *How Children Think and Learn*, 2nd edn. Oxford: Blackwell, 1998.
14. Arthur W, Bennett W, Stanush PL, McNelly TL. Factors that influence skill decay and retention: A quantitative review and analysis. *Hum Perform* 1998; **11**: 57–101.
15. Wenger E. *Communities of Practice. Learning, Meaning, and Identity*. Cambridge: Cambridge University Press, 1998.
16. Lave J, Wenger E. *Situated Learning. Legitimate Peripheral Participation*. Cambridge: Cambridge University Press, 1991.
17. Guile D, Young M. Apprenticeship as a conceptual basis for a social theory of learning. In: Paechter C, Preedy M, Scott D, Soler J. (eds) *Knowledge, Power and Learning*. London: Paul Chapman, 2001; 56–73.
18. Kneebone R, Scott W, Darzi A, Horrocks M. Simulation and clinical practice: strengthening the relationship. *Med Ed* 2004; **38**: 1095–1102.
19. Boon JM, Abrahams P, Meiring JH, Welch T. *The Virtual Procedures Clinic*. CD-ROM from Primal Pictures, ISBN 1904369006, 2004 (www.primalpictures.com).
20. John NW, Riding M, Phillips NI. Web-based surgical educational tools. *Stud Health Technol Inform* 2001; **81**: 212–217.
21. Christenson J, Parrish K, Barabe S *et al*. A comparison of multimedia and standard advanced cardiac life support learning. *Acad Emerg Med* 1998; **5**: 702–708.
22. Rosser JC, Herman B, Risucci DA, Murayama M, Rosser LE, Merrell RC. Effectiveness of a CD-ROM multimedia tutorial in transferring cognitive knowledge essential for laparoscopic skill training. *Am J Surg* 2000; **179**: 320–324.
23. Brisbourne M, Chin S, Melnyk E, Begg D. Using web-based animations to teach histology. *Anat Rec* 2002; **269**: 11–19.
24. Foster I, Kesselman C, Tuecke S. The anatomy of the Grid: enabling scalable virtual organisations. *Int J Supercomput Appl* 2001; **15**: 200–222.
25. Kneebone R, Kidd J, Nestel D, Asvall S, Paraskeva P, Darzi A. An innovative model for teaching and learning clinical procedures. *Med Educ* 2002; **36**: 628–634.
26. Kneebone R, Nestel D, Moorthy K *et al*. Learning the skills of flexible sigmoidoscopy – the wider perspective. *Med Educ* 2003; **37 (Suppl 1)**: 50–58.
27. <www.limbsandthings.com>.
28. <www.mentice.com>.
29. <www.surgical-science.com>.
30. <www.simsurgyer.no>.

31. <www.reachin.se>.
32. <www.xitact.com>.
33. <www.simbionix.com>.
34. <www.immersion.com>.
35. <www.haptica.com>.
36. <www.meti.com>.
37. <www.laerdal.com>.
38. <www.medsim.com>.
39. Moorthy K, Munz Y, Sarker SK, Darzi A. Objective assessment of technical skills in surgery. *BMJ* 2003; **327**: 1032–1037.
40. Martin JA, Regehr G, Reznick R *et al*. Objective structured assessment of technical skill (OSATS) for surgical residents. *Br J Surg* 1997; **84**: 273–278.
41. Datta V, Mackay S, Chang A, Darzi A. Electromagnetic motion analysis in the assessment of surgical technical skill. *Br J Surg* 2001; **88**: 79.
42. Hanna GB, Drew T, Cuschieri A. Technology for psychomotor skills testing in endoscopic surgery. *Semin Laparosc Surg* 1997; **4**: 120–124.
43. Seymour NE, Gallagher AG, Roman SA *et al*. Virtual reality training improves operating room performance: results of a randomized, double-blinded study. *Ann Surg* 2002; **236**: 458–463.
44. Johnston R, Bhoyrul S, Way L *et al*. Assessing a virtual reality surgical skills simulator. *Stud Health Technol Inform* 1996; **29**: 608–617.
45. Taffinder N, Sutton C, Fishwick RJ, McManus IC, Darzi A. Validation of virtual reality to teach and assess psychomotor skills in laparoscopic surgery: results from randomised controlled studies using the MIST VR laparoscopic simulator. *Stud Health Technol Inform* 1998; **50**: 124–130.
46. Grantcharov TP, Kristiansen VB, Bendix J, Bardram L, Rosenberg J, Funch-Jensen P. Randomized clinical trial of virtual reality simulation for laparoscopic skills training. *Br J Surg* 2004; **91**: 146–150.

Plate I Basic skills simulator using abstract scenes.

Plate II Basic skills simulator using procedure-related tasks.

Plate III Simulation of laparoscopic cholecystectomy.

Plate IV Simulated operating theatre with patient mannequin.

Plate V Endoscopy simulator in patient–practitioner setting.

Marcel Gatt John MacFie

2

Bacterial translocation in surgical patients

Recent years have seen an increasing recognition of the fact that the gastrointestinal tract has functions other than simply the digestion and excretion of foodstuffs. The gut is also a metabolic and immunological organ that serves as a barrier against living organisms and antigens within its lumen. This role is termed 'gut barrier function'. The fact that luminal contents in the caecum have a bacterial concentration of the order of 10^{12} organisms/ml of faeces,[1] whilst portal blood and mesenteric lymph nodes are usually sterile, dramatically illustrates the efficacy of this barrier function.

The idea that the alimentary tract, teeming with its own bacterial flora, could represent a source of sepsis under certain conditions has interested clinicians for many years. This theory, usually referred to as the 'gut origin of sepsis' hypothesis, is not new. In the late 19th century, the idea evolved that peritonitis could result from the passage of bacteria from organs adjacent to the peritoneal cavity. In Germany this was referred to as *durchwanderungs-peritonitis*, literally translated as 'wandering through peritonitis'. In 1891 and 1895, two separate investigators hypothesised that viable bacteria could pass through the intact gut wall *in vivo*.[2,3] It was Berg and Garlington in 1979 who defined this phenomenon as 'bacterial translocation'.[4]

'Translocation' is used to describe the passage of viable resident bacteria from the gastrointestinal tract to normally sterile tissues such as the mesenteric lymph nodes and other internal organs.[4] The term also applies to the passage of inert particles and other macromolecules, such as lipopolysaccharide endotoxins, across the intestinal mucosal barrier.

Marcel Gatt MD, MRCSEd
Surgical Research Registrar, Combined Gastroenterology Unit, Scarborough Hospital, Woodland Drive, Scarborough, North Yorkshire YO12 6QL, UK

John MacFie MB ChB MD FRCS
Consultant Surgeon, Combined Gastroenterology Unit, Scarborough Hospital, Woodland Drive, Scarborough, North Yorkshire YO12 6QL, UK (for correspondence)
E-mail: Johnmacfie@aol.com

BACTERIAL TRANSLOCATION

Bacterial translocation does occur in humans.[5] It has a prevalence of about 15% in elective surgical patients and occurs more frequently in patients with intestinal obstruction and those who are immunocompromised.[5–7] There is good evidence to show that translocation is associated with an increased incidence of septic complications but not mortality. Many studies have established an association between gastrointestinal microflora and nosocomial infection supporting the concept of the gut as a reservoir of bacteria and endotoxins.[8,9] However, the evidence that bacterial translocation is the mechanism which accounts for this association between enteric organisms and subsequent sepsis remains, at least in humans, largely circumstantial. This might reflect the methodological and ethical difficulties involved in obtaining samples of portal venous blood or mesenteric lymph nodes, which is necessary to confirm unequivocally the occurrence of translocation. To date, only one clinical study has been reported that provided compelling evidence of a mechanistic link between translocation and the development of late sepsis. O'Boyle *et al.*[5] were able to show that septic complications in 448 surgical patients were significantly more prevalent in those who showed bacterial translocation when compared to patients with no organisms in their mesenteric lymph nodes collected at laparotomy ($P < 0.001$). Furthermore, organisms responsible for septic morbidity were similar in spectrum to those observed in the mesenteric lymph nodes, many being from enteric strains. These data strongly support the 'gut origin of sepsis' hypothesis.

> **Key point 1**
>
> - Translocation refers to the passage of bacteria, inert particles and other macromolecules from the gut to normally sterile tissues.

Whilst it is tempting to think that any bacteria or endotoxin passing through the intestinal barrier might cause septic complications in the host, there is growing evidence to suggest that translocation may in fact be a normal phenomenon. It is possible that translocation occurs to allow the alimentary tract to be exposed to and sample antigens within the lumen such that the gut can mount a controlled local immune response helping to keep these antigens away from the internal milieu, a process known as oral tolerance. It is then only when the host's immune defences are overwhelmed that septic complications arise. Others go further and depict translocation not as the

> **Key point 2**
>
> - The gastrointestinal tract may represent an untreated source of sepsis that could trigger the systemic inflammatory response syndrome and eventually lead to multi-organ dysfunction, the so called 'undrained abscess' of multiple organ failure.

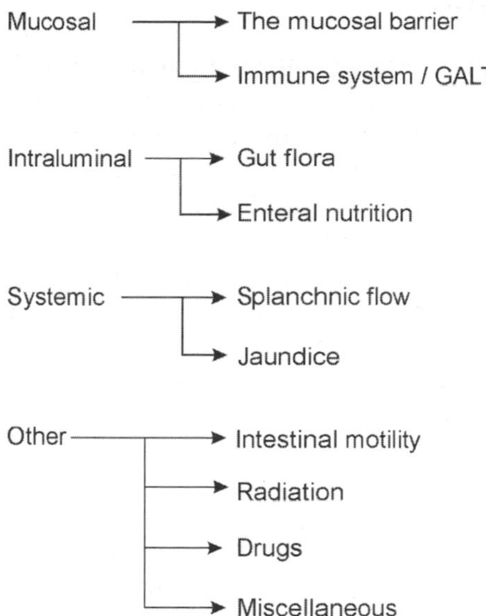

Fig. 1 Predisposing factors to translocation.

initiator of septic complications, but as a result of other insults, which have triggered a systemic inflammatory response, one of its effects being manifest as deterioration or breakdown of gut barrier function.[10]

PREDISPOSING FACTORS TO TRANSLOCATION

Numerous factors have been shown to influence translocation[11] as summarised in Figure 1.

THE MUCOSAL BARRIER

The intestinal epithelium is a polarised monolayer of enterocytes covered by mucus, a glycocalyx brush border, and secretory immunoglobulin A (sIgA). It represents a specialised anatomical barrier limiting the luminal contents of the bowel from the internal milieu. Physical breaches in this barrier, as can occur following ulceration, may predispose to translocation. A rapid rate of cellular turn over, specialisation and migration help the intestinal mucosa maintain physical integrity. Translocation may occur via either transcellular or paracellular routes, or a combination of the two (Fig. 2). Transcellular translocation is under the control of specific membrane pumps and channels, whereas paracellular translocation is permitted (at least theoretically) by breakdown of tight junctions. Transcellular migration has been shown to occur in rats where various organisms including *Escherichia coli* and *Proteus mirabilis* were visualised within intact enterocytes.[12] There is *in vitro* evidence that opening up the gaps between enterocytes by loosening the intercellular tight junctions may increase bacterial translocation.[13] Tight junctions can adjust their degree of 'leakiness' to meet physiological needs, and are also susceptible to numerous pathological stimuli that may change the intestinal permeability.

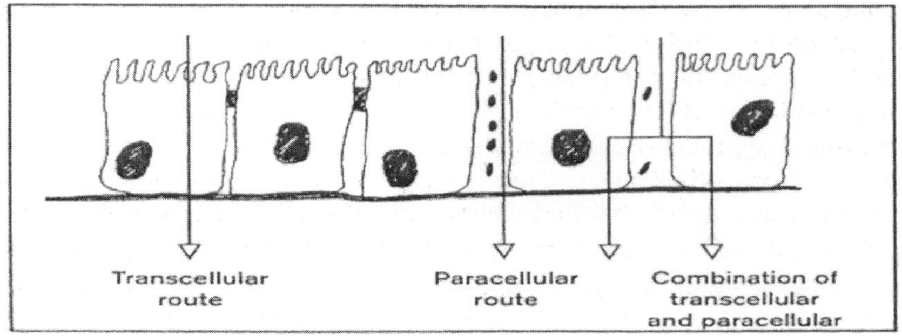

Fig. 2 Possible routes for bacterial translocation through the intestinal mucosa.

It is important to emphasise, however, that there is, as yet, no data in animal or human studies that directly confirm a causative relationship between changes in permeability and bacterial translocation. Similarly, there is no evidence to confirm that gross changes in villus morphology are causally related to increased rates of translocation.

HOST IMMUNE DEFENCES

The immune system is an extremely complex arrangement of cellular and humoral components, which interact in a closely orchestrated fashion to permit interaction with the outside whilst maintaining the internal milieu.[14] The gut harbours the largest number of mucosal-associated lymphoid tissue cells of any organ in the body.[15] These tend to be concentrated in Peyer's patches, but are also distributed widely in the lamina propria. The function of the gut-associated lymphoid tissue (GALT) is primarily to release sIgA. Oral tolerance is an additional important function of GALT and can be described as the decreased ability to stimulate a systemic immune response to antigens previously encountered in the gut.[16] Loss of oral tolerance, resulting in an uncontrolled inflammatory response, is thought to be important in the pathogenesis of numerous diseases primarily inflammatory bowel diseases. There is evidence that translocation in humans is associated with an increase in gut immune function. Woodcock *et al.*[17] showed that translocators had higher semiquantitatively scored IgA and IgM values ($P = 0.006$ and 0.016, respectively) in the small bowel mucosa. They were also able to demonstrate a significant increase in plasma cells ($P < 0.01$) and IgA positive cells ($P < 0.05$) in the lamina propria of translocators, along with an increased frequency of IgM positive cells which, however, was not statistically significant.[17]

BACTERIAL FLORA

The gut harbours more than 400 different species of bacteria. Absolute bacterial counts vary along the length of the bowel, being present at a concentration of about 10^8 organisms/ml in the region of the distal ileum, increasing to around 10^{12} organisms/ml in the region of the caecum.[1] Aerobes translocate much more readily to mesenteric lymph nodes despite the fact that anaerobes outnumber them 1000-fold beyond the ileo-caecal valve. Some members of the resident commensal flora are thought to cause bacterial antagonism by limiting the populations of more pathological and virulent microbial strains and competing with these organisms for adhesion with the gastrointestinal tract.[18,19] Attachment to enterocytes is considered an early step in translocation; therefore, bacterial antagonism may help to confine bacteria to the gastrointestinal tract. One rationale for the use of probiotics (live microbial feed supplements that beneficially affects the host by improving its microbial balance) and prebiotics (non-digestible foods, mainly plant fibres, consumed and used by gut bacteria as substrates for fermentation that selectively stimulate the growth and activity of beneficial strains) is to try and increase the numbers of non-pathogenic organisms while at the same time decreasing the sites of possible attachment of pathogens and by doing so, increase this bacterial antagonism against more virulent strains.

Efforts to decrease the bacterial load of the GI tract should theoretically decrease sepsis, consequently decreasing mortality. This is achieved by selective gut decontamination (SGD), the key word being 'selective', as it is considered important to diminish the counts of Gram-negative microbes in preference to anaerobic bacteria for the reasons already outlined. Selective decontamination is achieved through the combined use of oral non-absorbable antibiotics, short-term systemic preparations and microbial surveillance. Whilst there is strong evidence to suggest that SGD is effective in reducing respiratory tract infections in the critically ill,[20] unfortunately studies to date have shown conflicting results in relation to the effects on septic complications and mortality. One possibility for this is the increased free endotoxin load (and subsequent endotoxin translocation) associated with the death of so many bacteria. Another possibility is that decontamination regimens are not specific enough to eliminate pathogens preferentially and, therefore, upset the balance of indigenous flora in such a way as to diminish the effects of bacterial antagonism.

Intestinal obstruction is associated with a high prevalence of translocation of 41%,[5–7] and recent evidence suggests that bacterial overgrowth in the stomach is also associated with increased rates of translocation.[8] However, the nature and type of bacteria found to translocate are such that concentrations of bacteria alone cannot explain the increased prevalence seen in obstructed conditions.

Key point 3

- The judicious use of antibiotics to treat established foci of infection must be weighed against the potentially deleterious effects these antibiotics may have on upsetting the resident gut flora.

NUTRITIONAL SUPPORT: ENTERAL VERSUS PARENTERAL

There is now a consensus that peri-operative nutritional support is of benefit, particularly to patients with severe malnutrition.[21] Not surprisingly, most reviewers of nutritional support therapy urge the use of enteral (EN) as opposed to parenteral (TPN) support. Parenteral nutrition, it is said, results in mucosal atrophy and increased intestinal permeability, which reflect damage to the intestinal barrier. This predisposes to bacterial translocation and may be one explanation for increased rates of septic complications observed in some studies investigating TPN.

Key point 4

- There is no evidence to support the use of enteral in preference to parenteral nutrition with regards to reported effects on surrogate measures of gut barrier function (villus architecture or intestinal permeability).

A number of assumptions are implicit in these commonly held views about TPN. First, that bacterial translocation does occur in man, occurs more readily if intestinal barrier function is impaired and is associated with increased incidences of sepsis. Second, that septic morbidity is proven to be significantly higher in patients receiving TPN. And third, that the absence of luminal nutrients as might occur during starvation, malnutrition or TPN is associated with deleterious consequences to the gut barrier which predispose to translocation. Bacterial translocation does occur on a frequent basis in humans. It is associated with increased septic morbidity supporting the concept of the 'gut origin of sepsis' hypothesis. However, it probably also occurs in healthy individuals but is not significant in the non-immunocompromised host. There is no evidence to suggest that bacterial translocation is reduced by the use of enteral nutrition or increased in patients receiving parenteral nutrition. There is no evidence to confirm that short-term TPN is associated with villus atrophy or significant changes in intestinal permeability.[22] There is no evidence in humans to support the view that alterations in intestinal barrier function as assessed from changes in mucosal architecture or from alterations in intestinal permeability will predispose to an increased prevalence of bacterial translocation. Starvation or malnutrition by themselves do not induce bacterial translocation. Alterations in mucosal architecture or intestinal permeability may indicate changes in intestinal barrier function but do not necessarily equate with alterations in the prevalence of bacterial translocation. With the exception of trauma patients, there is no firm evidence that septic morbidity is increased in patients receiving parenteral as opposed to enteral nutrition.

The nature of the nutritional support that should be provided to patients should be determined by their tolerance to enteral nutrition and not by unjustified assumptions concerning the role of gut barrier function.

GUT-SPECIFIC NUTRIENTS

There is an increasing body of knowledge that suggests that certain nutrients have specific effects on gut function. Glutamine, for example, is known to be the preferred fuel source of the enterocyte and has been shown to impact on intestinal permeability[23] and may, in animal studies, reduce rates of translocation.[24] Other 'gut-specific nutrients' include arginine,[25] pre- and probiotics,[26,27] and certain anti-oxidants such as vitamin A.[28] These are extensively reviewed elsewhere.[29]

> **Key point 5**
>
> - The use of gut-specific nutrients such as probiotics, prebiotics, glutamine or antioxidants may yet prove to be important modalities for critically ill patients if these enhance a return to normal gut function.

SPLANCHNIC BLOOD FLOW

Diminished splanchnic blood flow, as seen in hypovolaemic shock and bowel ischaemia, is associated with translocation and septic complications in animal models. Oxygenation to the villi in man is dependent on a counter-current exchange mechanism such that oxygen saturation at the tip of the villi is lower than that of arterial blood. This makes the villus very susceptible to ischaema–reperfusion damage. The potential importance of splanchnic flow as a determinant of outcome was illustrated by a recent study, which showed that the use of the splanchnic vasodilator dopexamine was associated with a significant reduction in postoperative mortality.[30] Whether this was a result of reduced translocation is unclear but it is interesting to note that Deitch who has published extensively on this topic has speculated that splanchnic hypoperfusion results in the gut becoming a major site of pro-inflammatory factor production.[10] He argues that splanchnic hypoperfusion can lead to an ischaemia-reperfusion injury to the gut with a resultant loss of gut barrier function and an ensuing gut inflammatory response, without the need for translocation of microbes as far as the mesenteric lymph nodes or beyond. Once bacteria or endotoxin cross the mucosal barrier, even if trapped within the gut wall, they can still trigger an immune response such that the gut becomes a pro-inflammatory organ, releasing chemokines, cytokines and other pro-inflammatory intermediates which affect both the local as well as the systemic immune systems, finally giving rise to the systemic inflammatory response syndrome (SIRS) and multi-organ failure (MOF). This he calls the three-hit model of gut inflammation, namely hypoperfusion, ischaemia–reperfusion injury, and the loss of gut barrier function in association with a markedly increased pro-inflammatory response.[10]

> **Key point 6**
>
> - The early identification and appropriate aggressive treatment of conditions known to promote translocation, such as hypovolaemic shock, intestinal obstruction and malnutrition may lead to a decline in septic complications and, hopefully, a decreased associated mortality.

MISCELLANEOUS

Many other factors have been shown to influence translocation, particularly in animals. These include stress,[31] jaundice,[32] radiation,[33] variations in intestinal motility and various drugs.[34,35] Prokinetic agents such as cisapride and propranolol have been shown to decrease translocation,[34] as have sucralfate, bile salts and prostaglandin analogues.[35] Other drugs have been shown to increase translocation including chemotherapeutic and immunosuppressive agents as well as certain antibiotics.

CONCLUSIONS

The 'gut origin of sepsis' hypothesis is an attractive and simple concept that presupposes that bacteria cross the intestinal barrier and cause sepsis at distant sites. There is now compelling evidence in human subjects to support this theory and which confirms that translocation predisposes to an increase in septic morbidity. Bacterial and endotoxin translocation probably also occurs to a limited extent on a regular basis in healthy individuals. In this situation, translocation serves to provide an antigenic stimulus but normal barrier function is preserved and morbidity does not ensue. Only if normal mechanisms of defence are overwhelmed does translocation occur. This serves to emphasise the importance of maintaining all aspects of gut function in the critically ill.

Key points for clinical practice

- Translocation refers to the passage of bacteria, inert particles and other macromolecules from the gut to normally sterile tissues.
- The gastrointestinal tract may represent an untreated source of sepsis that could trigger the systemic inflammatory response syndrome and eventually lead to multi-organ dysfunction, the so called 'undrained abscess' of multiple organ failure.
- The judicious use of antibiotics to treat established foci of infection must be weighed against the potentially deleterious effects these antibiotics may have on upsetting the resident gut flora.
- There is no evidence to support the use of enteral in preference to parenteral nutrition with regards to reported effects on surrogate measures of gut barrier function (villus architecture or intestinal permeability).
- The use of gut-specific nutrients such as probiotics, prebiotics, glutamine or antioxidants may yet prove to be important modalities for critically ill patients if these enhance a return to normal gut function.
- The early identification and appropriate aggressive treatment of conditions known to promote translocation, such as hypovolaemic shock, intestinal obstruction and malnutrition may lead to a decline in septic complications and, hopefully, a decreased associated mortality.

References

1. Simon GL, Gorbach SL. The human intestinal microflora. *Dig Dis Sci* 1986; **31**: 147S–162S.
2. Fraenkel A. Ueber peritoneale infection. *Wein Klin Wochenschr* 1891; **4**: 241, 265, 285.
3. Flexner S. Peritonitis caused by the invasion of the *Micrococcus lanceolatus* from the intestine. *John Hopkins Hosp Bull* 1895; **6**: 64–67.
4. Berg RD, Garlington AW. Translocation of certain indigenous bacteria from the gastrointestinal tract to the mesenteric lymph nodes and other organs in the gnotobiotic mouse model. *Infect Immun* 1979; **23**: 403.
5. O'Boyle CJ, MacFie J, Mitchell CJ, Johnstone D, Sagar PM, Sedman PC. Microbiology of bacterial translocation in humans. *Gut* 1998; **42**: 29–35.
6. Deitch EA. Simple intestinal obstruction causes bacterial translocation in man. *Arch Surg* 1989; **124**: 699–701.
7. Sagar PM, MacFie J, Sedman P, May J, Mancey-Jones B, Johnstone D. Intestinal obstruction promotes gut translocation of bacteria. *Dis Colon Rectum* 1995; **38**: 640–644.
8. Macfie J, O'Boyle C, Mitchell CJ, Buckley PM, Johnson D, Sudworth P. Gut origin of sepsis: a prospective study investigating associations between bacterial translocation, gastric microflora, and septic morbidity. *Gut* 1999; **45**: 223–228.
9. Marshall JC, Christou NV, Meakins JL. The gastrointestinal tract: the undrained abscess of multiple organ failure. *Ann Surg* 1993; **218**: 111–119.
10. Deitch EA. Bacterial translocation or lymphatic drainage of toxic products from the gut: what is important in human beings? *Surgery* 2002; **131**: 241–244.
11. Weist R, Rath HC. Gastrointestinal disorders of the critically ill. Bacterial translocation in the gut. *Best Prac Res Clin Gastroenterol* 2003; **17**: 397–425.
12. Wells CL, Erlandsen SL, Bacterial translocation: intestinal epithelial permeability. In: Rombeau JL, Takala J. (eds) *Update in Intensive Care and Emergency Medicine (26): Gut Dysfunction in Critical Illness*. Berlin: Springer, 1996; 137–145.
13. Wells CL, van de Westerlo EMA, Jechorek RP *et al.* Exposure of the lateral enterocyte membrane by dissociation of calcium-dependent junctional complex augments endocytosis of enteric bacteria. *Shock* 1995; **4**: 204–210.
14. Parkin J, Cohen B, An overview of the immune system. *Lancet* 2001; **357**: 1777–1789.
15. Baumgart DC, Dignass AU. Intestinal barrier function. *Curr Opin Clin Nutr Metab Care* 2002; **5**: 685–694.
16. Kagnoff MF. Immunological unresponsiveness after enteric antigen administration. In: Strober W, Hanson LA, Sell KW. (eds) *Recent Advances in Mucosal Immunity*. New York: Raven, 1982; 95–111.
17. Woodcock NP, Robertson J, Morgan DR, Gregg KL, Mitchell CJ, MacFie J. Bacterial translocation and immunohistochemical measurement of gut immune function. *J Clin Pathol* 2001; **54**: 619–623.
18. Berg RD. Mechanisms confining indigenous bacteria to the gastrointestinal tract. *Am J Clin Nutr* 1980; **33**: 2472–2484.
19. Bernet MF, Brassart D *et al. Lactobacillus acidophilus* LA1 binds to cultured human intestinal cells and inhibits attachment and cell invasion by enterovirulent bacteria. *Gut* 1994; **35**: 483–489.
20. D'Amico R, Pifferi S, Leonetti C *et al.* Effectiveness of antibiotic prophylaxis in critically ill patients: Systematic review of randomized controlled trials. *BMJ* 1998; **316**: 1275–1285.
21. Satyanarayana R, Klein S. Clinical efficacy of perioperative nutrition support. *Curr Opin Clin Nutr Metab Care* 1998; **1**: 51–58.
22. Sedman PC, MacFie J, Palmer MD, Mitchell CJ, Sagar PM. Preoperative total parenteral nutrition is not associated with mucosal atrophy or bacterial translocation in humans. *Br J Surg* 1995; **82**: 1663–1667.
23. Tremel H, Kienle B, Weilemann L, Stehle P, Furst P. Glutamine dipeptide-supplemented parenteral nutrition maintains intestinal function in the critically ill. *Gastroenterology* 1994; **107**: 1595–1601.
24. Gianotti L, Alexander J, Gennari R, Pyles T, Babcock G. Oral glutamine decreases bacterial translocation and improves survival in experimental gut-origin sepsis. *J Parenter Enteral Nutr* 1995; **19**: 69–74.
25. Alican I, Kubes P. A critical role for nitric oxide in intestinal barrier function and

dysfunction. *Am J Physiol* 1996; **270**: G225–G237.
26. McNaught CE, MacFie J. Probiotics in clinical practice: a critical review of evidence. *Nutr Res* 2001; **21**: 343–353.
27. Bengmark S. Pre-, pro- and synbiotics. *Curr Opin Clin Nutr Metab Care* 2001; **4**: 571–579.
28. Thurnham DI, Northrop-Clewes CA, McCullough FS, Das BS, Lunn PG. Innate immunity, gut integrity, and vitamin A in Gambian and Indian infants. *J Infect Dis* 2000; **182 (Suppl)**: S23–S28.
29. Duggan C, Gannon J, Allan Walker W. Protective nutrients and functional foods for the gastrointestinal tract. *Am J Clin Nutr* 2002; **75**: 789–808.
30. Wilson J, Woods I, Fawcett J *et al*. Reducing the risk of major elective surgery: randomized controlled trial of preoperative optimization of oxygen delivery. *BMJ* 1999; **318**: 1099–1103.
31. Soderholm JD, Perdue M. Stress and gastrointestinal tract II. Stress and intestinal barrier function. *Am J Physiol* 2001; **280**: G7–G13.
32. Kale IT, Kuzu MA, Col C, Tekeli A, Tanik A, Koksoy C. Obstructive jaundice promotes bacterial translocation (BT) in humans. *Br J Surg* 1997; **84**: 8.
33. Guzman-Stein G, Bonsack MS, Liberty J, Delaney JP. Abdominal radiation causes bacterial translocation. *J Surg Res* 1989; **46**: 104–107.
34. Pardo A, Bartoli R, Lorenzo-Zuuiga V *et al*. Effect of cisapride on intestinal bacterial overgrowth and bacterial translocation in cirrhosis. *Hepatology* 2000; **31**: 858–863.
35. Fukushima R, Gianotti L, Alexander W, Pyles T. The degree of bacterial translocation is a determinant factor for mortality after burn injury and is improved by prostaglandin analogs. *Ann Surg* 1992; **216**: 438–445.

Owen Boyd

3

Optimisation of the high-risk surgical patient – the use of 'goal-directed' therapy

In the 1980s and early 1990s, the treatment of the critically ill patient was seen to be becoming increasingly expensive with little evidence that this expensive care improved outcome. This applied particularly to surgical patients in whom techniques originally pioneered in a healthy population are expanded to include patients who are more elderly with co-existing diseases. These high-risk patients have a higher mortality and morbidity rate and frequently die from multiple organ dysfunction syndrome (MODS), a syndrome that once established has proved largely resistant to therapeutic intervention. New evidence suggests that treatment targeted towards optimising cardiovascular function might improve outcome. To understand the principles involved, this paper discusses normal physiological changes around the time of surgery, surgical mortality, and the pathophysiology of MODS, before discussing evidence that manipulating cardiac function to increase blood flow reduces mortality and morbidity, this manipulation is known generically as 'goal-directed' therapy.

PHYSIOLOGICAL CHANGES IN THE PERI-OPERATIVE PERIOD

It has been known for some time that there are changes in cardiovascular function at the time of surgery. In patients undergoing thoracotomy,[1] low cardiac index and arterial hypoxia were indicators of non-survival. Following the development of the balloon-tipped, flow-directed pulmonary artery catheter, it was shown that patients who survived major surgery had higher cardiac index, lower systemic vascular resistance, and higher oxygen delivery than non-survivors.[2] It was found that the commonly monitored vital signs (heart rate, temperature, central venous pressure and haemoglobin) were the

Owen Boyd FRCA FRCP MD
Lead Consultant in Intensive Care Medicine, ITU, Royal Sussex County Hospital, Eastern Road, Brighton BN2 5BE, UK. (E-mail: owen.boyd@bsuh.nhs.uk)

poorest predictors of survival, while perfusion-related variables (such as oxygen delivery and oxygen consumption) and cardiac index (which express the interrelationship between oxygen transport and red cell volume and flow) were the best.[3] Furthermore, oxygen transport values change before the more commonly monitored variables; and, in patients who die or have complications,[4] vital signs usually remain in the normal range until the terminal event, while oxygen transport variables had started to change some hours previously.

It has been hypothesised that a rise in oxygen transport requirements after surgery may be necessary to pay back an oxygen debt that has accumulated during the surgical procedure. Furthermore, if the cumulative tissue oxygen debt is calculated during the period of operation, it is found that patients who survive have the smallest oxygen debt and patients who fail to survive have the biggest; patients with organ failure who survive have intermediate oxygen debts.[5]

In summary, cardiovascular changes around the time of surgery produce an increase in tissue perfusion; if this compensatory mechanism fails, patients are more likely to die and have complications.

Key point 1

- In the immediate postoperative period, a normal physiological response requires an increase in cardiac output and blood flow to the tissues. If this response fails, patients are more likely to have postoperative morbidity and mortality.

SURGICAL MORTALITY AND MORBIDITY

Assessing mortality rates in higher risk patients is difficult; the 1991 *Acute Physiology and Chronic Health Evaluation* database gives a 10.3% mortality for patients admitted directly to intensive care from the operating theatre in US centres;[6] in the *South West Thames ICU* database mortality was higher (9.4% for elective surgery and 28.7% for emergency surgery in 1993–1994),[7] and this is similar to data from the *Intensive Care National Audit and Research Council* database. Furthermore, the National Confidential Enquiry into Peri-Operative Deaths (NCEPOD) in England and Wales 1992–1993 showed that the median day of death was day 6 and that patients did not usually die soon after operation. Postoperative mortality is increased in older patients with pre-existing disease and more severe surgery, and this has recently been highlighted by the Society of Cardiothoracic Surgeons of Great Britain and Ireland.[8] Studies have also shown that thoracic and abdominal procedures have higher mortality and complication rates;[9] in elderly patients undergoing non-cardiac surgery, mortality is more related to factors such as a history of cardiac disease and signs of low CI around the time of surgery than factors such as the type of operation performed.[10]

In general, patients with non-elective admissions (mortality rate 30% versus 5% for elective admissions), ASA grade 3+ (mortality rate 27% versus 8% for

ASA < 3), age over 75 years (mortality rate 20% versus 11% for patients aged 65–74 years) and major surgery (mortality rate 25% versus 10% for non-major surgery) are associated with much higher mortality, and these factors are more important than the type of surgery.

Key point 2

- Postoperative mortality rates are higher than expected in patients who are elderly, have premorbid disease conditions, such as cardiac and respiratory failure, and are having urgent operative procedures.

MODS AND THE SURGICAL PATIENT

A syndrome in which there was multiple failure of a number of organ systems was first described in the 1970s in a group of surgical patients. This was initially termed multiple organ failure syndrome (MOF), but recently the terminology has been standardised and it is now called multiple organ dysfunction syndrome (MODS).[11] MODS carries a high mortality which increases as the number of organ systems fail.[12] The incidence of MODS in surgical intensive care unit (ICU) patients can be as high as 44.3%, and is associated with prolonged illness, death and increased cost. It is currently estimated that MODS accounts for 60–80% of all surgical ICU deaths,[13] and disappointingly there appears to have been little improvement in prognosis of established MODS over the last 20 years.

Key point 3

- Most surgical mortality in the sickest patients in the hospital being treated in intensive care units is usually due to multiple organ dysfunction syndrome.

There are a number of factors which acting independently or in combination trigger the onset of MODS but the final common pathway is that of cytokine activation; first, a local production of cytokines in response to an injury or infection which is a physiological response, then a release of a small amount of cytokines into the body's circulation, and finally a massive systemic reaction where cytokines turn destructive by compromising the integrity of the capillary walls and flooding end-organs. The triggers that lead from a normal response to an unregulated pathological response probably involve genetic factors and the priming of the inflammatory system by other stimulants. One can imagine in the surgical situation multiple stimulants to the inflammatory pathways been present in any one individual; these could include trauma, ischaemia, reperfusion injury, and infective and chemical insults. One of the major factors initiating cytokine activation appears to be alterations in microcirculatory flow,[14] and others are related to tissue damage and the stimulation of inflammatory mediators. Shoemaker and colleagues reported the link between failure of the normal postoperative responses of increased cardiac index and oxygen delivery maintaining flow and perfusion, and the development of MODS and death.[15] This is probably the result of the activation of nuclear factor-κB, but demonstrating this in humans undergoing surgery and then relating this to the pathogenic processes of MODS and patient outcome has been more complicated. However, the frequency and magnitude of postoperative organ dysfunction after thoraco-abdominal aneurysm[16] and abdominal aneurysm repair[17] is associated with an increased concentration of the cytokines tumor necrosis factor-α and interleukin-6, and this is related to extended visceral ischaemia times.

In summary, pathophysiological evidence shows a direct link between surgery and trauma and the development of MODS in some patients; there is also an implication that the degree of surgery makes this chain of events more likely. Moreover, evidence above suggests that this is also more likely to occur when physiological reserve is limited.

Key point 4

- Multiple organ dysfunction syndrome has a multifactorial pathophysiology, which includes reduced cardiac output and reduced tissue oxygenation.

HYPOTHESIS FOR THE MANAGEMENT OF HIGH-RISK SURGICAL PATIENTS

Sometime before all the scientific observations described above, Shoemaker and his colleagues had proposed a pragmatic treatment approach to the high-risk surgical patient.[18] They proposed that all patients should be treated to targets of cardiac index, oxygen consumption and oxygen delivery as defined by the values seen in the survivors; the value chosen, again on a pragmatic basis, was the median value for these parameters demonstrated by the survivors of surgery.[18] This hypothesis now fits elegantly into the scientific context. By pre-emptively influencing one of the major potential factors causing and stimulating cytokine release and resulting in MODS, that of tissue hypoperfusion, treatment based on the hypothesis would be expected to limit the degree of inflammatory activation and reduce the incidence and severity of MODS. Although it is conjecture, it is likely that the hyperdynamic circulatory responses observed by Shoemaker and colleagues[19] in their survivors of surgery may have reduced the inflammatory response in these patients to those of a normal and healthy physiological response to injury.

This was a hugely important idea combining, as it did, invasive monitoring technology, raised expectations for surgical intervention, a new confidence in fluid therapy and inotropic medication, and a preventative approach to medical care. The terms 'supra-normal goal-directed therapy' and simply 'goal-directed therapy' and 'optimisation' have arisen from this hypothesis, and are used almost synonymously. In 1978 when this was first suggested it

Table 1 A technique for optimising the surgical patient (after Boyd *et al.*[20])

Identify patient as being at higher risk
Admit to intensive care pre-operatively for placement of pulmonary artery catheter
Give fluids and inotropes if needed to achieve therapeutic goals (*e.g.* oxygen delivery index greater than 600 ml/min/m^2) while avoiding significant side effects such as tachycardia
Patient undergoes surgery
Patient returned to intensive care postoperatively and treatment continued to predefined targets until end-point (*e.g.* normal lactate) is achieved
Patient well enough to move to general ward
Patient discharged home

was just a hypothesis, but it has spawned a huge body of literature and considerable controversy, which remains to this day.

Although Shoemaker and colleagues laid down a very proscribed approach in their first descriptions of the goal-directed therapeutic approach using a PA catheter. The evolution of new technologies and a deeper understanding of the subject have meant that one now has to take a broader approach, and the terms are now applied to treatment whereby specific physiological goals, specifically related to aspects of tissue perfusion, are set and therapy is then given to the patient with the aim of attaining these goals of treatment. Table 1 shows a possible technique for applying goal-directed therapy in a surgical patient.

TRIALS TO INCREASE CARDIAC OUTPUT AND OXYGEN DELIVERY

There are a number of published studies investigating the role of goal-directed therapy in high-risk peri-operative patients and other patient groups. These studies followed a pre-emptive approach where targets for treatment are set with a specific goal of increasing tissue perfusion. The studies have used the monitoring tool of the PA catheter to provide treatment targets for increasing cardiac output and oxygen delivery, or have used the oesophageal Doppler monitor to provide treatment targets for increasing stroke volume. In addition, a number of studies have used mixed venous oxygen saturation as the target for treatment. The details of the studies and the patients enrolled are shown in Table 2. These trials have studied patients who have been considered to be at higher risk of postoperative morbidity and mortality due to nature of the surgery to be undertaken, or because of a number of risk factors related to pre-operative disease states that have been identified in the pre-operative assessment.

Healthcare economies are becoming increasingly financially constrained and it is essential to identify the cost-effectiveness of all new treatments. A number of studies shown in Table 1 also include a cost analysis as part of the original study protocol or as a separate publication; these cost analyses show reduced costs in patients treated in a 'goal-directed' fashion.[21–23]

Table 2 Randomised, controlled studies of peri-operative goal-directed therapy

First author	Criteria for study admission	*n*	Target for treatment in the 'protocol' group	Odds ratio for reduction in mortality (95% confid. interval)
Schultz	Fractured neck of femur	70	General 'optimised' physiological profile. Fluid. Vasodilators and inotropes used	0.07 (0.01–0.61)
Shoemaker	List of high-risk criteria for general surgical patients	58	CI > 4.5 l/min/m²; DO_2I > 600 ml/min/m²; VO_2I > 170 ml/min/m² using fluids, vasodilators and inotropes	0.07 (0.01–0.63)
Berlauk	Limb salvage arterial surgery	89	CI > 2.8 l/min/m²; PAOP 8–15 mmHg; SVR < 1100 dyne/s/cm⁵. Analysis based on treatment groups combined versus control	0.14 (0.01–1.65)
Fleming	Trauma specific diagnostic criteria	67	CI > 4.52 l/min/m²; DO_2I > 670 ml/min/m²; VO_2I > 166 ml/min/m² using fluid infusion and dobutamine if targets not met	0.41 (0.14–1.15)
Boyd	List of high-risk criteria for general surgical patients	107	DO_2I > 600 ml/min/m² using dopexamine	0.21 (0.06–0.79)
Bishop	Trauma specific diagnostic criteria	115	CI > 4.5 l/min/m²; DO_2I > 600 ml/min/m²; VO_2I > 170 ml/min/m²	0.38 (0.16–0.90)
Mythen	Elective cardiac surgery	60	Maximise SV and raise CVP by 3 mmHg with fluid challenges (200 ml hydroxyethyl starch) assessed by oesophageal Doppler	Not able to calculate
Durham	Trauma specific diagnostic criteria	58	DO_2I > 600 ml/min/m² and/or VO_2I > 150 ml/min/m² using fluid therapy and dopamine or dobutamine if targets not met	1.17 (0.22–6.33)
Bender	Infrarenal aortic reconstruction, lower limb revascularisation	104	PAOP 8–14 mmHg; CI > 2.8 l/min/m²; SVR < 1100 dyne/s/cm⁵	1.04 (0.06–17.08)
Sinclair	Fractured neck of femur	40	Maximise SV with fluid challenges and increase corrected flow time > 0.35 s assessed by oesophageal Doppler	0.47 (0.04–5.69)
Ziegler	Aortic reconstruction, limb salvage surgery	72	PAOP > 12 mmHg; S_vO_2 > 65% using fluid boluses, vasodilators and dobutamine	1.97 (0.31–12.54)

Table 2 *(continued)* Randomised, controlled studies of peri-operative goal-directed therapy

First author	Criteria for study admission	*n*	Target for treatment in the 'protocol' group	Odds ratio for reduction in mortality (95% confid. interval)
Ueno	Partial hepatectomy for hepatocellular carcinoma	34	CI > 4.5 l/min/m^2; DO_2I > 600 ml/min/m^2; VO_2I > 170 ml/min/m^2	Not able to calculate
Valentine	Aortic surgery	120	PA catheter placed in protocol patients, PAOP 8–15 mmHg; CI > 2.8 l/min/m^2; SVR < 1100 dyne/s/cm^5	3.11 (0.31–30.73)
Wilson	List of surgical or medical criteria for general surgical patients	138	PAOP > 12 mmHg using 4.5% human albumin; DO_2I > 600 ml/min/m^2 using fluids and adrenaline (*n* = 92) or dopexamine (*n* = 92). Analysis based on treatment groups combined vs control	0.16 (0.04–0.64)
Polonen	Elective cardiac surgery	393	PA catheter; S_vO_2 > 70%; serum lactate < 2 mmol/l	0.38 (0.08–1.81)
Takala	List of surgical or medical criteria	412	No specific additional targets. Dopexamine given in two doses. Analysis is treatment groups combined versus control	0.84 (0.45–1.57)
Lobo	List of surgical or medical criteria	37	DO_2I > 600 ml/min/m^2 using additional dobutamine	0.33 (0.07–1.65)
Venn	Fractured neck of femur	90	CVP group of patients had fluid boluses. Doppler group of patients had fluid boluses to maximise SV. Analysis is Doppler group versus control and CVP combined	0.72 (0.18–2.95)
Gan	Major elective surgery (anticipated blood loss > 500 ml)	100	Fluid boluses given to maximise SV	Unable to calculate
Sandham	Age > 60 years, major elective surgery, ASA III or IV	1994	PA catheter in the treatment group to target DO_2I 500 to 600 ml/min/m^2; CI > 3.5 to 4.5 l/min/m^2; MAP 70 mmHg; PAOP 18 mmHg	1.01 (0.73–1.41)
Stone	Age > 60 years, major elective abdominal surgery	100	Dopexamine infusion at 0.25 mcg/kg/min (double blind)	1.53 (0.24–9.59)

Details of references are available from the author of this review.
PA, pulmonary artery; PAOP, pulmonary artery occlusion pressure; DO_2I, oxygen delivery index; VO_2I, oxygen consumption index; CI, cardiac index; SVR, systemic vascular resistance; CVP, central venous pressure; SBP, systolic blood pressure; HR, heart rate; UO, urine output; SV, stroke volume; S_vO_2, mixed venous oxygen saturation; MAP mean arterial pressure; confid. interval, confidence interval.

> **Key point 5**
>
> - Careful monitoring with a pulmonary artery catheter or oesophageal Doppler allows fluid and inotropic therapy to be given immediately pre-operatively with a goal of increasing and maximising cardiac output, blood flow and tissue oxygenation. This has been turned 'goal-directed' therapy and it has been suggested that they should be applied to all higher risk surgical patients.

SYSTEMIC REVIEWS OF THE EFFECTS OF GOAL-DIRECTED THERAPY

As well as this review article, a number of other publications over the last 10 years have also reviewed the results of goal-directed therapy in surgical patients. The literature is complicated because some reviews have primarily addressed possible effectiveness of right heart catheterisation,[24,25] and others have included studies enrolling patients at a later stage of their illness[26,27] although separating those in the peri-operative period for the purposes of analysis.

When considering peri-operative patients specifically, Ivanov and colleagues[24] gave a combined odds ratio (OR) for the studies that they analysed of 0.58 (95% confidence interval [CI], 0.36–0.94) for improved outcome following early goal-directed therapy, and Heyland and colleagues[26] gave a combined OR of 0.20 (95% CI, 0.07–0.55); both reviews including slightly different studies. A similar analysis by Kern and colleagues showed that in higher risk patients and in patients treated early in the course of their disease, mortality was significantly reduced by as much as 23%.[28]

One systematic review has specifically addressed the issue of a possible reduction in complications, rather than mortality, following therapeutic alterations guided by information for a pulmonary artery catheter.[29] Twelve trials, including patients in the peri-operative period as well as those with general critical illness, defined major morbidity as organ failures; these studies enrolled a total of 1610 patients. Morbidity events showed a statistically significant reduction using pulmonary artery catheter guided strategies, 62.8% of the pulmonary artery catheter treatment group displayed organ failure morbidity, and 74.3% of the control group (relative risk ratio 0.78; 95% CI, 0.65–0.94; $P < 0.02$).

A recent analysis using Cochrane methodology, identified 12 published and peer-reviewed papers, which used goal-directed peri-operative targeting of global flow values: oxygen delivery and oxygen consumption, stroke volume, lactate and mixed venous oxygen. The studies include 1252 patients with an overall mortality of 6.2%. The mortality in the control group was 56/587 (9.5%) versus 21/665 (3.2%) in the protocol group, and the Peto odds ratio was 0.3 (95% CI, 0.19–0.49) for a reduction in mortality.[30]

A similar analysis for this review has identified 21 peri-operative studies enrolling 4258 patients. Overall, the mortality of the protocol patients was 7.06% and of the control patients 10.25% (OR, 0.67; 95% CI, 0.54–0.83). The studies can be further subdivided based on the severity of illness as defined by the control group mortality. Studies with a control group mortality ≤ 10% include 11 studies enrolling 3130 patients, the mortality of the protocol patients is 6.01% and the mortality of the control patients is 6.26% (OR, 0.96; 95% CI, 0.71–1.28). Studies with a control group mortality > 10% include 10 studies enrolling 1128 patients; the protocol mortality was 9.7% and the control mortality was 22.6% (OR, 0.37; 95% CI, 0.26–0.52).

In summary, reviews that have included a systematic, combined analysis have all shown improvement in outcome measurements.

> **Key point 6**
>
> - Twenty-one randomised controlled studies in surgical patients been conducted to test the hypothesis that 'goal-directed' therapy may improve outcome. Overall, the mortality of the protocol patients is 7.06% and of the control patients is 10.25% (OR 0.67; 95% confidence intervals 0.54–0.83).

OTHER INDICATORS OF INADEQUATE TISSUE OXYGENATION

INTRAMUCOSAL pH MEASUREMENT

Hollow viscus tonometry has had a resurgence of interest in the last 20 years as a method of measuring perfusion in end-organs, specifically the gastrointestinal tract.[31] The information from the technique has been used for the calculation of intramucosal pH (pH_i), or the gap between arterial pCO_2 and the tonometric pCO_2. There are several important reasons why attention has focused on the gastrointestinal tract: first, splanchnic organs suffer vasoconstriction in response to hypovolaemia; second, the critical level of oxygen delivery in the gastrointestinal tract is higher than in other organs systems; and thirdly, gastrointestinal tract hypoxemia may increase endotoxin and micro-organism translocation fuelling the inflammatory reaction.

A number of studies have noted a relationship between low pH_i and morbidity and mortality in surgical patients. But whether this can be used for treatment or is simply a marker of disease is open to debate as some studies have not even confirmed the predictive value of pH_i measurements in compromised patients following cardiac surgery.[32] In contrast. Lebuffe *et al.*[33] reported that automated air tonometry might be able to identify patients at risk of circulatory failure after cardiac surgery better that conventional haemodynamic variables. Similarly, a study of patients having elective repair of infra-renal abdominal aortic aneurysms confirmed that low pH_i values (< 7.32) and their persistence were predictors of major complications; however, treatment to elevate low pH_i values did not improve post-operative outcome.[34] In a recent European study of 290 surgical patients, the arterial-tonometric pCO_2 gap was a useful prognostic index of postoperative morbidity.[35]

Despite the possible usefulness of pH_i to provide a monitor of the adequate nature of resuscitation, it does not fit well with a pre-emptive goal-directed approach to surgical patients, and appears to be more useful as a guide monitor the adequacy of resuscitation.

Key point 7

- Evidence suggests that 'goal-directed' therapy should be considered in all high-risk patients undergoing surgery. Evidence from randomised controlled trials shows that this is likely to lead to reduced postoperative mortality, reduced postoperative morbidity, and reduced costs.

LESS INVASIVE MONITORS OF TISSUE OXYGENATION

Most of the monitoring that has been discussed in this paper relies on invasive techniques. These have been criticised due to the risk of side-effects and difficulty in placing the monitoring equipment in terms of location, equipment and expertise. A few less invasive techniques are available but have tended to be used on emergency and trauma patients, but may become, with further development, suitable for surgical patients. Measurements of transcutaneous pO_2 and pCO_2 is accurate and useful in shock resuscitation,[36] and other studies have shown that placement of extremely small probes with pO_2, pCO_2, and pH sensors directly in skeletal muscle can also successfully monitor resuscitation responses.[37]

Another technology that might be useful in the future is near-infrared spectroscopy which monitors haemoglobin O_2 saturation in skeletal muscle and subcutaneous tissue. During shock resuscitation, it was found to correlate with oxygen delivery[38] but it has not been investigated in peri-operative surgical patients.

CONCLUSIONS

This paper has reviewed the scientific basis and recent studies in the area of goal-directed therapy. The normal postoperative response of increasing cardiac output and tissue perfusion immediately postoperatively is lacking in some patients and this results in increased postoperative morbidity and mortality. This is more likely to occur in patients who are elderly, have pre-existing disease states, and are undergoing emergency operations. Most of the sick patients will die from multiple organ dysfunction syndrome rather than from a discrete cause related to the surgery. One of the major determinants in the pathophysiology of multiple organ dysfunction syndrome is reduced blood flow to tissues and tissue hypoxia. New monitoring techniques in association with accurate fluid infusions, and inotropic medication to improve cardiac function, can allow cardiac output and peripheral blood flow to be targeted towards predesignated levels, this has been termed 'goal-directed' therapy. Evidence from randomised controlled trials shows that 'goal-directed' therapy reduces postoperative morbidity, mortality, and costs. 'Goal-directed' therapy should be considered in all higher risk operative patients.

Key points for clinical practice

- In the immediate postoperative period, a normal physiological response requires an increase in cardiac output and blood flow to the tissues. If this response fails, patients are more likely to have postoperative morbidity and mortality.
- Postoperative mortality rates are higher than expected in patients who are elderly, have premorbid disease conditions, such as cardiac and respiratory failure, and are having urgent operative procedures.
- Most surgical mortality in the sickest patients in the hospital being treated in intensive care units is usually due to multiple organ dysfunction syndrome.
- Multiple organ dysfunction syndrome has a multifactorial pathophysiology, which includes reduced cardiac output and reduced tissue oxygenation.
- Careful monitoring with a pulmonary artery catheter or oesophageal Doppler allows fluid and inotropic therapy to be given immediately pre-operatively with a goal of increasing and maximising cardiac output, blood flow and tissue oxygenation. This has been turned 'goal-directed' therapy and it has been suggested that they should be applied to all higher risk surgical patients.
- Twenty-one randomised controlled studies in surgical patients been conducted to test the hypothesis that 'goal-directed' therapy may improve outcome. Overall, the mortality of the protocol patients is 7.06% and of the control patients is 10.25% (OR 0.67; 95% confidence intervals 0.54–0.83).
- Evidence suggests that 'goal-directed' therapy should be considered in all high-risk patients undergoing surgery. Evidence from randomised controlled trials shows that this is likely to lead to reduced postoperative mortality, reduced postoperative morbidity, and reduced costs.

References

1. Clowes Jr GHA, Del Guercio LRM. Circulatory response to trauma of surgical operations. *Metabolism* 1960; **9**: 67–81.
2. Shoemaker WC. Cardiorespiratory patterns of surviving and non-surviving post-operative surgical patients. *Surg Gynecol Obstet* 1972; **134**: 810–814.
3. Shoemaker WC, Czer LSC. Evaluation of the biologic importance of various haemodynamic and oxygen transport variables. *Crit Care Med* 1979; **7**: 424–429.
4. Kusano C, Baba M, Takao S *et al.* Oxygen delivery as a factor in the development of fatal postoperative complications after oesophagectomy. *Br J Surg* 1997; **84**: 252–257.
5. Shoemaker WC, Appel PL, Kram HB. Tissue oxygen debt as a determinant of lethal and nonlethal postoperative organ failure. *Crit Care Med* 1988; **16**: 1117–1120.
6. Knaus WA, Wagner DP, Draper EA *et al.* The APACHE III prognostic system: risk prediction of hospital mortality for critically ill hospitalized adults. *Chest* 1991; **100**: 1619–1636.

7. Pappachan JV, Millar B, Bennett ED, Smith GB. Comparison of outcome from intensive care admission after adjustment for case mix by the APACHE III prognostic system [see comments]. *Chest* 1999; **115**: 802–810.
8. Society of Cardiothoracic Surgeons of Great Britain and Ireland. Risk Factors: Incidence and impact on operative mortality. National Adult Cardiac Surgical Database of the Society of Cardiothoracic Surgeons of Great Britain and Ireland, 2000.
9. Pedersen T, Eliasen K, Henriksen E. A prospective study of mortality associated with anaesthesia and surgery: risk indicators of mortality in hospital. *Acta Anaesthesiol Scand* 1990; **34**: 176–182.
10. Wirthlin DJ, Cambria RP. Surgery-specific considerations in the cardiac patient undergoing noncardiac surgery. *Prog Cardiovasc Dis* 1998; **40**: 453–468.
11. Bone RC, Balk RA, Cerra FB *et al.* Definitions for sepsis and organ failure and guidelines for the use of innovative therapies in sepsis. The ACCP/SCCM Consensus Conference Committee. American College of Chest Physicians/Society of Critical Care Medicine [see comments]. *Chest* 1992; **101**: 1644–1655.
12. Beal AL, Cerra FB. Multiple organ failure syndrome in the 1990s. *JAMA* 1994; **271**: 226–233.
13. Noble JS, MacKirdy FN, Donaldson SI, Howie JC. Renal and respiratory failure in Scottish ICUs. *Anaesthesia* 2001; **56**: 124–129.
14. Kirkpatrick CJ, Bittinger F, Klein CJ, Hauptmann S, Klosterhalfen B. The role of the microcirculation in multiple organ dysfunction syndrome: a review and perspective. *Virchows Archiv* 1996; **427**: 461–476.
15. Shoemaker WC, Appel PL, Kram HB. Role of oxygen debt in the development of organ failure, sepsis and death in high risk surgical patients. *Chest* 1992; **102**: 208–215.
16. Welborn MB, Oldenburg HS, Hess PJ *et al.* The relationship between visceral ischemia, proinflammatory cytokines, and organ injury in patients undergoing thoracoabdominal aortic aneurysm repair. *Crit Care Med* 2000; **28**: 3191–3197.
17. Bown MJ, Nicholson ML, Bell PR, Sayers RD. Cytokines and inflammatory pathways in the pathogenesis of multiple organ failure following abdominal aortic aneurysm repair. *Eur J Vasc Endovasc Surg* 2001; **22**: 485–495.
18. Bland RD, Shoemaker WC, Shabot MM. Physiologic monitoring goals for the critically ill patient. *Surg Gynecol Obstet* 1978; **147**: 833–841.
19. Shoemaker WC, Montgomery ES, Kaplan E, Elwyn DH. Physiologic patterns in surviving and non-surviving shock patients. Use of sequential cardiorespiratory parameters in defining criteria for therapeutic goals and early warning of death. *Arch Surg* 1973; **106**: 630–636.
20. Boyd O, Grounds RM, Bennett ED. A randomized clinical trial of the effect of deliberate perioperative increase of oxygen delivery on mortality in high-risk surgical patients [see comments]. *JAMA* 1993; **270**: 2699–2707.
21. Shoemaker WC, Appel PL, Kram HB, Waxman K, Lee T-S. Prospective trial of supranormal values of survivors as therapeutic goals in high-risk surgical patients. *Chest* 1988; **94**: 1176–1186.
22. Boyd O, Grounds RM, Bennett ED. A randomized clinical trial of the effect of deliberate perioperative increase of oxygen delivery on mortality in high-risk surgical patients. *JAMA* 1993; **270**: 2699–2707.
23. Fenwick E, Wilson J, Sculpher M, Claxton K. Pre-operative optimisation employing dopexamine or adrenaline for patients undergoing major elective surgery: a cost-effectiveness analysis. *Intensive Care Med* 2002; **28**: 599–608.
24. Ivanov RI, Allen J, Sandham JD, Calvin JE. Pulmonary artery catheterization: a narrative and systematic critique of randomized controlled trials and recommendations for the future. *New Horiz* 1997; **5**: 268–276.
25. Leibowitz AB, Beilin Y. Pulmonary artery catheters and outcome in the perioperative period. *New Horiz* 1997; **5**: 214–221.
26. Heyland DK, Cook DJ, King D, Kernerman P, Brun-Buisson C. Maximizing oxygen delivery in critically ill patients: a methodologic appraisal of the evidence [see comments]. *Crit Care Med* 1996; **24**: 517–524.
27. Boyd O, Hayes M. The oxygen trail – the goal. *Br Med Bull* 1999; **55**: 125–139.
28. Kern JW, Shoemaker WC. Meta-analysis of hemodynamic optimization in high-risk patients. *Crit Care Med* 2002; **30**: 1686–1692.

29. Ivanov R, Allen J, Calvin JE. The incidence of major morbidity in critically ill patients managed with pulmonary artery catheters: a meta-analysis. *Crit Care Med* 2000; **28**: 615–619.
30. Grocott M, Hamilton M, Bennett ED, Rowan K. Peri-operative increase in global blood flow to explicit defined goals and outcomes following surgery. The Cochrane Library. 2003: Oxford.
31. Fiddian-Green RG, Gantz NM. Transient episodes of sigmoid ischemia and their relation to infection from intestinal organisms after abdominal aortic operations. *Crit Care Med* 1987; **15**: 835–839.
32. Bams JL, Mariani MA, Groeneveld AB. Predicting outcome after cardiac surgery: comparison of global haemodynamic and tonometric variables. *Br J Anaesth* 1999; **82**: 33–37.
33. Lebuffe G, Decoene C, Pol A, Prat A, Vallet B. Regional capnometry with air-automated tonometry detects circulatory failure earlier than conventional hemodynamics after cardiac surgery. *Anesth Analg* 1999; **89**: 1084–1090.
34. Pargger H, Hampl KF, Christen P, Staender S, Scheidegger D. Gastric intramucosal pH-guided therapy in patients after elective repair of infrarenal abdominal aneurysms: is it beneficial? *Intensive Care Med* 1998; **24**: 769–776.
35. Lebuffe G, Vallet B, Takala J *et al*. A European, multicenter, observational study to assess the value of gastric-to-end tidal pCO_2 difference in predicting postoperative complications. *Anesth Analg* 2004; **99**: 166–172.
36. Tatevossian RG, Wo CC, Velmahos GC, Demetriades D, Shoemaker WC. Transcutaneous oxygen and CO_2 as early warning of tissue hypoxia and hemodynamic shock in critically ill emergency patients. *Crit Care Med* 2000; **28**: 2248–2253.
37. McKinley BA, Ware DN, Marvin RG, Moore FA. Skeletal muscle pH, $P(CO_2)$, and $P(O_2)$ during resuscitation of severe hemorrhagic shock. *J Trauma* 1998; **45**: 633–636.
38. McKinley BA, Marvin RG, Cocanour CS, Moore FA. Tissue hemoglobin O_2 saturation during resuscitation of traumatic shock monitored using near infrared spectrometry. *J Trauma* 2000; **48**: 637–642.

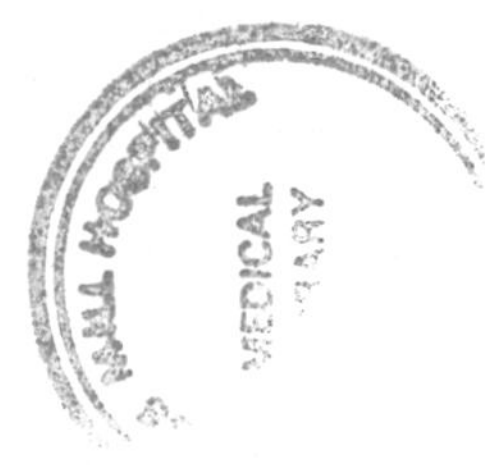

Sunil Kumar Hari I. Pandey Prabhjot Saggu

4

Abdominal tuberculosis

Tuberculosis continues to be a major problem, being responsible for 7–10 million new cases and 6% of deaths world-wide.[1] Abdominal tuberculosis is a common extrapulmonary manifestation of tuberculosis. Its incidence is also increasing in the west due to an increase in the immigrant population, ageing population, and an increasing incidence of human immunodeficiency virus (HIV) infections. Of non-HIV patients, 10–15% have extrapulmonary manifestations of tuberculosis and 50% of HIV-infected patients have extrapulmonary manifestations of tuberculosis. There is also a re-emergence of tuberculosis in India, especially the extrapulmonary (intestinal) variant, due to incomplete treatment, occurrence of multidrug-resistant strains, and an increasing incidence of HIV-AIDS.[2] The wide spectrum of presentation makes abdominal tuberculosis a difficult disease to recognise,[3] sometimes only made on postmortem.[2] In the last few years, advances in genetic tests, better imaging modalities, endoscopy and laparoscopic facilities have increased the detection of gastrointestinal tuberculosis.

*Colour figures (plates) referred to in this chapter are to be found in the 'Colour plates section' at the front of this volume (p1–8).

Sunil Kumar MS DNB FRCS(Ed), FRCS(Eng)
Senior Consultant, Department of Surgery, Tata Main Hospital, Jamshedpur, India
(for correspondence)
E mail: sunilvinita42@hotmail.com

Hari I. Pandey MS MCh
Consultant Surgeon, Tata Main Hospital, Jamshedpur, India

Prabhjot Saggu MBBS DNB(Std)
Resident Surgeon, Tata Main Hospital, Jamshedpur, India

> **Key point 1**
>
> - There is a resurgence of abdominal tuberculosis due to multidrug resistance and co-existence of HIV-AIDS.

PATHOLOGY AND PATHOGENESIS

Ingestion of infected sputum, unpasteurised milk (*Mycobacterium bovis*), haematogenous spread from miliary disease and direct spread from adjacent organs such as the fallopian tube may lead to infection of the gastrointestinal tract (Table 1).

After ingestion, the organisms are trapped in the Peyer's patches of the small and large intestines, which then undergo inflammatory enlargement leading to transverse mucosal ulcerations. An element of endarteritis is also present. Bowel perforation rarely occurs, but is usually confined by the surrounding inflammation. The mesenteric lymph nodes enlarge, may caseate leading to intra-abdominal abscesses. Fibrosis may follow leading to the typical 'napkin-ring strictures'.[4] Extensive inflammation of submucosa and subserosa mainly of the ileocaecal area gives rise to the hyperplastic form. Adjacent bowel loops, mesentery and nodes may adhere forming a mass, the 'intestinal cocoon'.

Peritoneal involvement takes the form of numerous miliary tubercles on the peritoneum and intestines (Plate VI, p3). The omentum thickens to form a mass leading to a 'rolled-up omentum'. Ascites is usually present.

Haematogenous involvement of the liver, spleen and pancreas may present as multiple parenchymal abscesses with organomegaly. Contiguous spread to the gastrointestinal tract may occur from disease present in the spine, genito-urinary system, parietal wall or the retroperitoneum (Plate VII, p3).

Histologically, involved tissue shows the typical granuloma which is a focus of epitheloid cells with a rim of fibroblasts, lymphocytes, histiocytes and Langhans' giant cells. Central caseation and acid-fast bacilli may be present (Table 2).

> **Key point 2**
>
> - The most common route for infection is ingestion of infected sputum.

Table 1 Sources and routes of abdominal infection

Direct ingestion
Infected sputum (*M. tuberculosis*)
Dairy products (unpasteurised milk, *M. bovis*)
Haematogenous spread: secondary to pulmonary tuberculosis
Direct extension from contiguous organ
Through fallopian tube

Table 2 Gross pathological types of tuberculosis

Intestinal
Ulcerative
Hyperplastic, plastic form – whole intestine plastered
Strictures
Perforative
Peritoneal
Wet type: ascites – generalised or loculated
Dry plastic: mesenteric thickening, caseous lymph nodes and fibrous adhesions
Fibrotic fixed type: mass formation of omentum, matting of bowel loops
Acute primary peritonitis
Mesenteric involvement
Mass
Abscess
Nodal
Solid organ: liver, spleen, pancreas involvement
Localised abscess
Multiple miliary form

CLINICAL PRESENTATION

Because of its varied presentation (Table 3) and its ability to mimic a variety of other abdominal conditions, a high index of suspicion is required.[5,6] Individuals aged 25–44 years are most commonly affected.[2]

The disease commonly presents insidiously with abdominal pain, fever, night sweats, weight loss, anorexia, nausea and vomiting, diarrhoea or constipation.[4,7–9] Rarer presentations are an acute abdomen, perianal abscess or fistulae, upper or lower gastrointestinal bleeding and dysphagia, if the oesophagus is involved.[10–15] The disease may also present as an entero-cutaneous fistula after bowel surgery, an umbilical abscess, a discharging sinus or as non-healing surgical wounds.

On examination, pallor, ascites, hepatomegaly or abdominal masses due to enlarged lymph nodes, adherent bowel loops or a cold abscess may be noted.[7–9] The classical doughy abdomen is considered non-specific.[2] Common complications are obstruction, perforation, fistulae and malabsorption.[4,12,14,16]

Key point 3

- Due to involvement of any intra-abdominal organ, the symptoms may be varied.

DIAGNOSIS

The diagnosis of abdominal tuberculosis is challenging. Even in highly endemic areas, the accuracy of clinical diagnosis is only 50%.[2] A clinical suspicion of tuberculous gastrointestinal infection should lead to a graded investigative work-up. A diagnosis at an early stage can lead to non-operative medical management.

Raised erythrocyte sedimentation rate, anaemia and hypoalbuminaemia are commonly seen.[7] Sputum for acid-fast bacilli (AFB), using Ziehl-Neilsen

Table 3 Common presentations of gastrointestinal tuberculosis

*	Abdominal pain	86% (77–94%)
*	Vomiting	46% (33–74%)
*	Abdominal distension	37% (28–45%)
*	Ascites	37% (19–60%)
*	Borborygmi	35% (26–50%)
*	Abdominal mass	33% (17–45%)
*	Diarrhoea	22% (11–48%)
*	Constipation	24% (12–46%)
*	Haematochezia	4% (2–13%)
*	Abdominal mass	30–35%
*	Constitutional symptoms	
	Weight loss	63% (35–87%)
	Fever	61% (29–100%)
	Anorexia	48% (10–100%)
	Amenorrhoea	23% (12–36%)
	Pulmonary	19% (4–51%)

Adapted from Rangabashyam *et al.*[4]

staining, may be positive in active pulmonary disease, and may provide indirect evidence of abdominal tuberculosis. Culture of mycobacteria can be done in liquid (BACTEC) or solid (Löwenstein-Jensen) media. In the BACTEC test, a fluorescent sensor in the vial reacts to depletion in oxygen dissolved in the broth growing the mycobacteria. Results are available in 10–14 days. Löwenstein-Jensen medium takes a longer time (4–6 weeks). However, if adequate bacterial load is not present, the culture may prove inconclusive. Ascitic fluid for AFB smear or culture gives a low yield.[4] The Mantoux test may be used as a screening test, but is of limited value in endemic areas because of high false-positive rates.[17]

BIOCHEMICAL INVESTIGATIONS

Biochemical investigations which are routinely used are the serum albumin to ascitic fluid gradient (SAAG), which is usually less than 1.1, reflecting an exudative ascites. The ascitic fluid has a high protein content (> 2.5–3 mg/dl), with a predominance of lymphocytes, and presence of neutrophils and monocytes.[7] Adenosine deaminase is an enzyme found in many cell types – macrophages, lymphocytes and erythrocytes. It is a marker for host immune response in cases of abdominal tuberculosis. Serum adenosine deaminase activity values of more than 42 IU/l are significant. Ascitic fluid adenosine deaminase levels > 33 U/l have a 100% and 95% sensitivity and specificity, respectively.[18] Its limitations are in patients with cirrhosis or patients with HIV infections. Another uncommonly used investigation is ascitic fluid interferon-γ levels, produced by T lymphocytes present in ascitic fluid;[4] its level measures severity of infection. Serum lactate dehydrogenase levels are elevated to over 90 U/l in patients with intestinal tuberculosis.[4]

Serological tests are based on detection of specific antibodies to mycobacterial tuberculosis. ELISA enables rapid diagnosis. The IgG component has high specificity for abdominal tuberculosis diseases. Monoclonal antibodies are prepared by hybridoma technology. Each can be used to detect surface or soluble cytoplasmic antigen as well as antibodies against surface antigen.

Genetic tests have come to play a very important role in the management of pulmonary and extrapulmonary tuberculosis. These are rapid, sensitive, specific and inexpensive methods of diagnosis and results are available in a few hours. TB-nested polymerase chain reaction (PCR) has the ability to detect as little as 8 fg of mycobacterial DNA, or 1 to 2 bacilli from a variety of sources.[19–21] Restriction fragment length polymorphism is also a very sensitive and specific test to detect very early cases of tuberculosis. Luciferase receptor assay is also a promising new modality.

Key point 4

- Rapid and specific diagnosis of gastrointestinal tuberculosis is possible with genetic tests.

RADIOLOGICAL TESTS

Chest X-ray is an important first investigation due to the fact that active pulmonary lesions may be present in up to 60% of patients with abdominal disease.[16] In patients presenting with an acute abdomen, an abdominal X-ray may show multiple air-fluid levels, dilated jejunum or ileum due to a distal stricture. A contrast study will show strictures with marked proximal dilation, thickening of the ileocaecal valve, a wide opened valve, accompanied by narrowing of the terminal ileum (Fleischner sign),[22] and a fibrotic terminal ileum opening into a contracted caecum (Stierlin's sign).[23] Enteroclysis or small bowel enema may also be used (Figs 1–3).

Ultrasonography of the abdomen may show lymph node involvement in the periportal, peripancreatic, mesenteric or retroperitoneal areas. The involved lymph nodes are usually matted together with hypo-echoic centres and occasionally may contain calcifications.[23,24] In early stage disease, a few regional lymph nodes and circumferential thickening of the wall of the caecum and terminal ileum may be seen.[24] In advanced ileocaecal tuberculosis, gross wall thickening, adherent bowel loops, larger regional nodes and mesenteric thickening may form a complex mass of varied echogenicity centred on the ileocaecal junction. These features are highly suggestive of ileocaecal tuberculosis.[24] Ultrasonography may also demonstrate free, loculated or focal ascites. Focal ascites is a fluid collection between bowel loops that appears as the 'club sandwich' sign.[24]

Peritoneal involvement presents as peritoneal or omental thickening. Multiple abscesses and homogenous organomegaly with focal lesions or calcification indicate visceral disease.[24]

Graded compression sonography is the most effective technique of evaluating mesenteric disease.[24] Ultrasound-guided FNAB of palpable masses has also given good results.[25]

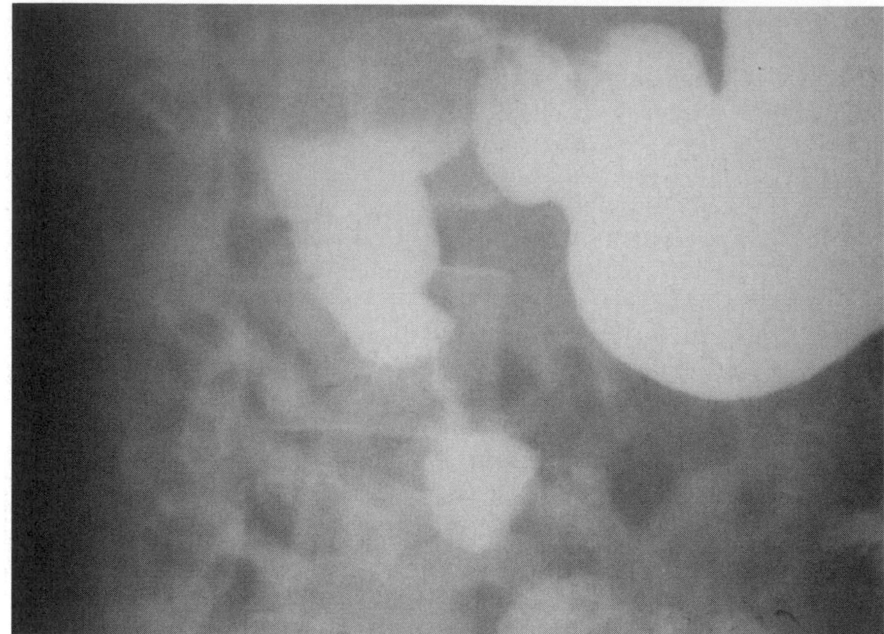

Fig. 1 Duodenal tuberculous stricture.

Abdominal CT is considered essential for the evaluation of extraluminal, peritoneal, nodal and visceral involvement.[26] Abdominal lymphadenopathy is the commonest manifestation of tuberculosis on CT. The nodes appear as

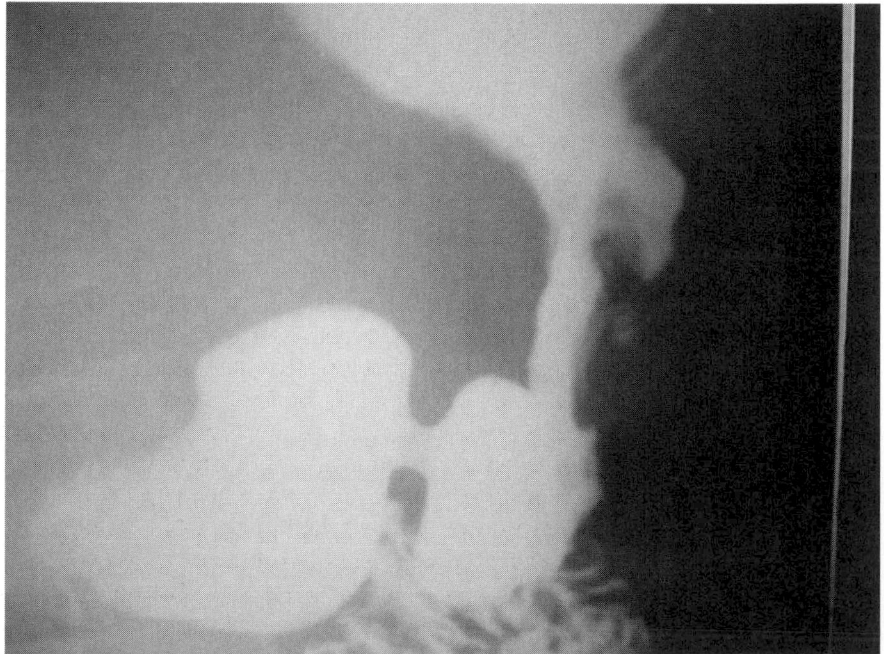

Fig. 2 Gastric tuberculous stricture.

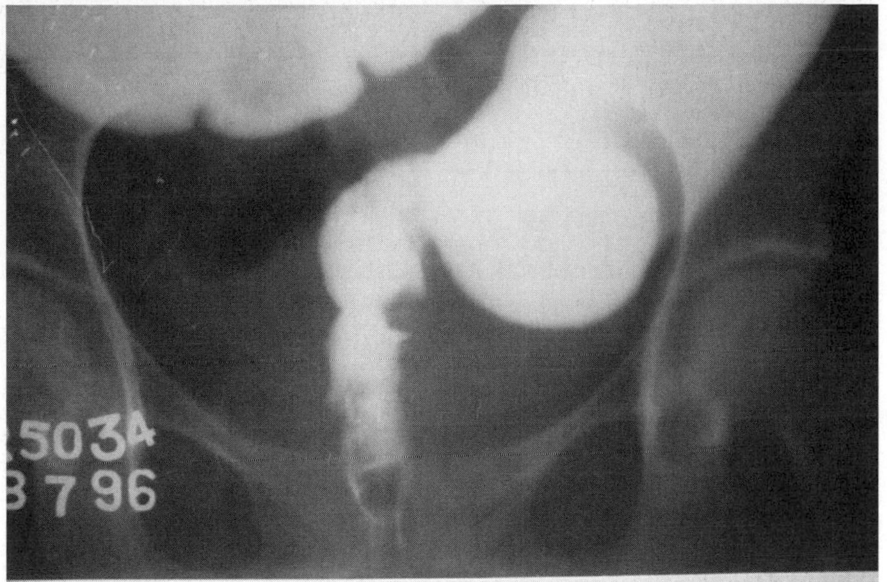

Fig. 3 Rectal tuberculous stricture.

hypodense centres with peripheral hyperdense enhancing rims. Ascitic fluid has high-density appearance due to high protein content. Thickening and nodularity of the peritoneum and mesentery can be easily detected. Thickening of bowel wall and ileocaecal valve, mesenteric or retroperitoneal lymph nodes seen may be confused with lymphoma, Crohn's disease or carcinoma. CT will also show solid visceral involvement.[27] Of late, CT enteroclysis is being used to detect small bowel tuberculosis.[28]

MRI depicts para-aortic, aortocaval and mesenteric nodes effectively. Macronodular tubercular liver abscesses appear on MR imaging, hypo-intense and minimally enhancing honeycomb-like lesions on T1W images. On T2W images, the lesions are hyperintense with a less intense rim relative to the surrounding liver.[22] FNAB or tissue specimen, may be obtained by direct, USG, CT, or laparoscopic biopsy.

ENDOSCOPIC EVALUATION

Endoscopy offers the advantage of minimal invasion and may help avoid surgery with upper gastrointestinal endoscopy for oesophageal, gastric, or duodenal disease, and colonoscopy and ileoscopy for rectal, colonic and ileocaecal disease. Endoscopic brush or needle cytology and biopsy are often diagnostic.[29] Capsule endoscopy for the small bowel may be helpful.[30]

Peritoneal biopsy has been reported to have high diagnostic accuracy for peritoneal tuberculosis. The peritoneal tissue can be obtained by blind needle biopsy, minilaparotomy, laparotomy and laparoscopy.[31] Laparoscopy is considered to be the most appropriate because of its ability to visualise the peritoneal cavity in detail and take biopsies from suspected lesions at the same time being minimally invasive and less morbid.[17,31,32]

> **Key point 5**
>
> - CT enteroclysis and capsule endoscopy are the newer tests that have been added to the diagnostic armamentarium.

DIFFERENTIAL DIAGNOSIS

Abdominal tuberculosis should be differentiated from primary gastrointestinal lymphoma, Crohn's disease, ulcerative colitis, disseminated carcinoma, amoebic colitis, chronic liver disease, fungal infection, sarcoidosis, peritoneal mesothelioma or acute appendicitis.[22,23,31] Tuberculosis may co-exist in a patient with malignancy. The presence of tuberculosis should prompt a search for a concomitant HIV infection[33] and *vice versa* due to the high incidence of tuberculosis in HIV patients.

MANAGEMENT OF GASTROINTESTINAL TUBERCULOSIS

The treatment of abdominal tuberculosis is primarily medical. A pathological diagnosis may not always be established. Hence, with given clinical, radiological or colonoscopic findings, a therapeutic trial may be indicated.[26] Evidence of tuberculosis elsewhere in the body in the presence of clinicoradiological features is also considered useful for the diagnosis. The World Health Organization guideline on antituberculous therapy recommends a 6-month course. Four drugs (Isoniazid, rifampicin, pyrazinamide, Ethambutol or streptomycin) for 2 months, followed by two-drug therapy (Isoniazid and rifampicin) for 4 months. Uncomplicated tuberculous enteritis can be managed with a 9–12-month chemotherapy,[35] with 2-month intensive four-drug treatment (Isoniazid, rifampicin, pyrazinamide, Ethambutol), followed by a 7-month, two-drug treatment (Isoniazid and rifampicin).[6] Supplementation with Pyridoxine, 10 mg daily, is necessary to counter peripheral neuritis due to Isoniazid (Table 4).

There have been numerous advances that allow better treatment of tuberculous enteritis, including intravenous streptomycin, rifampicin, and quinolones, which can be administered parenterally. In India, the Directly Observed Therapy (DOTS), wherein the patient takes the pills in the presence of a family member and a health professional, during the initial 2 months, has much improved compliance and ensured adequate treatment.

Table 4 Chemotherapy and common adverse effects

Drug	Daily dosage (mg/kg)	Adverse effects
Isoniazid	5	Peripheral neuritis, mental disturbances, hepatitis, rashes, acne, fever, drug interactions
Rifampicin	10	Orange urine, hepatitis, skin rashes, purpura, 'flu syndrome', drug interactions
Ethambutol	15	Optic neuritis, hyperuricaemia
Pyrazinamide	25	Hepatotoxicity, hyperuricaemia, arthralgia, rashes
Streptomycin	15	Ototoxicity, nephrotoxicity

Table 5 Second-line drugs

Second-line drugs
Amikacin
Kanamycin
Para-aminosalicylic acid (PAS)
Ciprofloxacin
Ofloxacin
Clarithromycin
Azithromycin
Rifabutin

[From Sheer and Coyle.[2]]

Medical therapy is considered successful when clinical signs improve (weight gain, good appetite, no fever, and no abdominal pain), and erythrocyte sedimentation rate and haemoglobin levels have returned to normal. Up to 70% response is seen in abdominal tuberculosis. In non-responders, drug resistance or associated pathology should be considered (malignancy or Crohn's disease). Single drug resistance is present in about 9.9% of cases, and multidrug resistance is seen in about 1.4% of patients. Drug resistance leads to a lower likelihood of cure, more expensive treatment; it warrants a culture and sensitivity analysis and recourse to second-line drugs (Table 5). The incidence of drug-related toxicity is also higher. The use of corticosteroids is controversial. While some decrease in the incidence of adhesions and intestinal obstruction (due to decreased fibrosis) may occur, in the absence of controlled trials evaluating its role, its routine use is not recommended.[4]

Key point 6

- Failure to improve on antituberculous therapy should warrant re-evaluation to rule out malignancy or Crohn's disease.

SURGERY IN ABDOMINAL TUBERCULOSIS

Surgery is indicated when there is doubt in the diagnosis, for mechanical complications,[35] severe intestinal haemorrhage,[13] or when the patient presents with an acute abdomen. Operative findings may include intestinal obstruction due to single or multiple strictures, which are managed with stricturoplasty or resection and anastomosis if multiple strictures are found in a short segment.[36,37] Accessible strictures may be dilated by endoscopic balloon.[36] Obstructed ileocaecal tuberculosis was earlier managed with ileotransverse bypass or extensive resection (right hemicolectomy). Due to high complication rates, a more conservative segmental resection, with a 5 cm margin, is considered adequate.[4] Perforation mandates a biopsy from the perforated gut, and resection of the involved segment and primary anastomosis. Primary repair of the perforation runs the risk of re-perforation or fistulisation.[38]

Several other procedures (gastrojejunostomy, duodenojejunostomy,[35] splenectomy, *etc.*) are being performed for tuberculous involvement of different organs.

Occasionally, one may come across the entire intestine being plastered, due to omental and bowel adhesions due to tubercular involvement. In such cases, little more than gentle exploration and tissue for diagnosis is possible because extensive adhesiolysis runs the risk of postoperative fistulation with prolonged morbidity and a higher mortality. Such cases are put on antituberculous treatment to which they respond well. Recurrent fistula-in-ano, or perianal abscess are a common presentation in tropical countries, which respond to antituberculous treatment after surgery.

Diagnostic laparoscopy has resulted in the avoidance of unnecessary exploratory laparotomy in a large number of patients. Laparoscopy is being increasingly used for definitive surgical treatment of abdominal tuberculosis.[39]

Key point 7

- Antituberculous therapy is the mainstay of treatment, the role of surgery is limited to diagnosis and the management of complications.

OUR EXPERIENCE WITH ABDOMINAL TUBERCULOSIS

At Tata Main Hospital there is a dedicated chest clinic, where all tuberculosis patients are registered and followed. Experience has shown that ileocaecal tuberculosis is the most common site of involvement in the abdomen, with the ascitic form being the next most common. Oesophageal, duodenal, gastric, colonic, pancreatic, hepatic and splenic involvement are also seen. We frequently see patients who present with an acute abdomen and are found to have ileal perforation or primary peritonitis. Mesenteric adenitis and strictures are also a common finding. Anorectal tuberculosis presents as ulcerative colitis, perianal abscess and recurrent fistula-in-ano. All patients are managed with antituberculous chemotherapy after diagnosis. With the inclusion of diagnostic laparoscopy for evaluation of non-specific pain abdomen, our detection rate of abdominal tuberculosis has increased.

CONCLUSIONS

The diagnosis of gastrointestinal tuberculosis is challenging as it presents with a variety of symptoms. A high index of suspicion is essential. The arrival of genetic tests, laparoscopy, improved endoscopy and radiology have aided the surgeon in arriving at an earlier diagnosis. Medical treatment is the mainstay of therapy. However, the high cost of treatment, the development of multidrug resistant strains, and infection with atypical mycobacteria in immunocompromised patients have all increased the incidence and severity of abdominal tuberculosis. The role of surgery is principally in diagnosis and the management of complications.

Key points for clinical practice

- There is a resurgence of abdominal tuberculosis due to multidrug resistance and co-existence of HIV-AIDS.
- The most common route for infection is ingestion of infected sputum.
- Due to involvement of any intra-abdominal organ, the symptoms may be varied.
- Rapid and specific diagnosis of gastrointestinal tuberculosis is possible with genetic tests.
- CT enteroclysis and capsule endoscopy are the newer tests that have been added to the diagnostic armamentarium.
- Failure to improve on antituberculous therapy should warrant re-evaluation to rule out malignancy or Crohn's disease.
- Antituberculous therapy is the mainstay of treatment, the role of surgery is limited to diagnosis and the management of complications.

References

1. Ahmed A, Pereira SP, Steger A, Starke I. Abdominal tuberculosis: the great mimic. *Hosp Med* 2001; **62**: XX–XX.
2. Sheer TA, Coyle WJ. Gastrointestinal tuberculosis. *Curr Gastroenterol Rep* 2003; **5**: 273–278.
3. Ismail Y, Muhamad A, Surg M. Protean manifestations of gastrointestinal tuberculosis. *Med J Malaysia* 2003; **58**: XX–XX.
4. Rangabashyam N, Anand BS, OmPrakash R. Abdominal tuberculosis. *Oxford Textbook of Surgery*, vol. 3, 2nd edn. Oxford: OUP, 2000; 3237–3249.
5. Badaoui E, Berney T, Kaiser L, Mentha G, Morel P. Surgical presentation of abdominal tuberculosis: a protean disease. *Hepatogastroenterology* 2000; **47**: 751–755.
6. Pulimood AB, Ramakrishna BS, Kurian G *et al*. Endoscopic mucosal biopsies are useful in distinguishing ganulomatous colitis due to Crohn's disease from tuberculosis. *Gut* 1999; **45**: 537–541.
7. Al Muneef M, Memish Z, Al Mahmoud S *et al*. Tuberculosis in the belly: a review of forty-six cases involving the gastrointestinal tract and peritoneum. *Scand J Gastroenterol* 2001; **36**: 528–532.
8. Ranger DS, Roskall T, Narward A-H *et al*. Abdominal tuberculosis: the problem of diagnostic delay. *Scand J Infect Dis* 1999; **31**: 517–XXX.
9. Bayramicli OU, Dabak G, Dabak R. A clinical dilemma: abdominal tuberculosis. *World J Gastroenterol* 2003; **9**: 1098–1101.
10. Candela F, Serrano P, Arriero J *et al*. Perianal disease of tuberculous origin: report of a case and review of literature. *Dis Col Rectum* 1999; **42**: 110–112.
11. Adhami S, Duthie G, Greenstone M. A tuberculous anal fistula. *J R Soc Med* 199X; **92**: 467–468.
12. Nagi B, Lal A, Kochhar R *et al*. Perforations and fistulae in gastrointestinal tuberculosis. *Acta Radiol* 2002; **43**: 501–506.
13. Kungeswaran E, Smith OJ, Quiason SG *et al*. Both massive upper and lower gastrointestinal hemorrhage secondary to tuberculosis. *Am J Gastroenterol* 1999; **94**: 270–272.
14. Wantabe T, Kudo M, Kayaba M *et al*. Massive rectal bleeding due to ileal tuberculosis. *J Gastroenterol* 1999; **34**: 525–529.

15. Prakash K, Kuruvilla K, Lekha V *et al*. Primary tuberculous stricture of the oesophagus mimicking carcinoma. *Trop Gastroenterol* 2001; **22**: 143–144.
16. Joy B, Gulshan B, Michael KC. Gastrointestinal tuberculosis: an eighteen patient experience and review. *J Clin Gastroenterol* 2000; **30**: 397–402.
17. Hassan I, Brilakis ES, Thompson RL, Que FG. Surgical management of abdominal tuberculosis. *J Gastrointest Surg* 2002; **6**: 862–867.
18. Petroianni A, Mugnaini I, Laurendi G *et al*. Abdominal tuberculosis mimicking Crohn's disease: a difficult diagnosis. *Panminerva Med* 2002; **44**: 155–158.
19. Shan YS, Yan JJ, Sy ED, Jin YT, Lee JC. Nested polymerase chain reaction in the diagnosis of negative Ziehl-Neilsen stained *Mycobacterium tuberculosis* fistula-in-ano. *Dis Colon Rectum* 2002; **45**: 1685–1688.
20. Gan HT, Chen YQ, Quyang Q, Bu H, Yang XY. Differentiation between intestinal tuberculosis and Crohn's disease in endoscopic biopsy specimens by polymerase chain reaction. *Am J Gastroenterol* 2002; **97**: 1446–1451.
21. Chan CM, Yuen KY, Chan KS *et al*. Single tube nested PCR in the diagnosis of tuberculosis. *J Clin Pathol* 1996; **49**: 290–294.
22. Buxi TBS, Sud S, Vohra R. CT and MRI in the diagnosis of tuberculosis. *Indian J Paediatr* 2002; **69**: 965–972.
23. Akhan O, Pringot J. Imaging in abdominal tuberculosis. *Eur Radiol* 2002; **12**: 312–323.
24. Batra A, Gulati MS, Sharma D, Paul SB. Sonographic appearance in abdominal tuberculosis. *J Clin Ultrasound* 2002; **28**: 233–245.
25. Malik A, Saxena NC. Ultrasound in abdominal tuberculosis. *Abdom Imaging* 2003; **28**: 574–579.
26. Nagi B, Kochar R, Bhasin DK, Singh K. Colorectal tuberculosis. *Eur Radiol* 2003; **13**: 1907–1912.
27. Suri S, Gupta S, Suri R. Computed tomography in abdominal tuberculosis. *Br J Radiol* 1999; **72**: 92–98.
28. Dean DT, Bender GN, Heitkamp DE, Lappas JE, Kelvin FM. Multidetector-row helical CT enteroclysis. *Radiol Clin North Am.* 2003; **41**: XX–XX.
29. Leung VKS, Tang WL, Cheung CH, Lai MS. Importance of ileoscopy during colonoscopy for the early diagnosis of ileal tuberculosis: report of two cases. *Gastrointest Endosc* 2001; **53**: XX–XX.
30. Reddy DN, Sriram PVJ, Rao GV, Reddy DB. Capsule endoscopy appearance of small bowel tuberculosis. *Endoscopy* 2003; **35**: 99.
31. Ibrarullah MD, Mohan A, Sarkari A *et al*. Abdominal tuberculosis: diagnosis by laparoscopy and colonoscopy. *Trop Gasteroenterol* 2002; **23**:150–153.
32. McLaughlin S, Jones T, Pitcher M, Evans P. Laparoscopic diagnosis of abdominal tuberculosis. *Aust NZ J Surg* 1998; **68**: 598–601.
33. Redyanly RD, Silverstein JE. Intraabdominal manifestation of AIDS. *Radiol Clin North Am* 1997; **35**: 1083–1125.
34. Lane JE, Barron TD, Solis MM, Tench DW, Stephens JL. Tuberculous enteritis: a case report. *Am Surg* 2000, **66**: 683–685.
35. Negi SS, Sachdev AK, Choudhary A, Kumar N, Ranjana. Surgical management of obstructive gastroduodenal tuberculosis. *Trop Gastroenterol* 2003; **24**: 39–41.
36. Akbar M. Stricturoplasty in tuberculous small bowel strictures. *J Ayub Med Coll Abbotabad* 2003; **15**: XX–XX.
37. Zafar A, Qureshi AM, Iqbal M. Comparison between stricturoplasty and resection anastomosis in tuberculous intestinal strictures. *JCPSP* 2003; **13**: 277–279.
38. Talwar S, Talwar R, Prasad R. Tuberculous perforations of the small intestine. *IJCP* 1999; **53**: XX–XX.
39. Chumber S, Samaiya A, Subramaniam R *et al*. Laparoscopy assisted hemi-colectomy for ileo-caecal tuberculosis. *Trop Gastroenterol* 2001; **22**: 107–112.

Plate VI Miliary tubercles.

Plate VII Tuberculous stricture and nodes.

Mohammed R.S. Keshtgar
Ursula B. McGovern David Chao

5

Malignant melanoma update

There is a rise in the incidence of malignant melanoma. The incidence is highest in Auckland, New Zealand, with an age-standardised rate of 56.2/100,000 and life-time cumulative risk of 5.7%.[1] The incidence has quadrupled in Australia and doubled in Britain, Norway, Canada and America. The lowest incidence is reported in Asian countries. It represents 5% of cutaneous malignancy but it is responsible for most skin cancer mortality.

Melanoma does not show any overall sex predilection. In men, the front and back of the trunk, and in women, the lower leg, are the commonest sites.

It is estimated that melanoma occurs 20 times more often in whites than blacks. Exposure to sunlight is an important aetiological factor and the incidence is higher in individuals with white complexion and blue eyes.

About 50–60% of melanomas arise from benign naevus or an area adjacent to it. The trigger factor is unknown. Malignant transformation in a mole should be suspected if there are changes in size, shape or colour. Other changes that are not as significant include, inflammation, crusting or bleeding, itching and diameter of 6 mm or more.

*Colour figures (plates) referred to in this chapter are to be found in the 'Colour plates section' at the front of this volume (p1–8).

Mohammed R.S. Keshtgar FRCSI FRCS(Gen) PhD
Senior Lecturer and Consultant Surgical Oncologist, Department of Surgery, University College London, 67–73 Riding House St, London W1W 7EJ, UK E-mail: m.keshtgar@ucl.ac.uk
(for correspondence)

Ursula B. McGovern BSc MBChB MRCP
SpR Medical Oncology, Department of Oncology, North Middlesex Hospital, Stirling Way, London N18 1QX, UK. E-mail: ursula.mcgovern@nmh.nhs.uk

David Chao BMBCh MRCP DPhil
Consultant Medical Oncologist, Department of Clinical Oncology, Royal Free Hospital, Gray's Inn Division, Pond St, London NW3 2QG, UK. E-mail: david.chao@royalfree.nhs.uk

Common features of melanoma include (A,B,C,D,E): (i) asymmetrical outline; (ii) border irregularity; (iii) colour variegation; (iv) diameter > 6 mm; and (v) elevation.

Familial malignant melanoma accounts for 8–12% of all melanomas, and tends to occur at a younger age. Between 3–5% of patients who have been diagnosed with melanoma go on to develop a second primary and this needs to be borne in mind during the patient follow-up.

Key point 1

- The incidence of melanoma is rising. Exposure to sunlight is a major aetiological factor. The majority of melanomas arise from pre-existing moles. Melanoma should be suspected if there are changes in size, shape or colour, bleeding, itching or moles more than 6 mm in diameter.

CUTANEOUS MELANOMA

TUMOUR TYPES

Lentigo maligna melanoma

This is the most benign form of melanoma and accounts for 10–15% of all cutaneous melanomas. It occurs in Hutchinson's freckle and mainly affects the areas heavily exposed to sun mainly the head and neck of the elderly.

Superficial spreading melanoma

This is the most common form of melanoma, which accounts for 70% of all cutaneous melanomas. The peak incidence is at the 5th decade of life, which is younger than for most cancers and has socio-economic considerations. It may occur at any anatomical site and affect any age group. Clinically, it has variable pigmentation with irregular border. The common site in men is the back and in women the legs. Histologically, this is associated with asymmetry, poor circumscription and lack of maturation.

Nodular melanoma

This is the most malignant type of malignant melanoma involving most exclusively the vertical growth phase. It usually present as a darkly pigmented raised nodule. It accounts for about 12% of all melanomas and is twice as common in men. Clinically, these lesions develop quickly.

Acral lentiginous melanoma

This type of melanoma occurs in palms, soles and subungal areas. It carries a worse prognosis than the superficial spreading melanoma but it is not as bad as the nodular variety.

Amelanotic melanoma

These lesions appear pink but close inspection may reveal some pigmentation. Lack of obvious pigmentation can lead to delay in diagnosis. It carries an even worse prognosis than nodular melanoma.

> **Key point 2**
>
> - Superficial spreading melanoma is the commonest form of melanoma and accounts for 70% of cases. Nodular melanoma accounts for 12% of cases and lentigo maligna melanoma for 10–15%. Pigmentation is not mandatory for the diagnosis of melanoma.

PROGNOSTIC FACTORS

There are several factors that are identified with direct impact on the patient's outcome. These factors are taken into consideration in the American Joint Committee on Cancer (AJCC) staging system. These factors can be subdivided into the clinical and histological prognostic factors.

Clinical prognostic factors

Age and gender: There are many studies that have demonstrated a relationship between age and prognosis. Older age is associated with worse prognosis as compared to younger age group.[2] Many studies have confirmed that female sufferers of melanoma have a better prognosis than male patients.[3]

Anatomical location: Primary melanomas located in the head and neck, trunk and acral regions are associated with worse prognosis those in extremity locations.[3,4]

Histological prognostic factors

Tumour thickness: Tumour thickness has been recognised as the most important prognostic factor in melanoma patients with stage I and II disease. There are two described methods of thickness measurement:

1. **Clark level** – In 1969, Clark and co-workers[5] described tumours based on the anatomical levels of involvement within the cutaneous and subcutaneous structures. They described 5 levels of invasion: level I, growth within the epidermis; level II, tumour growth extending to papillary dermis; level III, tumour involvement filling the papillary dermis and invading the junction between the papillary and reticular dermis; level IV, invasion of reticular dermis; and level V, invasion of the tumour within subcutaneous fat.
2. **Breslow thickness** – In 1970, Breslow described an alternative method of measuring the tumour thickness.[6] With the aid of an ocular micrometer, he measured the thickness of tumours in millimetres, starting from the top of the granular layer up to the base of the tumour.

Tumour thickness based on the Breslow classification is accepted as the most reliable, independent prognostic indicator in malignant melanoma. Additionally, it assists in therapeutic decision making with regards to the clearance margin for tumours and indication for sentinel node biopsy. In general, a tumour with thickness less than 1 mm is regarded as thin with good prognosis and overall survival rate of more than 95%. Tumours with thickness of 1–4 mm are regarded as intermediate thickness and more than 4 mm are regarded as thick melanomas.

Multivariate analysis has confirmed that Breslow thickness is statistically a more significant predictor of outcome as compared to Clark's level. However, Clark's level of invasion, is regarded as an independent prognostic indicator in thin melanomas (< 1 mm in thickness). In this subgroup, invasion of deeper anatomical levels is associated with a surprisingly higher rate of metastases as compared to primary tumour of the same thickness with more superficial levels.[7]

Key point 3

- Primary melanomas in the head and neck and acral regions carry a worse prognosis. Breslow tumour thickness expressed in millimetres is the most important prognostic factor. Presence of ulceration has a negative prognostic impact as does angiogenesis and vascular invasion.

The AJCC staging system was revised in 2002 (Table 1) and 10 key improvements were made including:

1. Ulceration is included in all T stages and classified as: (a) without ulceration; and (b) with ulceration.
2. Clark's micro-anatomical level of invasion is used only to define T1 melanomas.
3. Threshold for thickness was adjusted to change at 1, 2 and 4 mm.
4. Thick melanomas larger than 4 mm are classified as stage IIC.
5. Stage III is reserved for regional nodal disease and thick melanomas without this are down-staged to IIC.
6. The dimension of the lymph nodes is no longer included, N stage is determined by the number of the lymph nodes.
7. Lung metastases are defined as a separate category of M1 disease as they are associated with longer survival as compared to other visceral metastases.
8. Sentinel node status is taken into consideration in the revised system with clear distinction between clinical (macroscopic) and pathologically (microscopic) disease.
9. Additionally, the number of nodes involved has been substituted for the dimension of nodal involvement.
10. In-transit and satellite metastases in classified under regional nodal disease.

Ulceration: Ulceration is defined as the loss of epidermis overlying melanoma lesion when inspected under the microscope. Presence of ulceration has a negative impact on relapse-free survival. Balch *et al.*[8] analysed 17,600 melanoma patients looking at the prognostic factors. They found that tumours

Table 1 AJCC staging system for cutaneous melanoma, revised in 2002

Stage	Tumour (T)	Node (N)	Metastases (M)
0	*In situ*	0	0
IA	< 1.0 mm without ulcer; and < Clark IV	0	0
IB	< 1.0 mm without ulcer; and > Clark IV or 1.1–2.0 mm without ulcer	0	0
IIA	1.1–2.0 mm with ulcer; or 2.1–4.0 mm without ulcer	0	0
IIB	2.1–4.0 mm with ulcer; or > 4.0 mm without ulcer	0	0
IIIA	Any thickness without ulcer	1–4 nodes clinically occult; pathology positive	0
IIIB	Any thickness with ulcer	1–4 nodes clinically occult; pathology positive or 2–3 nodes	0
	Any thickness without ulcer	2-3 nodes clinically apparent	0
	Any thickness with or without ulcer	0 nodes + in-transit/satellite metastasis	0
	Any thickness with ulcer	1–3 nodes – clinically apparent	0
IIIC	Any thickness without ulcer	3 metastasis nodes or > 3 matted nodes or > 3 in-transit metastasis/satellite with nodal metastases	0
IV	Any thickness	Any nodal status	Any metastasis to skin, subcutaneous distant node, lung or visceral or any distant metastasis with elevated LDH

with ulceration carried survival rates comparable to those of the next higher tumour classification. Ulceration is, therefore, included as a second determinant for the T classification and as the only factor that has a negative impact in survival in node-negative patients.

Angiogenesis and vascular invasion: The formation of new microvessels is associated with poor clinical outcome. The process of neovascularisation is a gradual process and occurs at the base of the primary melanoma. A study conducted by Kashani-Sabet *et al.*[9] on 417 invasive melanoma cases, confirmed that the relapse rate and mortality were directly related to increasing tumour vascularity. The mortality in patients without vascularity was 12.3% as compared to 40% in patients with prominent vascularity ($P < 0.00005$).

Involvement of microvasculature is also associated with poor prognosis with increased incidence of relapse and death.

SURGICAL STRATEGY

Excision biopsy of suspected lesions is the mainstay of diagnosis of malignant melanoma. It is usually performed with a 1–2 mm margin and has to be full thickness.

PRIMARY MELANOMA

Surgery remains the most effective treatment modality for melanoma. The aim of surgery in cutaneous melanoma is to excise not only the primary tumour but also sufficient surrounding tissue. This approach will ensure that clinically invisible cells within the cutaneous lymphatics are also excised en-block to minimise local recurrence. The concept of wide, local excision is based on Handley's description of centrifugal spread of melanoma.[10] There has been some controversy on the appropriate margin of excision as an inadequate excision margin can lead to an increased risk of local and in-transit metastases which, in turn, are associated with worse prognosis. On the other hand, an unnecessarily wide excision margin is associated with more complex tissue closures and increased morbidity, hospital stay and additional cost.

Up to the 1970s, excision margins of 3–5 cm were the standard but subsequent trials demonstrated that narrower margins are safe. In a randomised, multicentre trial, Thomas *et al.*[11] investigated the effect of the excision margin on outcome in patients with high-risk melanoma (as defined by a thickness of 2 mm or greater). Between 1993–2001, 900 patients were recruited who were randomly allocated to undergo surgery either with 1-cm or 3-cm excision margins. Patients with palpable regional lymph nodes were excluded. None of the patients in this trial were allowed to undergo sentinel node biopsy (SLNB) or regional lymph node dissection (RLND). Patients were followed up for a median of 60 months. Overall, 453 patients were assigned to the 1-cm excision margin group and 447 to the 3-cm excision margin group. There were 168 local recurrences in the group with the 1-cm excision margin as compared to 142 in the 3-cm excision margin group. As far as mortality is concerned, there were 128 deaths attributed to the 1-cm and 105 to the 3-cm groups, respectively. There was no differences in overall survival. The authors concluded that a 1-cm excision margin is associated with significantly greater risk of regional recurrence than the 3-cm excision margin. This study does not address whether the 3-cm margin is better than 2-cm excision margin.

As far as thinner melanomas are concerned, a prospective, multicentre, randomised study by Khayat *et al.*[12] looked at 2-cm versus 5-cm excision margins on melanomas of 2.1 mm or smaller. Over a 5-year period, 337 patients were studied. The median follow-up period was 16 years. There were 22 recurrent cancers in the 2-cm arm as compared to 33 in the 5-cm arm. Ten-year, disease-free survival rates were 85% in the 2-cm margin group and 83% in the 5-cm group. The authors concluded that a 2-cm excision margin in this group of patients is adequate and a greater excision margin has no impact on recurrence rate or survival. In patients with tumours less than 1-mm thick, a 1-cm excision margin is adequate.

Key point 4

Tumour thickness (mm)	Excision margin (cm)
< 1	1
1–2	2
> 2	3

TREATMENT OF THE REGIONAL LYMPHATIC BASIN

ELECTIVE LYMPH NODE DISSECTION (ELND)

Although there have been a number of retrospective studies suggesting a distinct survival advantage of patients who undergo ELND as compared to observation and delayed therapeutic lymph node dissection (TLND), the result of early prospective randomised trials does not suggest this view, since no survival advantage was observed in these patients.[13,14]

SENTINEL NODE BIOPSY IN MALIGNANT MELANOMA

Morton and colleagues[15] introduced the concept of sentinel node biopsy to allow minimally invasive staging of the regional lymph node basin. They defined the sentinel lymph node (SLN) as 'the initial lymph node upon which the primary tumor drains'. As the first lymph node to meet the tumour cells, it has the highest chance of harbouring metastatic disease; its histological status would predict the status of the remainder of the lymphatic basin.

This procedure can allow the surgeon to select patients who would potentially benefit from regional lymphadenectomy. Although it remains to be seen whether the application of this concept will translate into a survival advantage or regional tumour control for stage I and II patients, the low morbidity and technical ease of the procedure has led to its increasing application in the management of patients with intermediate thickness malignant melanoma.

Lymphoscintigraphy is an essential first step in lymphatic mapping. The importance of pre-operative lymphoscintigraphy has been emphasised by many authors.[16,17] In addition to dynamic imaging, static acquisition needs to be performed in two views. In head and neck melanoma, lymphoscintigraphy and sentinel node biopsy can be a technically demanding procedure. During surgery, a combination of probe-guided surgery and blue dye mapping is the recommended approach, which complement each other (Plate VIII, p4).

The therapeutic benefit of SLNB is being evaluated by the Multicentre Selective Lymphadenectomy Trial (MLST) in which the primary outcome measure is melanoma-related mortality with secondary outcomes being disease-free survival, local, regional and distant recurrence rate. Patients with melanoma more than 1 mm underwent WLE alone or with SLNB. Those patients with positive SLN subsequently underwent completion lymphadenectomy. Over 2000 patients have been recruited in this trial and recruitment ended in March 2002. A second large-scale trial that is examining the value of SLNB is the Sunbelt Melanoma Trial, which is on-going. In this trial, all patients with melanoma greater than 1 mm in thickness undergo SLNB. Those patients with positive SLN based on hematoxylin/eosin, immunohistochemistry (HMB-45 and S-100) or reverse transcriptase polymerase chain reaction (RT-PCR) are randomised into surgery (completion lymphadenectomy) and/or adjuvant interferon therapy.

Key point 5

- Sentinel node biopsy is the staging investigation of choice in intermediate thickness melanoma. It is associated with low morbidity but its impact on survival and regional tumour control is unknown at present.

MANAGEMENT OF IN-TRANSIT MELANOMA METASTASIS

The incidence of in-transit metastasis in patients with high-risk primary melanoma (> 1.5 mm) is 5–8%. These metastases are lymphatic in nature and present as single or multiple nodules in close proximity to the primary tumour or scattered across the limb. There are different treatment options depending on the size and the number of lesions. These include simple excision, laser ablation, intralesional injection of bacille Calmette-Guerin (BCG) or cytokines, radiotherapy and isolated limb chemotherapy.

ISOLATED LIMB PERFUSION

Creech *et al.*,[18] at Tulane University in New Orleans, first described the technique of isolated limb perfusion in 1958. This procedure is described for management of inoperable in-transit limb metastasis and should be regarded as a palliative strategy. High concentrations of chemotherapeutic agents (15–25 times higher than systemic concentrations) are delivered to the extremity affected and the limb is isolated from the rest of the body using a tourniquet and by clamping the collateral vessels.[19] The major artery and vein in the limb is canulated and connected to an oxygenated extracorporeal circuit. Melphalan is the chemotherapeutic agent of choice due to its high efficacy and low limb toxicity. The commonly administered dosage is 10 mg/l perfused tissue for the leg and 13 mg/l tissue for the arm. Melphalan may be combined with tumour necrosis factor-α which increases the response rate and can sometimes prove effective where single-agent melphalan has previously failed, although there is an increased risk of toxicity.

ISOLATED LIMB INFUSION

Isolated limb infusion (ILI) was first described by Thompson *et al.*[20] at the Sydney Melanoma Unit in 1993. It involves placing small-bore vascular catheters in the femoral vessels and passing these into the contralateral affected leg, or ipsilateral affected arm, at the level of the knee or elbow (Fig. 1). The limb is warmed, and the patient anaesthetised 2–3 h later. After heparinisation, papaverine is injected into the arterial catheter and a

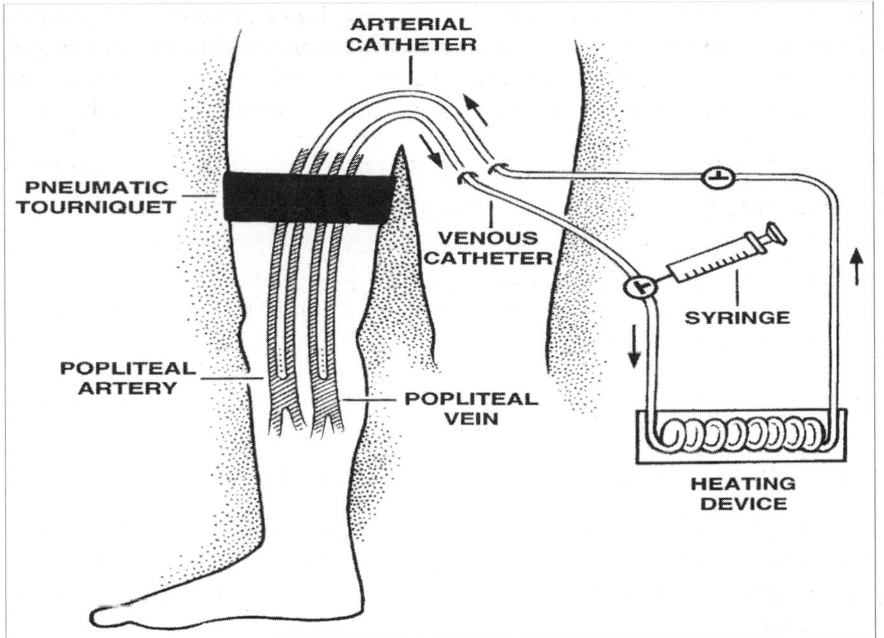

Fig. 1 Isolated limb infusion set-up.

pneumatic tourniquet is placed around the affected limb at a predetermined level above the catheters. A predetermined dose of chemotherapy (melphalan and actinomycin D, 7.5 mg/l and 75 mcg/l, respectively, in 400 ml saline for a lower limb, and 10 mg/l melphalan and 100 mcg/l actinomycin D, respectively, in 300 ml saline for an upper limb) is infused into the isolated limb over 4–6 min. The chemotherapy/blood mixture is then pumped around the progressively hypoxic limb for 30 min, and the drugs are then washed out of the limb using a litre of Hartmann's fluid. The tourniquet is then removed and the circulation re-established. Heparin is reversed with protamine, and the catheters removed from the groin. The patient is kept on bed rest with DVT prophylaxis for 6–7 days (Plate IX, p5).

ADJUVANT TREATMENT

Many patients present with high-risk primary melanomas (stage IIB or IIC/stage III), these patients can have a poor outlook, with 5-year survival ranging from 30–70%.[21] This reflects the biology of the disease rather than failure of surgical therapy, and also the lack of effective adjuvant therapy. There is now good evidence for the role of cytotoxic chemotherapy in the adjuvant setting for bowel and breast cancer and also emerging evidence in lung cancer. However, despite more that 100 clinical trials, adjuvant treatment in malignant melanoma remains controversial and opinions differ significantly between North America and Europe.

It is known that melanoma is susceptible to attack by the host's immune system and this has led to the use of immunostimulants, cytokines and vaccine therapies in an attempt to reduce the risk of recurrent melanoma in high-risk patients. Most studies have involved the use of interferon-α (IFN-α), a cytokine with diverse immunomodulatory effects on tumour cells. The exact mechanism of action of IFN-α remains poorly understood, but it is known to have a stimulatory effect on natural killer (NK) cells and also anti-angiogenic activity. In previous phase I and II trials in metastatic disease, IFN-α has demonstrated a response rate of 15% and this has prompted its use in multiple clinical trials in the adjuvant setting. Results have either been inconclusive or conflicting.

Kirkwood *et al.*[21] examined the use of high-dose interferon in a randomised trial for the Eastern Co-operative Oncology Group (ECOG) – E1684. This involved an induction phase of IFN-α at 20 mU/m^2 intravenously three times weekly for 4 weeks, followed by a maintenance phase of 10 mU/m^2 subcutaneously three times weekly for the remaining year. This is a highly toxic regimen, with significant fatigue, weight loss, myelosuppression and depression. In over half of the patients in the trial, treatment was reduced or discontinued and there were two toxic deaths from fulminant liver necrosis.[21] The trial initially showed an increased relapse-free survival rate when compared to observation alone, and this lead to FDA approval of high dose IFN-α for the post-surgical adjuvant therapy of high-risk melanoma. This remains the standard of care in many centres in North America. However, when the data were re-analysed at a median follow-up of 12.6 years, any advantage was no longer apparent and, in view of the toxicity of treatment, high dose IFN-α remains non-standard adjuvant therapy in Europe and the rest of the world.

In an effort to improve the efficacy and reduce toxicity of IFN-α, low-dose regimens have been looked at, particularly in Europe. Once again, several trials have not shown any benefit when compared to observation alone. The AIM-HIGH study[22] compared low dose IFN-α (3 mU three times weekly) for 2 years or until recurrence compared with observation alone. There was no significant difference between either arm in terms of overall survival and disease-free survival and 15% of patients withdrew due to toxicity. A meta-analysis[23] provided the most reliable consensus on the current data available, concluding there is currently no clear benefit of IFN-α in overall survival at any dose scheduling. Therefore, controversies remain. As IFN-α remains the only adjuvant treatment to have any impact on the natural history of the disease, it may be reasonable to discuss this as a treatment option with high-risk patients, informing them of the potential toxicity and the lack of consensus amongst oncologists regarding efficacy and benefit. Further randomised controlled trials are required to address the role of IFN-α in the adjuvant setting.

Key point 6

- The standard of care for adjuvant therapy in the UK and the rest of the world outside the US is close follow-up or clinical trial. The US standard of care for adjuvant treatment, is based on high dose IFN-α, but it has considerable toxicity and there is no significant overall survival benefit.

Various tumour-specific vaccines have been investigated as potential adjuvant treatment for high-risk melanoma, aiming to modulate the host's immune response against tumour cells as many melanoma carry distinct tumour-associated antigens that can be recognised by the immune system. These vaccines include a GM_2-ganglioside-based vaccine, stimulating production of IgM antibodies. Melacine, a vaccine comprising melanoma cell lysates,[24] and CancerVax where whole melanoma cells from three different cell lines are irradiated prior to vaccination. Vaccines are less toxic than other adjuvant treatments but their efficacy and ability to synergise with IFN-α remains to be established and current trials are on-going.

METASTATIC DISEASE

The prognosis of malignant melanoma is closely related to the stage at which it presents. The outlook for patients with disseminated disease is poor, with median survival of 6–10 months and less than 5% of patients surviving more that 5 years.[26]

Malignant melanoma is characterised by a poor response to chemotherapy. The mainstay of cytotoxic treatment is dacarbazine, an alkylating agent, with a response rate in the order of 20%. The median duration of response is 4 months but it is reasonably well tolerated. Temozolamide is an oral analogue of dacarbazine. There is 100% absorption after oral administration and it appears to have equivalent action to dacarbazine.[27] However, temozolamide is able to cross the blood–brain barrier and achieves significant CNS penetration. Studies have recently shown a trend towards decreased frequency of cerebral metastases during and following treatment with temozolamide.[28] Although currently not licensed in the UK, temozolamide, with its ease of administration and efficacy has clear advantages and is the subject of on-going trials.

Key point 7

- Disseminated malignant melanoma is characterised by a poor response to existing drugs. The mainstay of treatment is with dacarbazine or IFN-α, with similar response rates of under 20%.

Several studies have looked at combinations of chemotherapy. Agents such as vindesine, cisplatin and carmustine have been given in combination with dacarbazine. Although some of these combinations may lead to higher response rates, none of these regimens have been shown to prolong survival when compared to decarbazine alone.[29] Tamoxifen has also been administered in combination with chemotherapy, targeting oestrogen receptor expression on melanocytes. However, these studies failed to show an increase in response rates or prolong overall survival.[30]

The failure of any significant breakthrough over the last 30 years with chemotherapy trials for melanoma has lead to alternative treatment strategies being sought. Single agent IFN-α has a response rate of 15–20% in metastatic disease, with tolerable toxicities. Patients are more likely to respond with skin, subcutaneous and lymph node metastases than with visceral disease. High-dose bolus interleukin-2 (IL-2) received US FDA approval in 1998 as the regimen led to a durable response in a meaningful proportion of patients. The median response has yet to be reached in those patients who achieved a complete response and disease progression has not been noted in any patients with a response lasting for more than 30 months.[31] However, high-dose bolus IL-2 is associated with severe toxic effects, including the capillary leak syndrome leading to hypotension and renal insufficiency. Many patients require HDU or ITU support during treatment, rendering it impractical for many centres.

The combination of chemotherapy with immunotherapy – 'biochemotherapy' – has been extensively trialed. This is based on the premise that cytoreduction and cell damage by cytotoxic agents may increase sensitivity of melanoma cells to immunotherapy. IFN-α and IL-2 have been studied combined with chemotherapy. Phase II studies have shown tumour responses in 40–50% of patients but larger phase III trials, including a recent study by the ECOG, showed no survival benefit when compared to single-agent dacarbazine. In view of the toxicity associated with these combinations, their use in the metastatic setting remains controversial and is probably restricted to neo-adjuvant situations where a reduction in the size of the tumour may allow salvage surgery.

In view of the poor response to chemotherapy in disseminated disease, a number of studies have looked at the role of novel, targeted therapies. Two-thirds of melanomas have an activating mutation in BRAF. This leads to elevated RAF kinase activity and cellular proliferation.[32] BAY 43-9006 is a potent signal transduction inhibitor that prevents tumour cell proliferation and angiogenesis by blocking the Raf pathway. Phase II studies have looked at its activity as single agent[32] and in combination with chemotherapy.[33] Results have confirmed some activity with a favourable safety profile and further studies are being undertaken.

The use of vaccines has also been studied in metastatic disease using dendritic cells and heat-shock proteins to deliver immunogenic treatment and induce specific T-cell response and overcome immune tolerance. However, tumour cells usually develop escape mechanisms; although responses have been seen, the role of vaccines in metastatic disease remains within the context of clinical trials only. Vaccines have tended to move to the adjuvant setting as the immune response can be compromised in patients with advanced cancer.

Key point 8

- With poor response to existing standard treatments, disseminated disease is best managed by encouraging participation in clinical trials.

In a disease with such poor response to standard treatments, the importance of palliative and best supportive care cannot be over-stated. Pain can be managed with opiate analgesia and steroids can be useful to improve tumour-related cachexia. Bisphosphonates can be helpful for bony disease, although their efficacy is not as great as with other solid tumour types. Although melanoma is not particularly radiosensitive, there is a role for palliative radiotherapy for symptomatic control of cerebral metastases and painful bony lesions.

CONCLUSIONS

Malignant melanoma continues to represent a challenge in developing effective treatment options. With its rising incidence, high recurrence rates, rapid progression and poor response to current standard treatments, more trials are needed to develop better outcomes in this aggressive and often fatal disease.

Key points for clinical practice

- The incidence of melanoma is rising. Exposure to sunlight is a major aetiological factor. The majority of melanomas arise from pre-existing moles. Melanoma should be suspected if there are changes in size, shape or colour, bleeding, itching or moles more than 6 mm in diameter.
- Superficial spreading melanoma is the commonest form of melanoma and accounts for 70% of cases. Nodular melanoma accounts for 12% of cases and lentigo maligna melanoma for 10–15%. Pigmentation is not mandatory for the diagnosis of melanoma.
- Primary melanomas in the head and neck and acral regions carry a worse prognosis. Breslow tumour thickness expressed in millimetres is the most important prognostic factor. Presence of ulceration has a negative prognostic impact as does angiogenesis and vascular invasion.
- Tumour thickness (mm) / Excision margin (cm)

Tumour thickness (mm)	Excision margin (cm)
< 1	1
1–2	2
> 2	3

Sentinel node biopsy is the staging investigation of choice in intermediate thickness melanoma. It is associated with low morbidity but its impact on survival and regional tumour control is unknown at present.

- The standard of care for adjuvant therapy in the UK and the rest of the world outside the US is close follow-up or clinical trial. The US standard of care for adjuvant treatment, is based on high dose IFN-α, but it has considerable toxicity and there is no significant overall survival benefit.
- Disseminated malignant melanoma is characterised by a poor response to existing drugs. The mainstay of treatment is with dacarbazine or IFN-α, with similar response rates of under 20%.
- With poor response to existing standard treatments, disseminated disease is best managed by encouraging participation in clinical trials.

References

1. Morton DL, Wen DR, Wong JH *et al*. Technical details of intra-operative lymphatic mapping for early stage melanoma. *Arch Surg* 1992; **127**: 392–399.

2. Austin PF, Curse CW, Lyman G *et al*. Age as a prognostic factor in malignant melanoma population. Ann Surg Oncol 1994; **1**:487–494.
3. Masback A, Olsson H, Westerdahl N *et al*. Prognostic factors in invasive cutaneous malignant melanoma: a population-based study and review. *Melanoma Res* 2001; **11**: 435–445.
4. Garbe C, Buttner P, Bertz J *et al*. Primary cutaneous melanoma. Identification of prognostic groups and estimation of individual prognosis for 5,093 patients. *Cancer* 1995; **75**: 2484–2491.
5. Clark Jr WH, From L, Bernardino EA. The histogenesis and biologic behaviour of primary human malignant melanomas of the skin. *Cancer Res* 1969; **29**: 705–727.
6. Breslow A. Thickness, cross-sectional areas and depth of invasion in the prognosis of cutaneous melanoma. *Ann Surg* 1970; **172**: 902–908.
7. Buttner P, Garbe C, Bertz J *et al*. Primary cutaneous melanoma: optimised cut off points of tumour thickness and importance of Clark's level for prognostic classification. *Cancer* 1995; **75**: 2499.
8. Balch CM, Snoog SJ, Gershenwald JE *et al*. Prognostic factor analysis of 17,600 melanoma patients: validation of American Joint Committee on Cancer melanoma staging system. *J Clin Oncol* 2001; **19**: 3622–3634.
9. Kashani-Sabet M, Sagebiel RW, Ferreira CM *et al*. Tumour vascularity in prognostic assessment of primary cutaneous melanoma. *J Clin Oncol* 2002; **20**: 1826–1831.
10. Handley WS. The pathology of melanotic growths in relation to their operative treatment. *Lancet* 1907; **1**: 927–996.
11. Thomas MJ, Newton-Bishop J, A'Hern R *et al*. Excision margins in high-risk malignant melanoma. *N Engl J Surg* 2004; **350**: 757–766.
12. Khayat D, Rixe O, Martin G *et al*. Surgical margins in cutaneous melanoma (2 cm versus 5 cm for lesions measuring less than 2.1-mm thick). Long term results of large European Multicentric phase III study. *Cancer* 2003; **97**: 1941–1946.
13. Veronesi U, Adamus J, Bandiera B *et al*. Delayed regional lymph node dissection in stage I melanoma of the skin of the lower extremities. *Cancer* 1982; **49**: 2420–2430.
14. Sim FH, Taylor WF, Prichard DJ *et al*. Lymphadenectomy in the management of stage I malignant melanoma: a prospective randomised study. *Mayo Clin Proc* 1986; **61**: 697–705.
15. Morton DL, Wen DR, Wong JH *et al*. Technical details of intra-operative lymphatic mapping for early stage melanoma. *Arch Surg* 1992; **127**: 392–399.
16. Alex JC, Weaver DL, Fairbank JT *et al*. Gamma-probe guided lymph node localization in malignant melanoma. *Surg Oncol* 1993; **2**: 303–308.
17. Pijpers R, Collet GJ, Meijer S *et al*. The impact of dynamic lymphoscintigraphy and gamma probe guidance on sentinel node biopsy in melanoma. *Eur J Nucl Med* 1995; **22**: 1238–1241.
18. Creech O, Krementz E, Ryan M *et al*. Chemotherapy of cancer: regional perfusion utilising an extracorporeal circuit. *Ann Surg* 1958; **148**: 616–632.
19. Benckhuijsen C, Kroon BB, van Geel AN *et al*. Regional perfusion treatment with melphalan for melanoma in a limb: an evaluation of drug kinetics. *Eur J Oncol* 1988; **14**: 157–163.
20. Thompson JF, Gianoutsos MP. Isolated limb perfusion for melanoma-effectiveness and toxicity of cisplatin compared with that of melphalan and other drugs. *World J Surg* 1992; **16**: 227–233.
21. Sabel M, Sondak V. Pros and cons of adjuvant interferon in the treatment of malignant melanoma. *Oncologist* 2003; **8**: 451–458.
22. Hancock BW, Wheatley K, Harris N *et al*. Adjuvant interferon in high-risk melanoma: The AIM-HIGH Study – United Kingdom Coordinating Committee on Cancer Research randomised study of adjuvant low dose extended duration interferon alpha 2a in high-risk resected malignant melanoma. *J Clin Oncol* XXXX; **22**: 53–61.
23. Wheatley K, Ives N, Hancock B, Gore M, Eggermont A, Suciu S. Does adjuvant interferon-alpha for high-risk melanoma provide a worthwhile benefit? A meta-analysis of the randomised trials. *Cancer Treat Rev* 2003; **29**: 241–252.
24. Tsao H, Atkins M, Sober M. Management of cutaneous melanoma. *N Engl J Med* XXXX; **351**: 998–1012.
25. Bystryn JC. Vaccines for melanoma. *Dermatol Clin* 2002; **20**: 717–725.

26. Manola J, Atkins M, Ibrahim J, Kirkwood J. Prognostic factors in metastatic melanoma; a pooled analysis of Eastern Cooperative Oncology Group Trials. *J Clin Oncol* 2000; **18**: 3782–3793.
27. Middleton M, Grob JJ, Aaronson N *et al*. Randomised phase III study of temozolamide versus dacarbazine in the treatment of patients with advanced metastatic melanoma. *J Clin Oncol* 2000; **18**: 158–166.
28. Summers Y, Middleton M, Calvert H *et al*. Effects of temozolamide on CNS relapse in patients with advanced melanoma. *Prog Proc Am Soc Clin Oncol* 1999; **18**: 531a.
29. Eigentler T, Caroli U, Radny P, Garbe C. Palliative therapy for disseminated malignant melanoma: a systematic review of 41 randomised clinical trials. *Lancet Oncol* 2003; **4**: 748–759.
30. Argawala S, Ferri W, Gooding W, Kirkwood J. A phase III randomised trial of dacarbazine and carboplatin with or without tamoxifen in the treatment of patients with metastatic melanoma. *Cancer* 1999; **85**: 1979–1984.
31. Atkins MB, Lee S, Flaherty LE, Sosman JA, Sondak VK, Kirkwood JM. A prospective randomised phase III trial of concurrent bio-chemotherapy with cisplatin, vinblastine, dacarbazine, IL-2 and IFN versus dacarbazine alone in patients with metastatic melanoma (E3695): an ECOG-coordinated intergroup trial. *Prog Proc Am Soc Clin Oncol* 2003; **22**: 708.
32. Ahmad T, Marais L, Pyle M *et al*. BAY 43-90006 in patients with advanced melanoma: the Royal Marsden experience. *J Clin Oncol* 2004; **22 (Suppl)**: 7506.
33. Flaherty K, Brose M, Schuchter L *et al*. Phase I/II trial of BAY 43-9006, carboplatin and paclitaxel demonstrates preliminary antitumour activity in the expansion cohort of patients with metastatic melanoma. *J Clin Oncol* 2004; **22 (Suppl)**: 7507.

Plate VIII (a) A lymphoscintigram showing the injection site of radiocolloid at the site of excision scar right thigh. (b) Injection of patent blue dye. (c) Intra-operative detection of SLN using combined technique.

Plate IX Inoperable satellite metastases: (a) before regional chemotherapy; (b) after regional chemotherapy.

Martin Kurzer Allan E. Kark

6

Inguinal hernia repair – an update

Inguinal hernia repair is the most frequently performed operation in general surgery with about 100,000 procedures being carried out in the UK, 700,000 in the US, and 20 million world-wide, annually. There has been a great upsurge in interest in hernias over the last 15–20 years sparked by the introduction and widespread use of prosthetic mesh closely followed by the advent of laparoscopic surgery. In this chapter, we have given an overview of the current state of inguinal hernia surgery, to highlight areas of debate and controversy and to indicate possible future directions.

DIAGNOSIS

The diagnosis of an inguinal hernia is made clinically – a groin swelling that appears on coughing, straining or standing and that disappears on lying. When there is doubt about the nature of an irreducible groin swelling, or in patients with groin pain but no swelling, ultrasound is the most appropriate investigation with a high degree of sensitivity and specificity in experienced hands.[1] Its accuracy is, however, operator dependent and MRI may provide a more objective alternative.

INDICATIONS FOR OPERATION

The aims of surgical repair are to eliminate the swelling, to relieve pain and discomfort, and to remove the risk of strangulation. The cumulative probability of

Martin Kurzer MBBS FRCS
Surgeon, British Hernia Centre, 87 Watford Way, London NW4 4RS, UK
E-mail: martin@kurzer.co.uk (for correspondence)

Allan E. Kark FRCS FACS
Surgeon, British Hernia Centre, 87 Watford Way, London NW4 4RS, UK

strangulation of an inguinal hernia has been estimated to be 2.8% at 3 months and 4.5% after 2 years,[2] and this complication carries a significant morbidity and mortality, particularly in the elderly.[3] At present, conventional wisdom is that all inguinal hernias should be repaired; however, based on clinical judgement, one may elect not to advise repair in an elderly patient with an asymptomatic, broad-based, direct hernia.

WHICH OPERATION?

Using prosthetic mesh for hernia repair gives the lowest incidence of recurrence, but should this be carried out using an open or laparoscopic technique? Is there in fact one single 'best' operation, or should the procedure be tailored to hernia and patient characteristics, and to patient and surgeon preference?

OPEN TENSION-FREE MESH REPAIR OF INGUINAL HERNIA

Inguinal hernia repair using a tension-free mesh technique gives a better result than a 'conventional' sutured repair. The best objective evidence comes from the EU Hernia Trialists Collaboration meta-analysis of 2002 which reported on 20 randomised trials (5016 patients).[4] Individual patient data were obtained from 11 of the 20 participating trials and re-analysed centrally to derive a more complete and reliable meta-analysis. Compared with sutured repair, patients having a mesh repair had a shorter hospital stay, a faster return to normal activities and a lower incidence of persisting pain. Open mesh repair was also associated with a 50–70% reduction in the risk of recurrence. Nation-wide surveys of surgical practice reveal that the open mesh technique has become the procedure of choice for primary inguinal hernia repair.[5–7]

METHODS OF OPEN MESH INGUINAL HERNIA REPAIR

Since Lichtenstein's classic description of using a flat piece of mesh as an onlay, there have been a number of variations in mesh placement or configuration. Placing a mesh plug or cone through the deep ring[8] has achieved popularity because of its ease and generally good results, though plug repairs have been associated with high incidences of postoperative pain. Other, more elaborate, systems have been devised and have given acceptable outcomes in the hands of their developers. However, they add expense and complexity (with the accompanying risk of increased complications) to what is a straight-forward, effective procedure which already achieves excellent results.

LAPAROSCOPIC INGUINAL HERNIA REPAIR

Laparoscopic inguinal hernia repair was first described by Ger in 1982 but was not seen as a viable alternative to open repair until prosthetic mesh started to be used in the early 1990s. It has been advocated by enthusiasts as the method of choice for inguinal hernia repair but its routine use is controversial.[9] The place of laparoscopic repair for inguinal hernias is currently the subject of intense debate.

METHODS OF LAPAROSCOPIC REPAIR: TAPP VERSUS TEP

Early techniques such as simple ring closure or intraperitoneal onlay of mesh (IPOM) had high rates of recurrence and complications and have been superseded. The two current methods are transabdominal preperitoneal (TAPP) and totally extraperitoneal (TEP) repair. TEP is considered to be technically more difficult, partly because of unfamiliarity with the anatomy. The use of a balloon can greatly facilitate dissection, particularly useful for surgeons on the early part of their learning curve, although it does add to the cost of the procedure. Although TEP is theoretically less prone to result in visceral injury, UK surgeons have preferred to use TAPP[10] and large series of TAPP repairs have been reported with good results.[11]

Fixing the mesh in place with staples and inadvertently trapping nerves may give rise to long-term postoperative pain. Using larger pieces of mesh, held in place by intra-abdominal pressure has been advocated but can be associated with an increased risk of recurrence.[12] Fibrin glue may have a role to play in this context, though the product at present is experimental and expensive.

Key point 1

- Meta-analysis of randomised controlled trials has shown that laparoscopic repair of inguinal hernia gives less postoperative discomfort and a faster return to normal activity than open mesh

COMPARISON OF LAPAROSCOPIC WITH OPEN MESH REPAIR

A large number of randomised controlled trials comparing open with laparoscopic inguinal hernia repair have been published. Many suffered from poor study design, small numbers of patients (underpowered) and heterogeneous control and study groups, *e.g.* mixing open sutured and open mesh repairs, or TEP and TAPP. In addition, subjective end-points (such as postoperative pain and return to work) were not reported in a standard, quantified manner making comparisons difficult.

Two recent meta-analyses had access to, and were able to pool and re-analyse, individual patient data (IPD), giving greater statistical power and hence greater reliability than relying on aggregated published trial data.[13,14] The authors found that return to normal activity was faster and the incidence of long-term discomfort and numbness was less after laparoscopic repair although operating time was longer. Laparoscopic repair was associated with fewer postoperative complications although the number of serious visceral or vascular injuries was greater (Memon *et al.*[14] felt that there may have been a tendency to under-report minor complications). There were less haematomas after laparoscopic repair (particularly with TEP), but more seromas (after TAPP). The EU Hernia Trialists found no difference in the (short-term) recurrence rate between laparoscopic and open mesh repair. Memon *et al.*[14] found a trend towards an increase in the relative odds of short-term recurrence of 50% after laparoscopic repair compared with open repair, though this did not reach statistical significance. There is, at present, little data in the literature on long-term recurrence rates following laparoscopic repair.

The majority of randomised controlled trials (RCTs) have been conducted by laparoscopic enthusiasts, with the procedures carried out by experienced surgeons or closely supervised surgeons in training. They demonstrate the efficacy of the procedure in the hands of enthusiasts. But what about its effectiveness in the hands of a general surgeon without a special interest? In a recent large multicentre study of open versus laparoscopic repair, intra-operative, immediate postoperative and life-threatening complications occurred significantly more frequently in the laparoscopic group.[15] Surgeons who had carried out less than 250 laparoscopic repairs had a greater than 10% recurrence rate. For open repairs, there was no significant difference in recurrence rate whether the surgeon had performed less or more than 250 cases. Currently, only 4.1% of hernias in the UK are repaired laparoscopically[16] and a survey of UK surgeons suggests that this figure is unlikely to change in the foreseeable future.[9]

Key point 2

- Laparoscopic repair is more difficult to learn than open repair and carries the risk of serious visceral (bowel, bladder) or vascular injury.

LEARNING CURVE OF LAPAROSCOPIC REPAIR

Laparoscopic repair of groin hernia is undoubtedly a more complex procedure with a longer learning curve than open repair.[17] It requires different skills, and a familiarity with pre-peritoneal anatomy. Two large series concluded that 250–300 cases are required to achieve expertise.[11,15] This figure is hard to achieve with current surgical programmes, but could be reduced with more intensive training and the use of simulators. It has been suggested that laparoscopic hernia repair should only be carried out in specialist centres (Table 1).[18]

TREATMENT OF RECURRENT HERNIAS

Repair of a recurrent inguinal hernia can present a significant technical challenge particularly if there has been previous infection or mesh has been used. Re-operation (by an experienced surgeon) via an anterior approach has been advocated.[19] However, a recent multicentre randomised trial[15] found that the re-recurrence rate after repair of a recurrent hernia, even by an experienced surgeon, was 3.6% in a laparoscopic group and 17.2% using an open anterior technique. As well as re-recurrence there is a risk of testicular vessel damage and testicular atrophy, a distressing and potentially avoidable complication with medicolegal repercussions. For small discrete recurrences after anterior repair there is a place for a limited dissection and placing a plug or a cone in

Table 1 Comparison of open with laparoscopic inguinal hernia repair

Open tension-free mesh	*Laparoscopic*
Easy to learn	Long or steep learning curve
Little risk of major complications	Potential for serious bowel or bladder injury
Good results obtainable by 'non-experts'	Needs high level of technical expertise for good results
Ideal for day surgery, especially under local anaesthesia	Needs general anaesthesia
Suitable for almost all inguinal hernias	Not suitable for elderly or if co-morbidity
	Not suitable if previous abdominal surgery (TAPP only)
	Indicated for recurrent and bilateral hernia
	Diagnose occult contralateral hernia
More postoperative discomfort than laparoscopic repair	Less postoperative discomfort than open repair
More long-term discomfort than laparoscopic repair	
Longer to return to normal activities	Quicker return to normal activities
Cost-effective	Greater costs than open repair

the defect.[20] If the previous repairs were open anterior then the recurrence should be dealt with either laparoscopically[10] or using an open pre-peritoneal technique.[21] Laparoscopic recurrences should be repaired using an open anterior approach. If both methods have failed, consideration should be given to referring the patient to a surgeon with a special interest in hernias!

Key point 3

- NICE guidelines recommend that laparoscopic repair should be reserved for recurrent and bilateral inguinal hernia. Laparoscopic repair is more expensive (for unilateral hernias) than open repair. The most cost-effective repair for primary unilateral inguinal is open tension-free mesh under local anaesthetic.

TREATMENT OF BILATERAL HERNIAS

Until relatively recently standard teaching was to advise staged repair of bilateral inguinal hernia. Modern techniques of mesh repair have made this advice obsolete. Both open tension-free and laparoscopic repair are appropriate for synchronous bilateral inguinal hernia repair, with less cost than two separate procedures and no increased morbidity. Laparoscopic repair will be quicker, though bilateral open repair can be carried out as a day-case procedure.[22]

> **Key point 4**
>
> - Open tension-free repair is less complex, more easily learned and (arguably) safer and more cost effective than laparoscopic repair; it is the procedure of choice for primary unilateral inguinal hernia.

CHOICE OF ANAESTHETIC FOR INGUINAL HERNIA REPAIR

At present laparoscopic repair requires a general anaesthetic (GA). For open repair, the alternative is local anaesthesia (LA). Regional (epidural or spinal) anaesthesia can be used in certain circumstances and is the routine at a number of dedicated hernia clinics.[23] It is not ideal for ambulatory surgery because prolonged motor block will delay discharge from hospital and there is a high incidence of urinary retention (Table 2).

> **Key point 5**
>
> - Day-case rates in the UK for hernia repair are improving but are still far below the recommended guidelines.

LA has considerable advantages over GA in terms of reduced cardiac, CNS, and respiratory complications, while the incidence of urinary retention after

Table 2 Comparison of local and general anaesthesia for inguinal hernia repair

Local anaesthesia (LA)	*General anaesthesia (GA)*
Most cost-effective method, shortest total time in operating room, shortest time to discharge	Costlier than LA; more infrastructure needed – equipment, pre-operative investigations, staffing levels
More demanding than GA repair	Hernia repair can be carried out by surgeons in training
Difficult to teach hernia repair under LA	Easy to learn and teach hernia repair
Procedure may take longer than under GA	Short 'on-table' time; longer time in operating room and hospital
No CVS, CNS or respiratory problems	Not suitable for elderly, unwell patients
No urinary retention or postoperative nausea and vomiting	Incidence of urinary retention and postoperative nausea and vomiting
Low immediate postoperative pain	May need postoperative opiates
Ideal for day-case surgery	More likely to need unplanned overnight stay
Not suitable for strangulated or incarcerated hernias	Indicated for repair of strangulated or irreducible hernia
Not suitable for very obese or excessively anxious patients	Best for obese or anxious patient

local anaesthetic hernia repair is negligible.[24,25] These advantages are particularly appropriate for elderly patients and those with co-existing disease. In addition, LA has been shown to result in less postoperative pain and the shortest admission time of all anaesthetic methods.[25,26] These features combined with the absence of postoperative nausea and vomiting, excessive drowsiness or urinary retention make LA ideal for day-case surgery. However, the technique is more demanding of the surgeon, requiring patience, gentle handling of tissues and familiarity with the anatomy. It is also difficult to teach trainees hernia repair if LA is used. A poorly administered LA, with excess inappropriate sedation is worse than a well-administered GA in terms of patient safety and effectiveness.

In the UK only 6% of hernias are repaired under LA.[27] Yet in NHS units where surgeons have expressed an interest the number of cases carried out under LA will rise to over 30%,[28] and in dedicated consultant-led units this figure can reach over 80%.[29]

While one recent study concluded that there were no major differences between GA and LA in terms of postoperative mental function, complications, overall recovery and safety, all these cases were in-patients.[30] Postoperative nausea and vomiting are the main reasons for a delay in discharge following a day-case procedure and urinary retention is the most common reason for an unplanned overnight stay. Both lead to greater cost and decreased quality of care. With increasing pressure to provide a reliable day-case hernia service, surgeons should be aiming to carry out more open mesh repairs under LA. It has been suggested that reluctance to adopt LA for routine hernia repair results from 'a combination of tradition, surgeon preference, inadequate technical proficiency, and little incentive to use cost-effective techniques'.[5]

LONG-TERM DISCOMFORT FOLLOWING INGUINAL HERNIA REPAIR

There is evidence from a number of studies that up to 30% of patients will have some degree of discomfort or pain one year or more after inguinal hernia repair.[5,31–35] In the majority of patients, this will subside with the time but in up to 6% of patients this pain will be severe and markedly interfere with the patient's ability to continue normal daily activities.

Key point 6

- Postoperative pain is now recognised as an important long-term complication of inguinal hernia repair which patients should be made aware of pre-operatively. Careful audit is required to assess the incidence and extent of long-term disability.

The aetiology of this pain is unclear and is probably multifactorial. Its close association with numbness in some patients suggests a neuropathic cause,[36] although some have proposed that the use of mesh itself may be to blame. However, in Cunningham's series virtually all the repairs were non-mesh, and two other studies[36,37] have reported no difference in the incidence of chronic pain between patients having either a prosthetic or a sutured repair. Chronic groin pain in patients who have had inguinal hernia repair may be unrelated to the operation in up to 15% of cases.[38] Long-term pain is a real issue although the benefits of a mesh repair in terms of recurrence and other outcomes outweigh these considerations for the majority of patients.

SHOULD ALL INGUINAL HERNIAS BE REPAIRED?

One of the aims of surgical repair of an inguinal hernia is to relieve pain and discomfort. A recent prospective study[39] found that pre-operatively the majority of hernia patients had only mild or no pain at rest (80%), or on movement (58%), and some patients who had no pain pre-operatively at rest reported having pain 1-year postoperatively. Others have found that 5–10% of patients have more discomfort after inguinal hernia repair than before.[32,36] This has prompted some surgeons to question whether every hernia should be repaired. A randomised clinical trial, at present underway, should hopefully provide an answer.[40]

MESH AS A BIOMATERIAL

A wide range of prosthetic biomaterials are available for hernia repair, the three most suitable being polypropylene, polyester and expanded polytetrafluoroethylene (ePTFE). Polypropylene, distributed under various trade names, is favoured in the US, the UK and most of Europe, and fulfils most of the criteria for the ideal mesh.

Prosthetic mesh has made such a difference to the results of inguinal hernia repair that the temptation is to advocate its universal use. Some have expressed concern over possible long-term complications and there is a tendency not to use it in the young; there is no consensus, but a cut-off age of 18 years has been suggested.

Standard polypropylene mesh may be over-engineered with a tensile strength much greater than is required.[41] Small pore size (< 1 mm) can give rise to rigid, inelastic, uncomfortable 'scar plates' within the abdominal wall. Light-weight, large pore (> 1 mm) meshes stimulate less inflammatory reaction and less scar tissue formation. However, the benefit of using light-weight mesh in inguinal hernia repair has not yet been proven clinically[42] and may be associated with a greater risk of recurrence. There is no evidence that polypropylene mesh causes sarcoma formation in humans.

RETURN TO WORK AND NORMAL ACTIVITIES AFTER INGUINAL HERNIA REPAIR

Patients should be advised clearly, both verbally and with written instructions, that an early return to normal activities and work not only has no adverse consequences but is positively beneficial. The majority of patients should be able to return to normal activities at one week whether after an open or laparoscopic repair.[24,43] Failure to do so may relate to surgical technique or to pain and wound problems, but may equally well be a result of conflicting GP advice and inadequate pre-operative counselling.[43]

PROPHYLAXIS FOR VENOUS THROMBOEMBOLISM (VTE) AND INFECTION

There is little objective evidence in the literature regarding the use of VTE prophylaxis following inguinal hernia repair and this is reflected in the variation and inconsistency of practice amongst UK surgeons.[7] Patients should undergo risk assessment and management should follow local guidelines for surgical patients. Mechanical methods such as graded compression stockings, calf muscle pumps and early mobilisation are to be preferred over formal anticoagulation, because of the high incidence of haematoma.

Early fears of an increase in infection rate associated with mesh have proved unfounded. There is conflicting evidence that prophylactic antibiotics reduce the incidence of wound infection, although they are favoured in clinical practice.[7] A single dose of intravenous antibiotics should be administered to higher risk patients (*e.g.* diabetic, elderly, obese or immunocompromised patients) and for recurrent hernias. The vast majority of wound infections will respond to appropriate antibiotic treatment. Chronic mesh infection is rare with an estimated incidence of 1 in 1000. Evidence suggests that long-term antibiotics and attempts to save the mesh are ineffective.[44]

COST OF INGUINAL HERNIA REPAIR AND DAY-CASE SURGERY

Debate surrounds the cost of open and laparoscopic repairs. Direct hospital costs relate to time in the operating room, time in hospital, the use of specialised equipment (disposable, or increased sterilisation costs for re-usables) and an obligatory need for general anaesthesia (GA). Laparoscopic hernia repair in the UK has an additional NHS cost of £300 over open repair,[10] similar to figures from other countries.[45] The argument that the additional cost of laparoscopic repair is offset by an earlier return to work has been questioned,[46] and a recent analysis concluded that laparoscopic repair was not cost effective in terms of cost per recurrence avoided.[47]

It is now widely recognised that an increasing proportion of inguinal hernia repairs should be carried out as day-cases. 'Day surgery provides a high quality, patient-centred treatment that is safe, efficient and effective (and) is accompanied by a lower incidence of hospital acquired infection and an earlier return to normal activity compared with in-patient treatment'.[48] This is already the norm in specialist hernia centres[24] and the US. The proportion of inguinal hernias repaired in Europe as day-cases is increasing,[7,28,49] although, with one or two exceptions,[29] the use of local anaesthetic remains disappointingly low at 5–6%. The open tension-free mesh technique is the most cost-effective method of unilateral primary repair, and the greatest savings will be achieved by increasing the proportion of day-case procedures.

CONCLUSIONS

Inguinal hernia surgery has entered the realm of evidence-based practice. Recurrence rates alone are no longer the sole criterion of a successful repair and analysis of outcomes will include the incidence and potential seriousness of complications, time to recovery of normal activities and cost.[50] Day-case surgery for hernia will continue to increase and open and laparoscopic techniques will each find their place in the treatment of hernia. There are likely to be major advances in mesh technology.

Key points for clinical practice

- Meta-analysis of randomised controlled trials has shown that laparoscopic repair of inguinal hernia gives less postoperative discomfort and a faster return to normal activity than open mesh repair.
- Laparoscopic repair is more difficult to learn than open repair and carries the risk of serious visceral (bowel, bladder) or vascular injury.
- NICE guidelines recommend that laparoscopic repair should be reserved for recurrent and bilateral inguinal hernia. Laparoscopic repair is more expensive (for unilateral hernias) than open repair. The most cost-effective repair for primary unilateral inguinal is open tension-free mesh under local anaesthetic.
- Open tension-free repair is less complex, more easily learned and (arguably) safer and more cost effective than laparoscopic repair; it is the procedure of choice for primary unilateral inguinal hernia.
- Day-case rates in the UK for hernia repair are improving but are still far below the recommended guidelines.
- Postoperative pain is now recognised as an important long-term complication of inguinal hernia repair which patients should be made aware of pre-operatively. Careful audit is required to assess the incidence and extent of long-term disability.

References

1. Bradley M, Morgan D, Pentlow B, Roe A. The groin hernia – an ultrasound diagnosis? *Ann R Coll Surg Engl* 2003; **85**: 178–180.
2. Gallegos NC, Dawson J, Jarvis M. Risk of strangulation in groin hernias. *Br J Surg* 1991; **78**: 1171–1173.
3. The Royal College of Surgeons of England. *Clinical Guidelines on the Management of Groin Hernia in Adults*. London: RCSE, 1993.
4. EU Hernia Trialists Collaboration. Open mesh versus non-mesh repair of groin hernia: meta-analysis of randomized trials based on individual patient data. *Hernia* 2002; **6**: 130–136.
5. Bay-Nielsen M, Kehlet H. Quality assessment of 26,304 herniorrhaphies. *Lancet* 2001; **358**: 1124–1128.
6. Nilsson E, Haapaniemi S. Hernia registers and specialization. *Surg Clin North Am* 1998; **78**: 1141–1151.
7. Hair A, Duffy L, McLean J *et al*. Groin hernia repair in Scotland. *Br J Surg* 2002; **87**: 1722–1726.
8. Robbins AW, Rutkow IM. The mesh plug hernioplasty. *Surg Clin North Am* 1993; **73**: 501–511.
9. Beattie DK, Foley RJE, Callam MJ. Future of laparoscopic inguinal hernia surgery. *Br J Surg* 2000; **87**: 1727–1728.

10. National Institute for Clinical Excellence. *Guidance on the use of laparoscopic surgery for inguinal hernia*. Technology Appraisal Guidance no. 18. London: NICE; 2001.
11. Bittner R, Schmedt CG, Schwarz J, Kraft K, Leibl BJ. Laparoscopic transperitoneal procedure for routine repair of groin hernia. *Br J Surg* 2002; **89**: 1062–1066.
12. Smith AI, Royston CMS, Sedman PC. Stapled and nonstapled laparoscopic transabdominal preperitoneal (TAPP) inguinal hernia repair. *Surg Endosc* 1999; **13**: 804–806.
13. EU Hernia Trialists Collaboration. Laparoscopic versus open groin hernia repair meta-analysis of randomised trials based on individual patient data. *Hernia* 2002; **6**: 2–10.
14. Memon MA, Cooper NJ, Memon B, Memon MI, Abrams KR. Meta-analysis of randomized clinical trials comparing open and laparoscopic inguinal hernia repair. *Br J Surg* 2003; **90**: 1479–1492.
15. Neumayer L, Giobbie-Hurder A, Jonasson O *et al*. Open mesh versus laparoscopic mesh repair of inguinal hernia. *N Engl J Med* 2004; **350**: 1819–1827.
16. Bloor K, Freemantle N, Khadjesari Z, Maynard A. Impact of NICE guidance on laparoscopic surgery for inguinal hernias: analysis of interrupted time series. *BMJ* 2003; **326**: 578.
17. Edwards CC, Bailey RW. Laparoscopic hernia repair: the learning curve. *Surg Laparosc Endosc Percut Tech* 2000; **10**: 149–153.
18. Jacobs DO. Mesh repair of inguinal hernias – redux. *N Engl J Med* 2004; **350**: 1895–1897.
19. Richards SK, Vipond MN, Earnshaw JJ. Review of the management of recurrent inguinal hernia. *Hernia* 2004; **8**: 144–148.
20. Shulman AG, Amid PK, Lichtenstein IL. The 'plug' repair of 1402 recurrent inguinal hernias. *Arch Surg* 1990; **125**: 265–267.
21. Kurzer M, Belsham PA, Kark AE. Prospective study of open preperitoneal mesh repair for recurrent inguinal hernia. *Br J Surg* 2002; **89**: 90–93.
22. Kark AE, Belsham PA, Kurzer M. Simultaneous repair of bilateral groin hernias using local anaesthesia: review of 199 cases with a five-year follow-up. *Hernia* 2005; In press.
23. Amado W. Anesthesia for groin hernia surgery. *Surg Clin North Am* 2003; **83**: 1065–1077.
24. Kark AE, Kurzer M, Belsham P. Three thousand one hundred seventy five primary inguinal hernia repairs: advantage of ambulatory open mesh repair using local anaesthesia. *J Am Coll Surg* 1998; **186**: 447–456.
25. Nordin P, Zetterstrom H, Gunnarsson U, Nilsson E. Local, regional, or general anaesthesia in groin hernia repair: multicentre randomised trial. *Lancet* 2003; **362**: 853–858.
26. Song D, Grelich NB, White PF *et al*. Recovery profiles and costs of anesthesia for outpatient unilateral inguinal herniorrhaphy. *Anesth Analg* 2000; **91**: 876–881.
27. O'Riordan DC, Kingsnorth AN. Audit of patient outcomes after herniorrhaphy. *Surg Clin North Am* 1998; **78**: 1129–1139.
28. Metzger J, Lutz N, Laidlaw I. Guidelines for inguinal hernia repair in everyday practice. *Ann R Coll Surg Engl* 2001; **83**: 209–214.
29. Kingsnorth AN, Bowlwy DMG, Porter CS. A prospective study of 1000 hernias: results of the Plymouth Hernia Service. *Ann R Coll Surg Engl* 2003; **85**: 18–22.
30. O'Dwyer P, Serpell JW, Millar K *et al*. Local or general anesthesia for open hernia repair: a randomized trial. *Ann Surg* 2003; **237**: 574–579.
31. Kumar S, Wilson R, Nixon S, Macintyre I. Chronic pain after laparoscopic and open mesh repair of groin hernia. *Br J Surg* 2002; **89**: 1476–1479.
32. Bay-Nielsen M, Nordin P, Kehlet H. Chronic pain after repair of inguinal hernia. *Br J Surg* 2004; **91**: 1372–1376.
33. Courtney C, O'Dwyer P. Outcome of patients with severe chronic pain following repair of groin hernia. *Br J Surg* 2002; **89**: 1310–1314.
34. Callesen T, Bech K, Kehlet H. Prospective study of chronic pain after groin hernia repair. *Br J Surg* 1999; **86**: 1528–1531.
35. Poobalan A, Bruce J, King PM, Chambers WA, Krukowski ZH, Smith WC. Chronic pain and quality of life following open inguinal hernia repair. *Br J Surg* 2001; **88**: 1122–1126.
36. Gillion JF, Fagniez PL. Chronic pain and cutaneous sensory changes after inguinal hernia repair: comparison between open and laparoscopic techniques. *Hernia* 1999; **3**: 75–80.

37. Haapaniemi S, Nilsson E. Recurrence and pain three years after groin hernia repair. Validation of postal questionnaire and selective physical examination as a method of follow-up. *Eur J Surg* 2002; **168**: 22–28.
38. Nilsson E, Haapaniemi S, Gruber G, Sandblom G. Methods of repair and risk for re operation in Swedish hernia surgery from 1992 to 1996. *Br J Surg* 1998; **85**: 1686–1691.
39. Page B, Paterson C, Young D, O'Dwyer P. Pain from primary inguinal hernia and the effect of repair on pain. *Br J Surg* 2002; **89**: 1315–1318.
40. Fitzgibbons RJ, Jonasson O, Gibbs J *et al*. The development of a clinical trial to determine if watchful waiting is an acceptable alternative to routine herniorrhaphy for patients with minimal or no hernia symptoms. *Am Coll Surg* 2003: **196**: 737–742.
41. Junge K, Klinge U, Rosch R, Klosterhalfen B, Schumpelick V. Functional and morphologic properties of a modified mesh for inguinal hernia repair. *World J Surg* 2002; **26**: 1472–1480.
42. Post S, Weiss B, Willer M, Neufang T, Lorenz D. Randomized clinical trial of lightweight composite mesh for Lichtenstein inguinal hernia repair. *Br J Surg* 2004; **91**: 44–48.
43. Bay-Nielsen M. Convalescence after inguinal herniorrhaphy. *Br J Surg* 2004; **91**: 362–367.
44. Taylor E, Duffy K, Lee K *et al*. Surgical site infection after groin hernia repair. *Br J Surg* 2004; **91**: 105–111.
45. Davis C, Arregui M. Laparoscopic repair for groin hernias. *Surg Clin North Am* 2003; **83**: 1141–1161.
46. Wantz GE. Laparoscopic Herniorrhaphy. *J Am Coll Surg* 1997; **184**: 521–522.
47. Vale L, Grant A, McCormack K, Scott N, EU Hernia Trialists Collaboration. Cost-effectiveness of alternative methods of surgical repair of inguinal hernia. *Int J Technol Assess Health Care* 2004; **20**: 192–200.
48. Cooke T, Fitzpatrick R, Smith I. *Achieving day surgery targets: a practical approach towards improving efficiency in day case units in the UK*. London: Advance Medical Publications; 2004.
49. Bay-Nielsen M, Kehlet H. The Danish Hernia Database. *Hernia* 1998; **3** (Suppl 2): S65–S66.
50. Burney RE, Jones KR, Wilson Coon J. Core outcomes measures for inguinal hernia repair. *J Am Coll Surg* 1997; **185**: 509–515.

Dominic Slade Nigel Scott

7

Intestinal fistula management

An intestinal fistula is an abnormal communication between two epithelialised surfaces. Gastrointestinal fistulas may form between the gastrointestinal tract and an adjacent viscus (entero-enteral) or the skin (enterocutaneous). They may be congenital but are usually acquired. Primary or Type I fistulas develop as a result of an underlying disease affecting the gut wall whereas secondary or Type II fistulas occur after injury to otherwise normal gut. This classification has practical implications for the surgical management of intestinal fistulas (Table 1).

Patients with intestinal fistulation have many associated health issues that must be addressed simultaneously whilst attempting to treat the fistula. Physical problems associated with leakage of enteric content include sepsis, skin excoriation, and electrolyte, fluid and protein depletion. Psychological problems include altered body image, fear of ostracism and often a complete lack of faith in a surgical resolution of their problems. Decision-making in these patients can be extremely difficult and requires involvement of the patient, their relatives and a multidisciplinary team often in the setting of a specialised unit to produce a successful outcome.

ASSESSMENT

Initial assessment should identify the metabolic and nutritional consequences of a fistula and a strategy can then be formulated to correct them. This may

Dominic Slade MBChB FRCS
Specialist Registrar in General Surgery, Hope Hospital, Stott Lane, Salford, Manchester M6 8HD, UK
E-mail: dom.slade@talktalk.net

Nigel Scott FRCS
Consultant Surgeon, Hope Hospital, Stott Lane, Salford, Manchester M6 8HD, UK (for correspondence)
E-mail: nigel.scott@srht.nhs.uk

Table 1 Classification of gastrointestinal fistulas

Examples	Classification	Management	
Congenital	Tracheo-oesophageal	Type I	Resection
Acquired Inflammatory	Peptic ulceration	Type I	Resection
	Crohn's disease	Type I	Resection
	Pancreatitis	Type I	Conservative or drainage
	Diverticular disease	Type I	Resection
Neoplastic	Small bowel	Type I	Resection
	Colon	Type I	Resection
	Ovarian	Type I	Resection
Traumatic	Surgery	Type II	Conservative or resection
	Penetrating trauma	Type II	Conservative or resection
	Radiation enteritis	Type I	Resection
Infective	Tuberculosis	Type I	Anti-microbials or resection
	Actinomycosis	Type I	Anti-microbials

After Scott.[35]

determine the time scale for any future surgical intervention. The probable anatomy of an intestinal fistula may be apparent after a detailed history and clinical examination.

Likely prognosis and strategies to treat the fistula can then be formulated from the answers to two inter-related questions: (i) is the fistula a consequence of pre-existing gastrointestinal disease or of damage to previously healthy tissue? and (ii) will this fistula close spontaneously or require surgical resection?

When answering these questions, we need to know the condition of adjacent bowel and whether there is any associated intra-abdominal sepsis. As a general rule of thumb, Type I fistulas require surgical resection of the diseased segment whereas Type II fistulas have the potential to close spontaneously with conservative management.[1]

Key point 1

- Spontaneous closure is related to whether the fistula has arisen from diseased bowel (Type I, unlikely) or injury to otherwise normal bowel (Type II, more likely).

PRIMARY OR TYPE 1 GASTROINTESTINAL FISTULAS

CROHN'S DISEASE

Crohn's disease is the classic fistulating disease of the gut. It is characterised by full-thickness granulomatous inflammation that is breached by a fissuring ulcer leading to abscess formation. This breaks through the skin or into an adjacent viscus establishing the fistula tract.

Some 6–40% of Crohn's cases develop fistulas; usually entero-enteral but frequently enterocutaneous. In some series, 20–30% of all external small bowel fistulas are secondary to Crohn's but the proportion is much higher if post-resection enterocutaneous fistulas are included.[2]

As the terminal ileum is most commonly affected, these patients often present with a right iliac fossa mass comprising fistulating disease in combination with an abscess cavity. They may also develop fistulation at the site of a previous ileocolic anastomosis that, in turn, can involve the second or third part of the duodenum.

Management – medical

There is little evidence that aggressive medical therapy with high-dose steroids, azathioprine and parenteral nutrition will close either an entero-enteric or an enterocutaneous fistula. Indeed, the vast majority of patients ultimately require surgical resection.[3] The same is true of immunomodulating therapies such as 6-mercaptopurine, where initial closure of an entero-cutaneous fistula is inevitably followed by a relapse on discontinuing the treatment. Tacrolimus failed to demonstrate any benefit over placebo in a randomised controlled trial of fistula closure in Crohn's disease.[4]

Infliximab by contrast, a chimaeric antibody (75% human, 25% mouse) to TNF-α, has demonstrated a fistula closure rate of 55% within 3 months of treatment but the duration of closure was short-lived.[5] However, less favourable results have been reported by others when infliximab therapy has been followed by resection of relapsed or resistant abdominal fistulas.[6]

Management – surgical

Radiological or surgical drainage of a Crohn's abscess may be an effective temporising measure to down-grade intra-abdominal sepsis, but definitive resection of the affected bowel segment with simultaneous drainage will inevitably be required in most patients.[7]

The presence of associated sepsis in Crohn's disease is a key factor in decisions surrounding surgical management of these patients. In a large series, 13% of all operations for Crohn's disease were complicated by leak, abscess and fistula formation. These complications were associated pre-operatively with a low serum albumin level, and steroid use, and intra-operatively with the presence of an abscess or fistula.[8]

The first step in surgical management should, therefore, be elimination of all intra-abdominal sepsis whilst correcting any nutritional depletion. This may require primary surgical resection with drainage of the abscess. In a normally nourished patient with a serum albumin level above 30 g/l and with no evidence of sepsis, it may be safe to perform resection and primary anastomosis away from the abscess cavity. Conversely, in patients who are malnourished, with an albumin level below 30 g/l and with evidence of sepsis, resection should be combined with exteriorisation of the bowel ends as an end stoma and mucous fistula. Laparoscopic or laparoscopic-assisted resection in patients with fistulating Crohn's disease has been described but a laparotomy approach is still probably most appropriate for complex fistulating disease.[9]

COLONIC DIVERITICULAR DISEASE

The most common fistula, seen in association with diverticular disease, is between the sigmoid colon and the dome of the bladder, with an incidence of about 8% amongst those patients requiring resection for diverticular disease.[10] The passage of air bubbles (pneumaturia), or faecal matter (faecaluria) in the urine is very suggestive. Cystoscopy allows exclusion of a neoplastic lesion and may show the fistula, seen as an oedematous patch surrounded by localised inflammation with polyps. Spiral CT with water soluble contrast and/or barium enema are useful in delineating the extent of the sigmoid diverticular change – the presence of barium in a urine sample after such studies confirming a colovesical fistula.

Management

Segmental resection of the diseased bowel is curative and it is uncommon to find any bladder defect requiring surgical repair. Postoperative management should include an in-dwelling urinary catheter left in place for 10 days. Women who have had a previous hysterectomy develop diverticular colovaginal fistulas from the diseased sigmoid colon coming into contact with the vault of the vagina; again, treatment is by surgical resection.

> **Key point 2**
>
> - Important risk factors for postoperative fistulation include low serum albumin (< 30 g/l), intraperitoneal sepsis and pre-operative steroid use – exteriorisation should be considered in these patients if feasible.

MALIGNANT INTESTINAL FISTULAS

Colorectal cancers may fistulate into any adjacent viscus producing urinary, enteral, colovaginal or rarely cutaneous fistulas.

Management

Careful pre-operative evaluation using examination under anaesthesia, cystoscopy, colonoscopy and multiple radiological modalities allows the surgeon(s) to plan radical clearance with curative intent. Contrary to popular belief, malignant fistulas from locally advanced colonic cancer are not necessarily indicative of a poorer prognosis and radical excision in the absence of nodal metastasis may offer a good chance of cure. Fistulas resulting from diffuse inoperable malignancy are better treated by non-surgical, palliative means.

NECROTISING PANCREATITIS

Gastrointestinal fistulas arise on a background of necrotising pancreatitis either directly through damage to the distal pancreatic duct with associated proximal stricture formation or through deliberate attempts to drain a pseudocyst percutaneously or transgastricaly. Collateral damage to small bowel with subsequent fistula formation may also follow multiple pancreatic necrosectomies.

Management

Octreotide (somatostatin analogue) therapy to reduce exocrine function and the maintenance of nutrition may lead to spontaneous closure of a pancreatic fistula. Surgical resolution may at times only be achieved by fistula drainage into a jejunal Roux loop.

RADIATION ENTERITIS

Increasing use of radiotherapy for the treatment of gynaecological, rectal, and genito-urinary malignancies has led to more patients presenting with radiation enteritis. This condition is characterised by an obliterative vasculitis and a reduction in the number of actively dividing cells. This may give rise to stricture formation and intestinal fistulation, usually entero-enteral.

Management

The prognosis for radiation fistulas is poor; they rarely close with conservative management and the only effective strategies for treating them are surgical associated with significant morbidity and mortality. Constructing a proximal loop stoma to the fistula is the simplest and safest strategy in poor-risk patients. If resection of the diseased segment and anastomosis is to be attempted, it must involve bowel which has been spared from the radiation field. Postoperative death, permanent stomas, intestinal failure, refistulation and intra-abdominal sepsis are seen frequently.

SECONDARY OR TYPE II GASTROINTESTINAL FISTULAS

Secondary fistulas arise in normal gut usually after laparotomy and occur as a result of unrecognised enteric injury and/or breakdown of an anastomosis or repaired serotomy. Enteric fistulae can also develop after the abdomen is deliberately left open – as a laparostomy in cases of severe wide-spread abdominal sepsis or for planned re-operation or delayed closure.[11] Management of patients with large postoperative abdominal wall defects can be extremely difficult and various techniques have been described for achieving temporary wound closure.

The modified sandwich-vacuum pack technique uses sub-atmospheric vacuum dressings to manage an open abdomen following sepsis, visceral oedema, abdominal compartment syndrome, or large wall defects.[12] An opened irrigation bag covers the viscera with loose approximation sutures to the rectus sheath, the whole defect being covered with an occlusive self-adhesive drape. Vacuum tubing is passed through the drape and attached to wall suction (125–150 mmHg). The dressing is kept in place until the viscera are covered with granulation tissue. This dressing technique is associated with a spontaneous fistula rate of 4–5% in reported series.[12,13] Purpose-built vacuum-assisted wound closure devices (VACs; 125 mmHg) have also been used in this setting with a fistula rate of 7%.[14] It remains uncertain how many of these fistulas would have occurred in the absence of vacuum therapy as secondary small bowel fistulas may arise in up to 25% of patients with laparostomies. They do not close spontaneously because healing of the abdomen by secondary intention leads to mucocutaneous continuity of the fistula.[15] In patients with established enterocutaneous fistulas, VACs device therapy appears useful in controlling the fistula effluent, and reducing skin excoriation, although there is no convincing evidence to suggest they accelerate postoperative fistula closure.[16,17]

With the increasing use of prosthetic mesh for repair of abdominal wall defects, fistulas may arise in association with a prosthetic mesh used electively or to achieve closure of large abdominal defects following laparotomy in critical illness. Fistulation rates for mesh prostheses in the acute setting have been reported ranging from 12–75%.[12] In a series of 274 consecutive critically ill patients managed by staged closure of their laparotomy wound with absorbable polygalactin 910 mesh, the spontaneous fistula rate was 8.4% and believed to have been the result of direct mesh erosion. The principles for secondary fistula management should still be followed in these patients but represent an additional problem because associated sepsis can often only be eliminated by removal of their mesh. Secondary fistulas remain the most common fistulas encountered in surgical practice today. Risk factors for postoperative fistulation include those associated with anastomotic failure such as age, nutritional status and site of the anastomosis as well as peritonitis, hepatic or renal insufficiency, previous surgery and immunocompromise.[18]

The presentation of a postoperative fistula depends on the degree of associated sepsis. A low-volume leak walled off from the peritoneal cavity may only produce minimal systemic upset and discharge of enteric contents through the abdominal wound. Alternatively, the presentation may be peritonitis, multiple organ failure, and complete dehiscence of the abdominal wound with discharge of litres of enteric fluid. The absence of severe systemic sepsis is an indication that the fistula is well localised and may heal spontaneously.

Key point 3

- A fistula will not close if there is chronic sepsis, discontinuity of the bowel ends, distal obstruction, mucocutaneous continuity, residual damaged or diseased bowel or in the presence of malnutrition.

FISTULA CHARACTERISTICS

A fistula may be simple or complex. Simple fistulas form a short, direct track from bowel to skin. Complex fistulas, by contrast, drain to the skin through long, often multiple tracks via an abscess cavity. Simple fistulas generally have a better prognosis and are more likely to close spontaneously.

Fistulas are conventionally described as high-output if they produce more than 200 ml in a 24-h period. High-output fistulas arise from proximal small bowel and may have a worse prognosis and lower rate of spontaneous closure than low-output fistulas.

Small bowel fistulas have a higher mortality and complication rate than colonic fistulas due largely to their higher output, associated sepsis and malnutrition.

Principal reasons why a fistula will not close include: (i) discontinuity of bowel ends; (ii) distal obstruction; (iii) chronic abscess; (iv) mucocutaneous continuity of fistula with skin; (v) damaged or diseased residual intestine; and (vi) malnutrition (after Alexander-Williams and Irving[19]).

> **Key point 4**
>
> - If a Type II fistula has not healed after 6 weeks of parenteral nutrition and bowel rest it is unlikely to close spontaneously.

MANAGEMENT

The over-riding principle of managing Type II fistulas is rigorous elimination of all sepsis by the most appropriate means with effective complication-free nutrition. Management should follow a staged plan and this can be summarised by the four 'R's – resuscitation, restitution, reconstruction, and rehabilitation.

> **Key point 5**
>
> - Management of Type II fistulas should adhere to the principles of the four 'R's – resuscitation, restitution, reconstruction and rehabilitation.

Resuscitation

Initial treatment is aimed not at the fistula but at the patient and correction of their fluid depletion and sepsis. Resuscitation with attention to airway, breathing and support of the circulation (ABCs) follows the same lines as any critically ill patient. Transfer to a high dependency or intensive care unit may be necessary to support organ dysfunction. Fluid resuscitation should be aimed at correcting sodium-rich fistula losses (enteric fluid sodium content is about 110 mmol/l) with equivalent volumes of normal saline. Measurement of urinary sodium losses as well as volume may be helpful in assessing adequate resuscitation with high-output fistulas. Patients with peritonitis require stabilisation and operative exteriorisation of bowel ends to manage uncontrolled intra-abdominal enteric leaks.

Attention to wound care is essential to protect the surrounding skin from destruction by the enteric contents and to collect them for accurate measurement of losses. This can be time-consuming and requires dedicated nursing resources.

The morale of the patient, relatives and staff requires attention for what may be a difficult, long-term problem. The surgeon may also require support and advice from colleagues sometimes best effected by referral to a specialised fistula unit.[20]

Restitution

This involves returning the patient to a state from which fistula closure may occur either spontaneously or surgically. This requires attention to SNAP: (i) sepsis elimination; (ii) nutrition, effective and complication free; (iii) anatomy of the fistula as well as the proximal and distal gut; and plan surgical resolution or wait for spontaneous closure.

Sepsis results from incompletely localised enteric contents discharging from the fistula. Sepsis prevents healing and leads to multiple organ failure with a mortality in excess of 50%.[21] Furthermore, sepsis drives catabolism rendering nutritional support ineffective and compounding the malnourished state. It is essential to locate and eliminate sepsis by whatever means necessary. Computed tomography (CT) scanning with intravenous and oral contrast is the most valuable tool for base-line evaluation. Percutaneous drainage may be effective in managing isolated collections but will do nothing for collections fed by the fistulating gut. In this situation, laparotomy is required with three surgical strategies in mind:

- Resect the fistula and exteriorise the ends.
- Left upper quadrant laparotomy with diversion of enteric contents to a high loop jejunostomy.
- Formation of a laparostomy when bowel cannot be exteriorised after multiple laparotomies in ICU patients.

Complex fistulas or persistent postoperative sepsis are indications for early re-operation allowing resection of the fistulous segment and drainage of the abscess cavity. In this early stage of management, an end stoma with mucous fistula is a safe strategy. If wide-spread intra-abdominal collections are excluded on CT imaging then the formation of a proximal loop jejunostomy above the fistula through a left upper quadrant laparotomy can control sepsis and avoid a full laparotomy with its attendant risk of further enterotomy. This approach is not without its problems as it immediately precipitates intestinal failure with stoma losses as high as 4 l/day. If there are multiple enterotomies in a gut fixed within the peritoneal cavity, then formation of a laparostomy allows multiple abscesses to drain and salvages patients with multiple organ failure in the intensive care setting.[22]

Nutrition: Malnutrition is a constant feature in high-output fistulas associated with persistent sepsis that impairs substrate utilisation. Nutrition as a therapy allows a steady supply of nutrients whilst 'resting the gut'.

Enteral nutrition is the preferred route of administration as long as the patient has enough accessible functioning gut. A useful technique in proximal enterocutaneous fistulas with accessible distal bowel shown to be of sufficient length and integrity by a distal contrast study is to tube feed the distal gut. Fistuloclysis, as this method is known, can also be utilised for feeding down the distal limb of a proximal jejunostomy brought out as part of sepsis elimination in the early stages of fistula management.[23] Not only does fistuloclysis allow weaning from parenteral nutrition but it also prevents the atrophy associated with defunctioned gut aiding subsequent surgical adhesiolysis, reconstruction and anastomosis.

Reduced oral intake with parenteral nutrition decreases fistula output volumes considerably. Indeed it has been suggested that parenteral nutrition might allow spontaneous fistula closure through 'gut rest', although there is no convincing evidence for this.[24] Parenteral nutrition must be used in patients who are unable to establish enteral feeding due to lack of available functioning gut – by definition, intestinal failure. To ensure line longevity in these patients, it is essential to establish a dedicated feeding line cared for by fully trained staff. Parenteral nutrition is not without its problems including complications from line placement (pneumothorax, vascular injury), line care (sepsis, endocarditis, thrombosis, occlusion) as well as the metabolic consequences of excessive calorie administration (hepatic dysfunction). A typical regimen would consist of 9 g nitrogen and 1400 calories with suitable additives and electrolytes. Feed administration should be over a nocturnal 12-h period to allow mobilisation during the day.

Anatomy: the anatomy of a postoperative fistula is ascertained through a series of contrast studies looking at proximal and distal bowel along with fistulography where contrast is injected directly into the fistula track. It is important to establish the fistula's relationship to the remaining bowel, to determine whether distal feeding can be initiated and to exclude distal obstruction, the presence of an abscess cavity, or remaining disease that may be preventing spontaneous fistula closure.

Plan or procedure: this stage is heralded by the successful elimination of sepsis and malnutrition and the clear delineation of the anatomy of the fistula and remaining bowel. Spontaneous closure is unlikely if the fistula is through diseased gut, *e.g.* colorectal cancer, residual Crohn's disease, or radiation enteritis.[25] Spontaneous closure often occurs within 6 weeks of the initiation of total parenteral nutrition in up to 70% of all cases; conversely, if there is no evidence of closure in this time, it is more likely that surgical reconstruction will be required.[26]

Key point 6

- Restitution of a patient to a state where fistula closure can occur requires attention to SNAP (sepsis, nutrition, anatomy and plan or procedure).

Somatostatin and gut rest: somatostatin-14, and its more potent analogue octreotide, reduce ileostomy diarrhoea and have been advanced as useful adjuncts to reducing fluid and electrolyte losses from high-output fistulas. Only six controlled studies have analysed the effect of these agents on gastrontestinal fistula output, three for each drug (see Table 2).[33] Of these, one somatostatin and two octreotide studies demonstrated a significant effect on output over conservative therapy. No study has demonstrated an increased number of patients achieving fistula closure. Therefore, it has to be concluded that the clinical role of these agents in closing small bowel fistulas remains unclear.

Reconstruction

This is a challenging surgical exercise with the key components of reconstruction including: (i) access to the peritoneal cavity; (ii) anastomosis of the gastrointestinal tract; and (iii) abdominal closure.

Table 2 Effect of somatostatin-14 and octreotide on fistula output

	Treatment	*n*	Output	1 day % output reduction	Effect on output
Torres *et al.* (1992)[27]	TPN	20	ND	ND	$P < 0.05$
	S + TPN	20		ND	
Nubiola-Calonge *et al.* (1987)[28]	Pl,O,O + PN	6	692	9	$P < 0.01$
	O,Pl,O + PN	8		53	
Scott *et al.* (1993)[29]	Pl	8	401	ND	NS
	O	11		ND	
Sancho *et al.* (1995)[30]	Pl + TPN	17	729	32	NS
	O + TPN	14		34	
Pederzoli *et al.* (1986)[31]	TPN	18	ND	39	NS
	S + TPN	8		82	
Planas *et al.* (1990)[32]	TPN	16	ND	ND	$P < 0.05$
	S + TPN	15		ND	

After Hesse *et al.*[33]
TPN, total parenteral nutrition; PN, parenteral nutrition; Pl, placebo; O, octreotide; S, Somatostatin-14 therapy; ND, not determined; NS, not significant.

It cannot be stressed too strongly that early operative intervention should always be avoided unless it is to drain sepsis, raise a stoma, resect ischaemic bowel or to exteriorise a fistula. Access to the peritoneal cavity for definitive reconstruction requires its reconstitution from the obliterative phase seen after intra-abdominal sepsis, fistulation and surgery. This may take up to 6 months to occur and can be assumed clinically by the prolapse of fistulas through the abdominal wound.

After entering the abdomen in the midline, the abdominal wall should be cleared out to the flanks to enable small bowel separation from the more pliable peritoneum encountered here. The entire bowel from duodenal–jejunal flexure distally should be carefully dissected to demonstrate the location of the fistula and to exclude distal obstruction. After resection of the fistula, a standard sutured anastomosis is performed in one or two layers.

Abdominal closure is mandatory after fistula reconstruction to cover the anastomosis and prevent the suture line from breaking down and refistulating. Relaxing incisions and the use of suture techniques such as 'near and far' closure help to bring the large abdominal wall defects encountered after laparostomy together.[34] The use of prosthetic mesh directly over the anastomosis should be avoided due to the risks of refistulation.

Rehabilitation

Postoperative fistulas that resolve spontaneously may only add days or weeks to a patient's hospital stay. However, postoperative fistulation associated with life-threatening illness, prolonged stays on intensive care with multiple organ failure and repeated surgical intervention have a significant impact on the well-being and morale of the patient, their family and friends. Specialised nursing care and support is essential for both the technical aspects of patient care and the holistic management of an individual having to adjust to the prolonged illness and alteration in body image that accompanies complicated postoperative fistulation.

Key points for clinical practice

- Spontaneous closure is related to whether the fistula has arisen from diseased bowel (Type I, unlikely) or injury to otherwise normal bowel (Type II, more likely).
- Important risk factors for postoperative fistulation include low serum albumin (< 30 g/l), intraperitoneal sepsis and pre-operative steroid use – exteriorisation should be considered in these patients if feasible.
- A fistula will not close if there is chronic sepsis, discontinuity of the bowel ends, distal obstruction, mucocutaneous continuity, residual damaged or diseased bowel or in the presence of malnutrition.
- If a Type II fistula has not healed after 6 weeks of parenteral nutrition and bowel rest it is unlikely to close spontaneously.
- Management of Type II fistulas should adhere to the principles of the four 'R's – resuscitation, restitution, reconstruction and rehabilitation.
- Restitution of a patient to a state where fistula closure can occur requires attention to SNAP (sepsis, nutrition, anatomy and plan or procedure).

References

1. Sansoni B, Irving M. Small bowel fistulas. *World J Surg* 1985; **9**: 897–903.
2. McIntyre P *et al*. Management of enterocutaneous fistulas; a review of 132 cases. *Br J Surg* 1984; **71**: 293–296.
3. Hawker P *et al*. Management of enterocutaneous fistulae in Crohn's disease. *Gut* 1983; **24**: 284–287.
4. Sandborn W *et al*. Tacrolimus for the treatment of fistulas in patients with Crohn's disease; a randomised placebo controlled trial. *Gastroenterology* 2003; **125**: 380–388.
5. Present D *et al*. Infliximab for the treatment of fistulas in patients with Crohn's disease. *N Engl J Med* 1999; **340**: 1398–1405.
6. Poritz L, Rowe W, Koltun W. Remicade does not abolish the need for surgery in fistulizing Crohn's disease. *Dis Colon Rectum* 2002; **45**: 771–775.
7. Ayuk P *et al*. The management of intra-abdominal abscesses in Crohn's disease. *Ann R Coll Surg Engl* 1996; **78**: 5–10.
8. Yamamoto T, Allen R, Keighley M. Risk factors for intra-abdominal sepsis after surgery in Crohn's disease. *Dis Colon Rectum* 2000; **43**: 1141–1145.
9. Hasegawa H *et al*. Laparoscopic surgery for recurrent Crohn's disease. *Br J Surg* 2003; **90**: 970–973.
10. McConnell E, Tessier D, Wolff B. Population-based incidence of complicated diverticular disease of the sigmoid colon based on gender and age. *Dis Colon Rectum* 2003; **46**: 1110–1114.

11. Mughal M, Bancewicz J, Irving M. Laparostomy. A technique for the management of intractable abdominal sepsis. *Br J Surg* 1986; **73**: 253–259.
12. Navsaria P *et al.* Temporary closure of open abdominal wounds by the modified sandwich-vacuum pack technique. *Br J Surg* 2003; **90**: 718–722.
13. Barker D *et al.* Vacuum pack technique of temporary abdominal closure: a 7-year experience with 112 patients. *J Trauma* 2000; **48**: 201–206.
14. Suliburk J *et al.* Vacuum-assisted wound closure achieves early fascial closure of open abdomens after severe trauma. *J Trauma* 2003; **55**: 1155–1160.
15. Tremblay L *et al.* Skin only or silo closure in the critically ill patient with an open abdomen. *Am J Surg* 2001; **182**: 670–675.
16. Cro C *et al.* Vacuum assisted closure system in the management of enterocutaneous fistulas. *Postgrad Med J* 2002; **78**: 364–365.
17. Alvarez A, Maxwell G, Rodriguez G. Vacuum-assisted closure for cutaneous gastrointestinal fistula management. *Gynecol Oncol* 2001; **80**: 413–416.
18. Falconi M, Pederzoli P. The relevance of gastrointestinal fistulae in clinical practice; a review. *Gut* 2001; **49 (Suppl IV)**: iv2–iv10.
19. Alexander-Williams J, Irving M. *Intestinal Fistulas*. Bristol: John Wright, 1982.
20. Scott N *et al.* Spectrum of intestinal failure in a specialised unit. *Lancet* 1991; **337**: 471–473.
21. Bosscha K *et al.* Open management of the abdomen and planned re-operations in severe bacterial peritonitis. *Eur J Surg* 2000; **166**: 44–49.
22. Carlson G, Scott N. Laparostomy and allied techniques. *Surgery* 1996; **14**: 102–105.
23. Teubner A *et al.* Fistuloclysis can successfully replace parenteral feeding in the nutritional support of patients with enterocutaneous fistula. *Br J Surg* 2004; **91**: 625–631.
24. Sitges-Serra A, Jaurrieta E, Sitges-Creus A. Management of postoperative enterocutaneous fistulas: the roles of parenteral nutrition and surgery. *Br J Surg* 1982; **69**: 147–150.
25. Reber H *et al.* Management of external gastrointestinal fistulae. *Ann Surg* 1978; **188**: 460–467.
26. Sternquist J, Bubrick M, Hitchcock C. Enterocutaneous fistula. *Dis Colon Rectum* 1978; **21**: 578–581.
27. Torres AJ, Landa JI, Moreno-Azcoita M *et al.* Somatostatin in the management of gastrointestinal fistulas. A multi-center trial. *Arch Surg* 1992; **127**: 97–99.
28. Nubiola-Calonge P, Badia JM, Sancho J *et al.* Blind evaluation of the effect of octreotide (SMS 201-995), a somatostatin analogue, on small bowel fistula output. *Lancet* 1987; **2**: 672–4.
29. Scott NA, Finnegan S, Irving MH. Octreotide and postoperative enterocutaneous fistulae: a controlled prospective study. *Acta Gastroenterol Belg* 1993; **56**: 266–270.
30. Sancho JJ, di Costanzo J, Nubiola P *et al.* Randomized double-blind placebo-controlled trial of early octreotide in patients with postoperative enterocutaneous fistula. *Br J Surg* 1995; **82**: 638–641.
31. Pederzoli P, Bassi C, Falconi M *et al.* Conservative treatment of external pancreatic fistulas with parenteral nutrition alone or in combination with continuous intravenous infusion of somatostatin, glucagon, or calcitonin. *Surg Gynaecol Obstet* 1986; **163**: 428-432.
32. Planas M, Porta I, Angles R *et al.* (Somatostatin and/or total parenteral nutrition for the treatment of intestinal fistulas). *Rev Esp Enferm Dig* 1990; **78**: 345–347.
33. Hesse U, Ysebaert D, Hemptinne BD. Role of somatostatin-14 and its analogues in the management of gastrointestinal fistulae: clinical data. *Gut* 2001; **42 (Suppl)**: iv11–iv21.
34. Malik R, Scott N. Double near and far Prolene suture closure: a technique for abdominal wall closure after laparostomy. *Br J Surg* 2001; **88**: 146.
35. Scott N. Intestinal fistulas. *Surgery* 2000; **18**: 167–171.

Colin D. Johnson

8

Standards in the treatment of pancreatic disease

Clinicians providing care for patients with acute pancreatitis or pancreatic cancer now have the benefit of clear guidelines to shape their practice. There have been numerous publications defining guidelines and standards in acute pancreatitis, and notably the British Society of Gastroenterology (BSG) guidelines published in 1998,[1] a consensus conference from an *ad hoc* group meeting at Santorini,[2] and a consensus document produced by the International Association of Pancreatology.[3] Recently, the BSG guidelines have been updated.[4] These documents provide full references for the present review.

ACUTE PANCREATITIS

INITIAL ASSESSMENT

Pancreatitis is a condition which ranges in severity from a mild, self-limiting disorder lasting 2 or 3 days, to a prolonged severe illness with multiple organ failure at death. Initial assessment includes correct diagnosis, initial treatment, and an attempt to identify patients with potentially fatal disease and others who will require intensive care management.

The diagnosis of acute pancreatitis should be considered when there is a clinical presentation with upper abdominal pain, usually associated with at least one episode of vomiting. This is associated with an elevation of pancreatic enzyme levels in plasma. Most clinicians look for an elevation of 2 or 3 times the upper limit of normal, of lipase or amylase, respectively. However,

*Colour figures (plates) referred to in this chapter are to be found in the 'Colour plates section' at the front of this volume (p1–8).

Colin D. Johnson MChir FRCS
Reader in Surgery, University Surgical Unit, Southampton General Hospital, Southampton SO16 6YD, UK. E-mail: c.d.johnson@soton.ac.uk

pancreatitis may present with raised levels below these thresholds, as a result of delay in blood sampling, or impaired pancreatic enzyme function.

The differential diagnosis of hyperamylasaemia with abdominal pain must include any condition which can allow escape of luminal material to gain access to the peritoneal cavity or general circulation. A high level of suspicion should be maintained for conditions such as perforated ulcer, intestinal ischaemia and infarction, and other conditions which lead to low flow state in the gut such as myocardial infarction or leaking aortic aneurysm. If any doubt about the diagnosis exists, urgent contrast enhanced CT scan should be obtained immediately.

Although amylase is widely used for the diagnosis of acute pancreatitis, both the BSG and the IAP guidelines conclude that lipase is a preferable test because it is more pancreas specific, and remains elevated for longer after onset of symptoms.

Other diagnostic tests are not helpful for diagnosis of acute pancreatitis.

Key point 1

- The diagnosis of acute pancreatitis is made by a combination of clinical features and elevated plasma lipase levels (or amylase levels if this is not available). In case of diagnostic doubt, urgent CT should be performed.

IDENTIFICATION OF THE CAUSE

About half the cases of acute pancreatitis are caused by gallstones. It is important to recognise this aetiology early in the course of disease, because important treatment decisions will follow from this diagnosis. Patients with severe acute pancreatitis secondary to gallstones should be considered for immediate endoscopic sphincterotomy, and all patients with gallstone pancreatitis should have definitive management of the gallstones before discharge from hospital. Accordingly, an ultrasound examination of the gallbladder should be performed within 24 h of admission to hospital, although this may be delayed until the next working day for patients with predicted mild disease admitted at the weekend. The presence of gallstones in the gallbladder is sufficient to make the diagnosis of biliary pancreatitis. Other features consistent with that diagnosis (but neither conclusive nor necessary) are a dilated common bile duct at ultrasonography, and elevation of plasma liver enzymes, especially transaminases. Ultrasound is not sensitive for detection of common bile duct stones, and it is not necessary to demonstrate bile duct stones in order to presume a biliary cause for the pancreatitis.

Key point 2

- Urgent ultrasonography is required for all patients with acute pancreatitis, to determine the presence or absence of stones in the gallbladder.

Table 1 Causes of acute pancreatitis (AP) and appropriate treatment strategies

Cause	Frequency	Treatment strategy
Gallstones	50–60%	Urgent endoscopic sphincterotomy for severe AP Cholecystectomy with cholangiography or endoscopic sphincterotomy for all cases before discharge from hospital
Alcohol abuse	15–25%	Supportive Avoid further alcohol consumption
Various drugs	< 5%	Supportive Avoid cause if possible
ERCP	< 5%	Supportive
Viral infections	< 5%	Supportive
Idiopathic	10–20%	Supportive

Other causes of pancreatitis should be sought, even if gallstones are present. However, there are few urgent interventions available to deal with these other causes of pancreatitis (see Table 1).

A single negative ultrasound examination does not exclude gallstone aetiology. If no other cause of the pancreatitis is found, ultrasonography should be repeated by a skilled operator under optimum conditions.

IMMEDIATE MANAGEMENT

Some patients present with organ failure already apparent at the time of admission to hospital. Such patients clearly require appropriate support. Others may appear initially well but deteriorate within hours or days of admission. It is difficult to identify these patients before evidence of organ failure appears. Accordingly, initial treatment should take account of the frequent occurrence of hypoxaemia and hypovolaemia in patients with acute pancreatitis. All patients should be given adequate analgesia, supplemental oxygen by nasal catheter, and adequate intravenous fluids including colloid if necessary to maintain blood pressure and urine output.

If there is any evidence of circulatory or respiratory insufficiency, patients should be managed in an HDU or ITU, using the SSC guidelines[5] to guide resuscitation goals.

Key point 3

- Early aggressive fluid replacement and supplemental oxygen, together with analgesia, may prevent or reverse organ failure. All patients should receive these treatments until it is clear they are no longer needed.

IDENTIFICATION OF SEVERE AND POTENTIALLY FATAL ACUTE PANCREATITIS

The Atlanta symposium[6] defined severe acute pancreatitis by the presence of any complication. Many methods exist for attempting to predict severe acute pancreatitis within the first 24–48 h of admission to hospital. The most popular are the Ranson[7,8] and the modified Glasgow scores,[9] and the APACHE-II score.[10] The APACHE-II score has the advantage that it can make as good a prediction as the pancreatitis scores, within 24 h of admission to hospital, rather than 48 h. Other clinical features independently associated with severe outcome include age and the presence of obesity (body mass index, BMI > 30).[11,12] Pleural effusion on initial chest X-ray is also a sign of severe disease. Aetiology is generally thought to have no effect, although some evidence suggests that first attacks of alcohol-related pancreatitis may be more severe. The confounding effect of obesity in that group has not been examined.

CT has been used for the identification of patients with local complications (although this technique is not widely used in the UK. The CT severity index described by Balthazar *et al.*[13] relies on the presence and extent of peripancreatic fluid infiltrates, and pancreatic hypoperfusion representing areas of necrosis (Table 2). Both the scoring systems and CT identify complications (organ failure, pancreatic necrosis) that are already present, and clearly such patients should be managed in an appropriate critical care setting. It is more important that the clinician attempts to identify severe disease, or the presence of complications, than to argue over which particular system should be used. When organ failure or local complications are present appropriate supportive treatment should be started immediately.

Recent evidence has shown that some patients with organ failure recover rapidly, and thereafter pursue an uncomplicated course. It seems that transient organ failure, present for less than 48 h is rarely associated with other complications or death, whereas the mortality rate amongst patients with

Table 2 CT grading of severity based on Balthazar *et al.*[13] and associated outcomes

CT grade		
A	Normal pancreas	0
B	Oedematous pancreatitis	1
C	B plus mild extrapancreatic changes	2
D	Severe extrapancreatic changes including one fluid collection	3
E	Multiple or extensive extrapancreatic collections	4
Necrosis		
None		0
< one-third		2
> one-third, < one-half		4
> half		6

CT severity index (CTSI) = CT grade + necrosis score

CTSI	Complications	Deaths
0–3	8%	3%
4–6	35%	6%
7–10	92%	17%

Table 3 Fators associated wit increased risk of death in acute pancreatitis

Age	>70	17%
Obesity	BMI>30	25%
Ranson score	5 or more	40%
APACHE-11 score	>10	20%
(within 24 h admission)	>18	75%
CT: necrosis	<50%	17%
	>50%	20%
CT: Balthazaar	7 or more	17%
Infected necrosis		38%

persistent organ failure is high.[14,15] Some consideration of the patient's response to therapy is useful in the assessment of severity.

A number of individual biochemical tests have been assessed for prognosticating severity. The only test routinely available at present is C-reactive protein. This reaches a peak at 96 h after onset of symptoms but it may be elevated earlier than this. A level > 150 mg/l is a marker of severe disease and is often associated with the presence of pancreatic necrosis.

Key point 4

- Severity stratification should be made in all patients within 48 h of diagnosis. A clear assessment of severity should be recorded in the notes.

Key point 5

- CT may be helpful in identification of patients with local complications, but early CT is unlikely to influence management during the first week (unless antibiotic prophylaxis is being considered).

POTENTIALLY FATAL ACUTE PANCREATITIS

Few studies have looked at identification of patients who are likely to die (as opposed to develop complications but survive). The features listed in Table 3 have been shown to select patients with increased risk of death. This potentially fatal group is of considerable interest and should be offered a full intensive supportive therapy. These patients represent an appropriate group for clinical investigation of potential therapies.

TREATMENT OF GALLSTONES

All patients with gallstone-related pancreatitis should have definitive management of the gallstones before discharge from hospital, unless a clear plan has been made for definitive treatment within the next 2 weeks. This is essential in order to prevent further potentially fatal attacks of pancreatitis, or other biliary complications. Evidence continues to accumulate to support this recommendation.[16]

Treatment of the gallstones will usually be by laparoscopic cholecystectomy (with on-table cholangiography) unless the patient is elderly or unfit for general anaesthesia. An acceptable alternative is endoscopic sphincterotomy. The aim of treatment is to prevent a further attack of pancreatitis; if the gallstones have been hitherto asymptomatic, laparoscopic cholecystectomy may not be necessary if an adequate sphincterotomy can be performed.

Key point 6

- Treatment of gallstones to prevent further attacks of pancreatitis should take place during the index admission, or within 2 weeks of discharge.

Patients with predicted severe acute pancreatitis, or those who have organ failure on or shortly after admission, and who have gallstones, should be offered endoscopic sphincterotomy. This ideally should be done with 72 h of admission to hospital, earlier if possible. The patient may need referral to a specialist centre in order to achieve this. The evidence supporting this recommendation is strong, but not unanimous. There are two consistent trials supporting this policy, from Leicester[17] and Hong Kong,[18] and a discordant trial from Germany[19] which has been heavily criticised because it included a majority of patients with mild pancreatitis, the recruitment rate was slow, suggesting inadequate experience of urgent ERCP in many hospitals, many of the excess complications in the sphincterotomy group were respiratory complications, and the numbers of patients in whom successful duct drainage was achieved were not stated. Therefore, the balance of evidence still favours urgent endoscopic sphincterotomy, particularly in patients with organ failure that has not resolved with initial treatment.

Key point 7

- Patients with biliary pancreatitis who have one or more organ failures that fail to resolve or improve within 24 h should be offered emergency endoscopic sphincterotomy.

PREVENTION OF COMPLICATIONS

Apart from the general measures outlined above (fluid resuscitation, oxygenation), and endoscopic sphincterotomy in gallstone pancreatitis, no specific treatment has been convincingly demonstrated to affect outcome in acute pancreatitis.

A number of small studies have suggested possible benefit for patients given enteral nutrition during the first week, in terms of a reduction of the inflammatory response, and perhaps of other complications. The rationale for this is that prolonged starvation facilitates endotoxin absorption or bacterial translocation from the gut and this inappropriately drives the systemic inflammatory response syndrome. However, differences were apparent only in studies comparing enteral and parenteral nutrition;[20–22] in a trial of enteral nutrition versus no treatment, no benefit was observed.[23] The role of enteral nutrition at present remains uncertain and more clinical trial evidence is required.

There have been a number of trials of antibiotic prophylaxis in severe acute pancreatitis. The rationale for prophylaxis is to prevent infection of pancreatic necrosis. However, disadvantages perceived by some authors include an increase in fungal and other resistant organism infections. The evidence is not clear cut, as different end-points have shown benefit for antibiotics in the different randomised trials conducted to date. All the trials have been too small to give a definitive answer about mortality, but a Cochrane review[24] concluded that antibiotic prophylaxis might reduce mortality in patients with pancreatic necrosis. Given that the rationale for antibiotic treatment is to prevent infected necrosis, it is inappropriate to use antibiotics in patients without CT evidence of hypoperfusion.

Since the Cochrane review, a further trial[25] has been published which has only served to inflame the controversy. This trial included 76 patients, but not all had pancreatic necrosis. The trial design included the option to begin antibiotics for the treatment of 'sepsis'. Inevitably, this meant that many patients with SIRS were deemed to have sepsis and were given open label antibiotics. It is of interest that this occurred much more frequently in the placebo-treated group than with active treatment. The trial was reported as showing no difference between placebo and antibiotics, but it has been interpreted by the supporters of antibiotic treatment as being strong evidence in favour of such treatment!

Another large trial including 100 patients, treated with meropenem or placebo has just closed to recruitment. The results of this trial are awaited with interest.

Key point 8

- Enteral nutrition may be given safely during the first week of acute pancreatitis. Parenteral nutrition should not be used during the first 5 days, and until it is evident that the enteral route is insufficient.

Key point 9

- There is currently no consensus on the value of prophylactic antibiotics for patients with pancreatic necrosis. Patients without pancreatic necrosis will not benefit from prophylactic antibiotics.

TREATMENT IN SPECIALIST UNITS

It is recommended that all patients with acute pancreatitis should be managed by a clinical team led by a consultant with an interest in pancreatic disease. Such a

Table 4 Features of a specialist unit for the treatment of severe acute pancreatitis

Clinicians	A multidisciplinary team of specialists in surgery, endoscopy, intensive care, anaesthesia, gastroenterology, nutrition and full support staff
Team leader	A surgeon or gastroenterologist with specific knowledge of and interest in pancreatico-biliary disease
Critical care	Facilities for HDU/ITU management of critically ill patients including renal and respiratory support
Radiology	Expertise permitting the use of dynamic helical or multislice CT, percutaneous needle aspiration and drainage procedures: MR and angiography are helpful but not essential
Endoscopy	Facilities for ERCP and all therapeutic endoscopy (on an emergency basis) by an experienced endoscopist. EUS available as an elective diagnostic procedure.

team should be present in every hospital receiving emergency admissions, but of necessity, not all these teams will contain sufficient expertise to provide specialist services. Patients with severe disease may need to be referred to a specialist centre which should have the attributes listed in Table 4.

TREATMENT OF PANCREATIC NECROSIS

Pancreatic necrosis is a consequence of a severe inflammatory event in the pancreas, and represents the most serious end of the spectrum of severity. Management strategies for pancreatic necrosis continue to evolve, but it is now clear that the presence of infection is the single most important determinant of outcome. Sterile necrosis can be managed in the majority of cases by appropriate supportive treatment, in the expectation that organ failure will resolve with a mortality rate close to 10%.[26] By contrast, the mortality rate for infected necrosis remains around 40%.

It is now clear that diagnosis of presence or absence of infection in necrotic areas in and around the pancreas can be reliably and safely achieved by fine needle aspiration under CT or ultrasound guidance. It is not clear when infection occurs, so FNA should not be undertaken too early. Furthermore, surgical intervention becomes easier and safer with increasing delay from onset of symptoms, so early diagnosis may not affect a decision to operate. Some patients who are initially unwell will recover and their condition will be improving by 7–10 days after onset of symptoms.

For these reasons, the search for necrosis and possible infection should begin 7–10 days after admission to hospital. Patients who at this time have persistent symptoms (pain, SIRS) should undergo contrast-enhanced CT. If this shows areas of hypoperfusion (*i.e.* necrosis) affecting > 30% of the pancreas, fine needle aspiration under appropriate imaging guidance should be performed. Samples of the necrotic area should be sent for microscopy, and culture. Fluid collections around the pancreas usually resolve spontaneously, and there is no benefit in aspiration or drainage of these collections. Fluid infiltrates in the retroperitoneal tissue may represent retroperitoneal fat necrosis. If a patient is systemically unwell, FNA and culture should be performed in these areas even if the pancreas itself remains well perfused.

Patients with infected necrosis will require intervention to debride the cavity containing necrotic material. The ideal approach for this is not agreed. Many surgeons believe that only surgical debridement can be effective in removing necrotic solid material from the pancreas and retroperitoneum (Plate X, p5). Others advocate aggressive courses of percutaneous drainage with or without irrigation. The absence of consensus about the choice between surgical, endoscopic, percutaneous or radiological procedures is in strong contrast to the wide-spread agreement that if infected necrosis is present, aggressive treatment of all necrotic areas is the key to successful outcome. Nevertheless, mortality rates are high, in the region of 20–40%, and concentration of such seriously ill patients in specialist units is clearly desirable in order to improve experience and expertise.

Key point 10

- Specialist units should be able to provide surgical radiological and endoscopic services whenever required.

Key point 11

- The manaqement of infected pancreatic necrosis is controversial, but there is agreement that aggressive therapy is needed to drain and/or debride all areas of necrosis.

Key point 12

- The identification of infected necrosis is based on contrast-enhanced CT demonstration of hypoperfusion on a scan performed 7–14 days after onset of symptoms, followed by FNA for culture of material from the necrotic areas.

PANCREATIC CANCER

INITIAL ASSESSMENT

Most patients with pancreatic cancer have epigastric pain; jaundice is present in about three-quarters of cases. Recent onset diabetes in a patient without family history or obesity may be the first sign of pancreatic cancer, and such patients should undergo high quality ultrasound imaging of the pancreas.

Patients with obstructive jaundice can be managed with a simple treatment algorithm. Initial assessment of the jaundiced patient should include ultrasonography before or on the first visit to hospital. Signs of pancreatic cancer include the presence of extra- and intrahepatic bile duct dilatation, the absence of gallstones, and the presence of a mass in the head of pancreas. Even when overlying bowel gas obscures the head of pancreas, the diagnosis may be made by inference from the other features.

Patients with findings suggestive of pancreatic cancer should have a planned urgent admission to hospital for further assessment. Our protocol is

Table 5 Advantages of obtaining CT before ERCP in the assessment of a patient with obstructive jaundice

Stent artefact may obscure a small ampullary or lower bile duct tumour
CT may demonstrate an operable tumour, and avoid the need for ERCP
CT may show hilar obstruction, leading to choice of percutaneous rather than endoscopic drainage
Evidence of duodenal obstruction may be helpful in deciding on surgical drainage

to arrange contrast enhanced helical CT on the day preceding planned ERCP. The advantages of a prior CT are shown in Table 5.

The majority of patients with pancreatic cancer will have inoperable disease, and will receive palliative treatment, usually at the admitting hospital. Increasingly, patients with inoperable disease will undergo percutaneous needle biopsy to obtain histological confirmation. Such biopsy should not be considered unless there are clear criteria that indicate an inoperable tumour. In cases of diagnostic doubt, biopsy should be performed only after consultation with a pancreatic surgeon, as most prefer to avoid pre-operative biopsy of respectable tumours.

If this algorithm is followed, patients with obstructive jaundice can be managed with a minimum of time in hospital. Emergency admission to hospital is unnecessary and may be wasteful of resources. With a little planning, it is possible to provide an efficient service on the basis of a single out-patient visit with ultrasound examination, and a short admission to hospital to include CT, ERCP and stent placement if appropriate.

Key point 13

- If initial ultrasound demonstrates dilated intrahepatic ducts, the patient probably has malignancy. A dilated common bile duct and the absence of gallstones suggest pancreatic cancer even if the pancreas cannot be visualised.

Key point 14

- CT should precede ERCP and stent, in order to confirm the diagnosis, and assist in staging and planning treatment.

PALLIATIVE TREATMENTS

Obstructive jaundice

Patients with peri-ampullary malignancy frequently develop obstruction of the lower common bile duct. In most cases, this can be adequately palliated by insertion of a biliary endoprosthesis or stent. The stent may be made either of plastic, or expanding metal mesh. The plastic stents have the advantages of ease of insertion and low cost, but the disadvantage of limited life (median duration of stent patency

3–4 months). Metal expanding stents may be placed either percutaneously or endoscopically; they open to a large lumen and they remain patent for much longer than plastic stents. They are also considerably more expensive.

Comparative trials of the endoscopic and percutaneous routes predate the era of expanding metal stents. It is generally agreed, however, that the endoscopic route is to be preferred, unless endoscopic cannulation cannot be achieved. The usual reason for this will be lack of endoscopic access as a result of duodenal invasion by tumour. Because the median duration of survival of patients with advanced pancreatic cancer is only 3–4 months, many patients will be adequately palliated by insertion of a plastic stent. The early occlusion of a plastic stent, particularly in a patient with a better than average prognosis, is an indication for insertion of a metal expanding prosthesis.

Most patients who require relief of obstructive jaundice are adequately treated by a stent. Surgical bypass may be preferred in patients who are likely to survive more than 6 months. Often this will be patients who are considered candidates for surgical resection, and who have small tumours with local invasion that precludes resection. Surgical bypass may be preferred in these patients, particularly if the decision of non-resectability can only be made at laparotomy.

Gastric outlet obstruction

Although there is some data concerning the use of expanding metal stents for duodenal obstruction, the consensus view at present is that these achieve poor palliation. Duodenal obstruction can be relieved by gastrojejunostomy. This may be performed by either open surgery, laparoscopic surgery or a laparoscopic-assisted approach.

When a patient is undergoing biliary bypass surgery a gastric drainage procedure should be performed.

The accumulated surgical experience over several decades indicates that drainage procedures which use the gallbladder have a higher risk of recurrent jaundice than those which achieve drainage by anastomosis to the bile duct. This is usually because tumour invasion along the common bile duct occludes the cystic duct. Although some authors advocate cholecystojejunostomy if there is wide separation of the cystic duct junction from the tumour, a more reliable policy for long-term relief of jaundice is always to use the bile duct for biliary drainage.

Key point 15

- Patients with advanced tumours and obstructive jaundice should have endoscopic plastic stent placement in the first instance. Failure of cannulation, or early stent occlusion may require placement of an expanding metal stent, by the percutaneous route if necessary.

Key point 16

- Surgical bypass is only appropriate in patients with a relatively good prognosis. Surgical treatment should include choledochojejunostomy, and gastrojejunostomy.

Palliative chemotherapy

Until very recently, most clinicians felt there was no effective treatment available for patients with pancreatic cancer. A large number of clinical trials had produced equivocal or negative results. The few positive trial results all included treatment regimens containing 5-fluorouracil (5-FU).[27] This was considered the most effective agent.

The introduction of gemcitabine has seen a complete change in the approach of most medical oncologists. Although the survival benefit is small (median increase of 3 weeks) and most patients survive less than 6 months,[28] gemcitabine is seen as an effective treatment. NICE guidelines recommend that if chemotherapy is to be given, gemcitabine should be used.[29] One possible reason for the enthusiasm for this agent is the perception that gemcitabine treatment is associated with a reduction in pain and an improvement in quality of life.

Treatment of pancreatic cancer remains a gloomy business, and further trials are in progress to investigate other agents in combination with gemcitabine such as the GEMCAP study, which compares gemcitabine alone with gemcitabine and capecitabine.

Key point 17

- The accepted chemotherapy treatment for pancreatic cancer is now gemcitabine. Investigation of new agents should use gemcitabine as the standard for comparison.

A large number of other treatments are under investigation. These include immunotherapy, directed towards receptors expressed by the pancreatic cancer cells, or hormonal regulation, treatments designed to induce susceptibility to chemotherapeutic agents using a variety of techniques such as viral vectors for gene transfer, or manipulation of gene expression using tumour specific promoters and other approaches such as nutritional manipulations. These approaches seem to be some way from clinical application at present.

RELIEF OF PAIN

Pain is a frequent symptom of pancreatic cancer, and may be severe. There should be no hesitation in prescription of adequate pain relief medication, with progression from mild analgesics and non-steroidal anti-inflammatory drugs to opiates if required. Although most patients are in fact pain-free at the time of diagnosis, the majority will have pain sufficiently severe to require morphine during the later stages of their illness. Adequate doses should be prescribed as there are no concerns about drug misuse or addiction in this patient group.

Pain relief may be enhanced by neurolytic procedures. There is considerable evidence from case series that celiac plexus block can provide good pain relief in patients with advanced pancreatic cancer. This may be achieved by a number of techniques depending on the precise siting of the needle tip, and the method of guidance. This includes the anterior approach guided by ultrasound, anterior or posterior CT guidance, and injection at endoscopic ultrasound. The best evidence for effectiveness of this treatment comes from a randomised trial[30] (with a placebo group receiving injection of saline) of celiac plexus block delivered at open bypass surgery for patients with inoperable tumours. This trial showed that patients with pain obtained substantial relief and reduction in morphine use, and that patients without pain had the onset of severe pain and requirement for morphine delayed by a block given at the time of bypass surgery.

Key point 18

- If bypass surgery is performed, celiac plexus block by injection of 50% ethanol should be part of the procedure.

Percutaneous celiac plexus block may be difficult if the anatomy is distorted by tumour invasion, and does depend on appropriate expertise for radiological guidance. An alternative is surgical division of the splanchnic nerves within the chest. This has been shown to be effective in pancreatic cancer patients when done by a transhiatal approach at open operation. Now it is usually offered using a bilateral thoracoscopic approach.[31] This procedure has been reported as giving good pain relief in patients with chronic pancreatitis.[32–34] Currently, a randomised trial is in progress to determine the relative merits of thoracoscopic splanchnicectomy and celiac plexus block (NaTTS Trial).

Painful bony metastases usually respond well to radiotherapy. As noted above, the pain from the primary tumour may improve with gemcitabine treatment, and for patients with continuing severe upper abdominal pain, resistant to other therapies, chemoradiotherapy may offer some benefit.

NUTRITIONAL MEASURES IN PANCREATIC CANCER

Pancreatic cancer is well recognised as a cause of cancer cachexia. A number of factors account for this association, which is only partly due to metabolic effects of the tumour. It is known that the cachexia is associated with an inappropriate enhanced inflammatory response, which promotes catabolism. In addition, patients with pancreatic cancer may have prolonged inadequate intake of nutrients because of abdominal pain, feeling of fullness, duodenal obstruction or opioid-related anorexia. These patients also frequently have impaired pancreatic function, because of obstruction of the pancreatic duct. This often overlooked deficiency can be easily remedied by prescription of regular preprandial pancreatic enzyme supplements. Trial evidence has shown that in patients with pancreatic cancer this will help maintain body weight and will improve quality of life.[35]

Key point 19

- Prescription of pancreatic enzyme supplements should be considered in all patients with inoperable pancreatic cancer.

The difficulties experienced by many patients in maintaining adequate dietary intake can be overcome by the use of dietary supplements. High-energy, high-protein supplements may help to replace inadequate intake. Furthermore, there is evidence that unsaturated fatty acids may help to diminish the immune response and may reverse the process of cachexia.[36,37] In patients with evidence of weight loss, specific treatment with unsaturated fat-rich supplements should be considered.

> **Key point 20**
>
> - Cancer cachexia is multifactorial. Attention should be given to general dietary measures, and enzyme supplements. In patients with weight loss, specific dietary supplements may be helpful.

SURGICAL RESECTION

Pre-operative assessment

Patients with potentially operable tumours should be assessed by a pancreatic surgical team. This will include evaluation of good quality pancreatic imaging, and assessment of the patient's fitness to withstand prolonged anaesthesia and an extensive surgical procedure.

High-quality, cross-sectional images are usually obtained by contrast-enhanced CT with high-dose, rapid infusion contrast, and image acquisition during the arterial and portal phases. Key points in CT assessment include extension of the tumour around the mesenteric or portal vein, and any arterial involvement, as well as careful evaluation for metastases. Extra-abdominal spread without local invasion or liver metastases is extremely rare, and chest CT is not part of the routine protocol.

Almost all pancreatic surgeons are happy to rely on cross-sectional imaging for diagnosis. There are concerns about percutaneous transabdominal biopsy. Although initial reports that suggested a risk of intra-abdominal seeding following needle biopsy have not been confirmed by an increased incidence of intraperitoneal recurrence, there remains the problem of sampling error, particularly when dealing with a small tumour. A biopsy that confirms malignancy may support a decision to resect, but a biopsy showing fibrosis or inflammation only cannot exclude malignancy, and should not prevent resection. If the result of a biopsy is unlikely to affect management, there seems little reason to perform the biopsy.

Recently, with wider availability of endoscopic ultrasound, it is possible to obtain transduodenal biopsies using endoscopic ultrasound guidance. These techniques are in development, but may offer a way of obtaining material for histological examination, by a route that will not compromise subsequent resectional surgery.

> **Key point 21**
>
> - In a patient suspected of having operable pancreatic cancer, transabdominal percutaneous biopsy should be avoided. Surgical resection will be performed on the basis of radiological assessment.

Pancreatic resection

Pancreatic surgery should be confined to specialist centres, and the decision that a patient is or is not operable should be made by the multidisciplinary team in these centres. In this way, resection rates will be appropriate, and the accumulation of expertise and experience is likely to reduce complication and mortality rates. Centralisation of cases also improves the opportunities for training.

Most patients will have a tumour in the head of the pancreas, and the appropriate operation for this is pancreaticoduodenectomy. There is no agreement on the value of preservation or excision of the pylorus. Randomised comparisons show little difference in clinical outcome both in terms of immediate postoperative recovery, the proportion of patients with delayed gastric emptying, or long-term cancer-free survival. The choice between a standard Whipple's, or pylorus preserving procedure can be according to the preference of the surgeon.

There is no evidence to support the routine resection of portal or mesenteric vein, or for doing a total pancreatectomy. Long-term survival rates are no better (and may be worse) after total pancreatectomy, and postoperative complications are greater with these more extended procedures.

However, extended resection to include portal or mesenteric vein, or total pancreatectomy, may be justified in a fit patient in whom the tumour distribution makes this necessary to achieve complete tumour clearance (R0 resection). It must be remembered, however, that venous involvement is a sign of advanced disease, and the results of such procedures are less good than the average.

Lymph node resection

Extended lymph node dissection is theoretically appealing, in that it should remove tissue which is potentially invaded at a microscopic level. However, it has been difficult to demonstrate any survival advantage for extended lymph node dissection, and there is little enthusiasm in the West for the very radical procedures proposed mainly by Japanese authors.

One difficulty with the few randomised trials that have been published is uncertainty about the extent of resection. For this reason, definitions of pancreatic and lymph node dissection were agreed at a consensus meeting held in Castelfranco, Italy.[38] That consensus was unable to recommend strongly the wide-spread adoption of extended lymph node dissection.[39]

A randomised trial in North America found no difference in outcome between standard and extended lymph node dissection.[40] However, the definitions used in that paper were not those agreed at Castelfranco, and it is not clear from the publication that the so called 'extended' group in fact had a radical dissection.

A multicentre Italian study[41] showed no difference overall in survival after pancreaticoduodenectomy with or without a radical lymph node dissection. However, in that study, the subgroup of patients with microscopically involved lymph nodes did show a survival benefit. The experience of that trial also confirmed the suspicion that more extensive dissection was associated with a greater risk of complications.

Key point 22

- Pancreaticoduodenectomy with or without pylorus preservation is the most appropriate procedure for resection of tumours of the pancreatic head.

Key point 23

- Extended resections such as total pancreatectomy or mesenteric/portal vein resection are unnecessary as a routine, but may be appropriate when necessary to achieve R0 resection.

Key point 24

- Extended and radical lymph node dissection may have some advantages but the case is not proven.

CONCLUSIONS

In the management of acute pancreatitis, and pancreatic and peri-ampullary malignancy, there is considerable benefit for specialisation of services. The majority of patients in both groups will be treated at the admitting hospital. They should be under the care of clinicians with an interest in the management of pancreatic disease, because such clinicians are more likely to provide care in accordance with national guidelines.[42] Patients who require surgical treatment or other specialised interventions not available locally should be transferred to a specialist centre where the full range of services and support are available. The UK guidelines sponsored by the British Society of Gastroenterology and other specialist organisations contain clear definitions of the level of service provided by specialist centres. They also have clear standards suitable for audit of the clinical service in local and specialist practice.

Key points for clinical practice

Acute pancreatitis

- The diagnosis of acute pancreatitis is made by a combination of clinical features and elevated plasma lipase levels (or amylase levels if this is not available). In case of diagnostic doubt, urgent CT should be performed.
- Urgent ultrasonography is required for all patients with acute pancreatitis, to determine the presence or absence of stones in the gallbladder.
- Early aggressive fluid replacement and supplemental oxygen, together with analgesia, may prevent or reverse organ failure. All patients should receive these treatments until it is clear they are no longer needed.

(continued on next page)

Key points for clinical practice

Acute pancreatitis (continued)

- Severity stratification should be made in all patients within 48 h of diagnosis. A clear assessment of severity should be recorded in the notes.
- CT may be helpful in identification of patients with local complications, but early CT is unlikely to influence management during the first week (unless antibiotic prophylaxis is being considered).
- Treatment of gallstones to prevent further attacks of pancreatitis should take place during the index admission, or within 2 weeks of discharge.
- Patients with biliary pancreatitis who have one or more organ failures that fail to resolve or improve within 24 h should be offered emergency endoscopic sphincterotomy.
- Enteral nutrition may be given safely during the first week of acute pancreatitis. Parenteral nutrition should not be used during the first 5 days, and until it is evident that the enteral route is insufficient.
- There is currently no consensus on the value of prophylactic antibiotics for patients with pancreatic necrosis. Patients without pancreatic necrosis will not benefit from prophylactic antibiotics.
- Specialist units should be able to provide surgical radiological and endoscopic services whenever required.
- The management of infected pancreatic necrosis is controversial, but there is agreement that aggressive therapy is needed to drain and/or debride all areas of necrosis.
- The identification of infected necrosis is based on contrast-enhanced CT demonstration of hypoperfusion on a scan performed 7–14 days after onset of symptoms, followed by FNA for culture of material from the necrotic areas.

Pancreatic cancer

- If initial ultrasound demonstrates dilated intrahepatic ducts, the patient probably has malignancy. A dilated common bile duct and the absence of gallstones suggest pancreatic cancer even if the pancreas cannot be visualised.
- CT should precede ERCP and stent, in order to confirm the diagnosis, and assist in staging and planning treatment.
- Patients with advanced tumours and obstructive jaundice should have endoscopic plastic stent placement in the first instance. Failure of cannulation, or early stent occlusion may require placement of an expanding metal stent, by the percutaneous route if necessary.

(continued on next page)

Key points for clinical practice

Pancreatic cancer (continued)

- Surgical bypass is only appropriate in patients with a relatively good prognosis. Surgical treatment should include choledochojejunostomy and gastrojejunostomy.
- The accepted chemotherapy treatment for pancreatic cancer is now gemcitabine. Investigation of new agents should use gemcitabine as the standard for comparison.
- If bypass surgery is performed, celiac plexus block by injection of 50% ethanol should be part of the procedure.
- Prescription of pancreatic enzyme supplements should be considered in all patients with inoperable pancreatic cancer.
- Cancer cachexia is multifactorial. Attention should be given to general dietary measures, and enzyme supplements. In patients with weight loss, specific dietary supplements may be helpful.
- In a patient suspected of having operable pancreatic cancer, transabdominal percutaneous biopsy should be avoided. Surgical resection will be performed on the basis of radiological assessment.
- Pancreaticoduodenectomy with or without pylorus preservation is the most appropriate procedure for resection of tumours of the pancreatic head.
- Extended resections such as total pancreatectomy or mesenteric/portal vein resection are unnecessary as a routine, but may be appropriate when necessary to achieve R0 resection.
- Extended and radical lymph node dissection may have some advantages but the case is not proven.

References

1. British Society of Gastroenterology. United Kingdom guidelines for the management of acute pancreatitis. *Gut* 1998; **42 (Suppl 2)**: S1–S13.
2. Dervenis C *et al*. Diagnosis, objective assessment of severity, and management of acute pancreatitis. Santorini Consensus Conference. *Int J Pancreatol* 1999; **25**: 195–210.
3. Toouli J *et al*. Guidelines for the management of acute pancreatitis. *J Gastroenterol Hepatol* 2002; **17 (Suppl)**: S15–S39.
4. British Society of Gastroenterology. UK guidelines for the management of acute pancreatitis: first revision. *Gut* 2005; In press.
5. Dellinger RP *et al*. Surviving Sepsis Campaign guidelines for management of severe sepsis and septic shock. *Crit Care Med* 2004; **32**: 858–873.
6. Bradley III EL. A clinically based classification system for acute pancreatitis. Summary of the International Symposium on Acute Pancreatitis, Atlanta, GA, September 11–13, 1992. *Arch Surg* 1993; **128**: 586–590.
7. Ranson JH *et al*. Prognostic signs and the role of operative management in acute pancreatitis. *Surg Gynecol Obstet* 1974; **139**: 69–81.

8. Ranson JH. Etiological and prognostic factors in human acute pancreatitis: a review. *Am J Gastroenterol* 1982; **77**: 633–638.
9. Blamey SL *et al*. The early identification of patients with gallstone associated pancreatitis using clinical and biochemical factors only. *Ann Surg* 1983; **198**: 574–578.
10. Larvin M, McMahon MJ. APACHE-II score for assessment and monitoring of acute pancreatitis. *Lancet* 1989; **2**: 201–205.
11. Funnell IC, Bornman PC, Weakley SP, Terblanche J, Marks IN. Obesity: an important prognostic factor in acute pancreatitis. *Br J Surg* 1993; **80**: 484–486.
12. Johnson CD, Toh SK, Campbell MJ. Combination of APACHE-II score and an obesity score (APACHE-O) for the prediction of severe acute pancreatitis. *Pancreatology* 2004; **4**: 1–6.
13. Balthazar EJ, Freeny PC, van Sonnenberg E. Imaging and intervention in acute pancreatitis. *Radiology* 1994; **193**: 297–306.
14. Buter A, Imrie CW, Carter CR, Evans S, McKay CJ. Dynamic nature of early organ dysfunction determines outcome in acute pancreatitis. *Br J Surg* 2002; **89**: 298–302.
15. Johnson CD, Abu-Hilal M. Persistent organ failure during the first week as a marker of fatal outcome in acute pancreatitis. *Gut* 2004; **53**: 1340–1344.
16. Cameron DR, Goodman AJ. Delayed cholecystectomy for gallstone pancreatitis: re-admissions and outcomes. *Ann R Coll Surg Engl* 2004; **86**: 358–362.
17. Neoptolemos JP *et al*. A prospective study of ERCP and endoscopic sphincterotomy in the diagnosis and treatment of gallstone acute pancreatitis. A rational and safe approach to management. *Arch Surg* 1986; **121**: 697–702.
18. Fan ST *et al*. Early treatment of acute biliary pancreatitis by endoscopic papillotomy. *N Engl J Med* 1993; **328**: 228–232.
19. Folsch UR, Nitsche R, Ludtke R, Hilgers RA, Creutzfeldt W. Early ERCP and papillotomy compared with conservative treatment for acute biliary pancreatitis. The German Study Group on Acute Biliary Pancreatitis. *N Engl J Med* 1997; **336**: 237–242.
20. Gupta R *et al*. A randomised clinical trial to assess the effect of total enteral and total parenteral nutritional support on metabolic, inflammatory and oxidative markers in patients with predicted severe acute pancreatitis (APACHE II > or =6). *Pancreatology* 2003; **3**: 406–413.
21. Kalfarentzos F, Kehagias J, Mead N, Kokkinis K, Gogos CA. Enteral nutrition is superior to parenteral nutrition in severe acute pancreatitis: results of a randomized prospective trial. *Br J Surg* 1997; **84**: 1665–1669.
22. Windsor AC *et al*. Compared with parenteral nutrition, enteral feeding attenuates the acute phase response and improves disease severity in acute pancreatitis. *Gut* 1998; **42**: 431–435.
23. Powell JJ, Murchison JT, Fearon KC, Ross JA, Siriwardena AK. Randomized controlled trial of the effect of early enteral nutrition on markers of the inflammatory response in predicted severe acute pancreatitis. *Br J Surg* 2000; **87**: 1375–1381.
24. Bassi C, Larvin M, Villatoro E. Antibiotic therapy for prophylaxis against infection of pancreatic necrosis in acute pancreatitis. *Cochrane Database System Rev* 2003; CD002941.
25. Isenmann R *et al*. Prophylactic antibiotic treatment in patients with predicted severe acute pancreatitis: a placebo-controlled, double-blind trial. *Gastroenterology* 2004; **126**: 997–1004.
26. Ashley SW *et al*. Necrotizing pancreatitis: contemporary analysis of 99 consecutive cases. *Ann Surg* 2001; **234**: 572–579.
27. Haycox A, Lombard M, Neoptolemos J, Walley T. Current treatment and optimal patient management in pancreatic cancer. *Aliment Pharmacol Ther* 1998; **12**: 949–964.
28. Burris III HA *et al*. Improvements in survival and clinical benefit with gemcitabine as first-line therapy for patients with advanced pancreas cancer: a randomized trial. *J Clin Oncol* 1997; **15**: 2403–2413.
29. National Institute for Clinical Excellence. *Gemcitabine for Pancreatic Cancer*. London: NICE, 2001.
30. Lillemoe KD *et al*. Chemical splanchnicectomy in patients with unresectable pancreatic cancer. A prospective randomized trial. *Ann Surg* 1993; **217**: 447–455.
31. Le Pimpec BF *et al*. Thoracoscopic splanchnicectomy for control of intractable pain in pancreatic cancer. *Ann Thorac Surg* 1998; **65**: 810–813.

32. Bradley III EL, Reynhout JA, Peer GL. Thoracoscopic splanchnicectomy for 'small duct' chronic pancreatitis: case selection by differential epidural analgesia. *J Gastrointest Surg* 1998; **2**: 88–94.
33. Buscher HC, Jansen JB, van Dongen R, Bleichrodt RP, van Goor H. Long-term results of bilateral thoracoscopic splanchnicectomy in patients with chronic pancreatitis. *Br J Surg* 2002; **89**: 158–162.
34. Ihse I, Zoucas E, Gyllstedt E, Lillo-Gil R, Andren-Sandberg A. Bilateral thoracoscopic splanchnicectomy: effects on pancreatic pain and function. *Ann Surg* 1999; **230**: 785–790.
35. Bruno MJ, Haverkort EB, Tijssen GP, Tytgat GN, van Leeuwen DJ. Placebo controlled trial of enteric coated pancreatin microsphere treatment in patients with unresectable cancer of the pancreatic head region. *Gut* 1998; **42**: 92–96.
36. Barber MD, Ross JA, Voss AC, Tisdale MJ, Fearon KC. The effect of an oral nutritional supplement enriched with fish oil on weight-loss in patients with pancreatic cancer. *Br J Cancer* 1999; **81**: 80–86.
37. Wigmore SJ, Barber MD, Ross JA, Tisdale MJ, Fearon KC. Effect of oral eicosapentaenoic acid on weight loss in patients with pancreatic cancer. *Nutr Cancer* 2000; **36**: 177–184.
38. Pedrazzoli S *et al*. A surgical and pathological based classification of resective treatment of pancreatic cancer. Summary of an international workshop on surgical procedures in pancreatic cancer. *Dig Surg* 1999; **16**: 337–345.
39. Fernandez-Cruz L, Johnson C, Dervenis C. Locoregional dissemination and extended lymphadenectomy in pancreatic cancer. *Dig Surg* 1999; **16**: 313–319.
40. Yeo CJ *et al*. Pancreaticoduodenectomy with or without extended retroperitoneal lymphadenectomy for periampullary adenocarcinoma: comparison of morbidity and mortality and short-term outcome. *Ann Surg* 1999; **229**: 613–622.
41. Pedrazzoli S *et al*. Standard versus extended lymphadenectomy associated with pancreatoduodenectomy in the surgical treatment of adenocarcinoma of the head of the pancreas: a multicenter, prospective, randomized study. Lymphadenectomy Study Group. *Ann Surg* 1998; **228**: 508–517.
42. Aly EA, Milne R, Johnson CD. Non-compliance with national guidelines in the management of acute pancreatitis in the United Kingdom. *Dig Surg* 2002; **19**: 192–198.

Plate X Solid material removed at necrosectomy. Radiological descriptions of necrosis often use terms such as 'fluid infiltrate' or 'fluid collections'. Percutaneous drainage of necrotic areas may release some pus, but the resolution of the infective process usually requires removal of solid material by a surgical approach.

Majid Hashemi

9

Laparoscopic gastric banding for obesity

The first open insertion of the adjustable silicon gastric band in humans was in 1991; the first laparoscopic insertion was in 1993.[1] Rapid popularisation, with a momentum in 1998–1999, was a result of the relative simplicity of the procedure, patient acceptability, low immediate morbidity and parallel advances in laparoscopy. Laparoscopic adjustable gastric banding (LGB or AGB), in turn, has led to increased awareness of bariatric surgical techniques such as gastric bypass and has itself been a catalyst for the investigation and treatment of obesity as a whole.

Despite this, many unknowns dominate current practice: the mechanism of action, the identification of good prognostic indicators, accurate and objective assessment of outcome, the most appropriate and efficient follow-up protocol and the management of late complications and band failures.

LGB AND OTHER PROCEDURES

The body's natural reaction is to defend vigorously against weight loss through compensation in energy intake and expenditure. This is why many attempts at weight loss are ultimately unsuccessful. Surgical manipulation to induce weight loss appears to be more sustainable. The band is a purely restrictive procedure and, as such, bears comparison with vertical banded gastroplasty (VBG). Although studies have shown less early weight loss following LGB compared to VBG,[2] the adjustable band has fewer early complications and appears safer.[3]

The Roux-en-y gastric bypass (RYGBP) and other bypass procedures such as the bilio-pancreatic diversion lead to even greater weight loss but are more complex.[4,5] In a comparison of two of the largest series to date, Biertho *et al.*[6]

Majid Hashemi FRCS
Senior Lecturer/Consultant in Upper Gastrointestinal and Bariatric Surgery, Department of Surgery, Royal Free and University College Medical School, Undergraduate Centre, Whittington Campus, London N19 5NF, UK. E-mail: m.hashemi@ucl.ac.uk

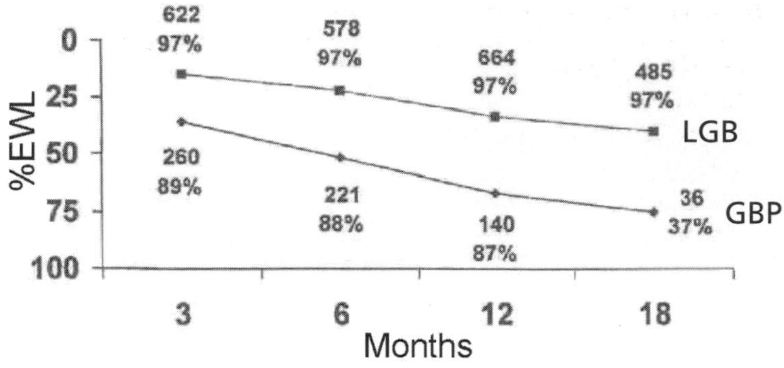

Fig. 1 Comparison of laparoscopic gastric banding and gastric bypass/RYGBP[6]

demonstrated greater weight loss in the GBP group when compared with LGB (Fig. 1). This study was flawed due to the lack of standardisation of most variables and because of disparity between the two populations, the bypasses having been performed on US residents, while the LGBs were placed in Switzerland.

Malabsorption is more common after bypass and deficiencies of vitamin D coupled with calcium malabsorption can lead to osteoporosis, often further accentuated in perimenopausal women. Although weight loss in the first 2 years is slower after LGB than after bypass surgery, mortality is 0.5% for RYGBP but only 0.1% after LGB; the rare deaths that do occur after banding usually result from pulmonary embolus.[5,6]

PATIENT SELECTION

Selection guidelines are based on the proposition that in appropriate patients the benefits gained from surgically assisted weight loss justify the risks and cost of surgery. Selection criteria in the UK have been guided by the National Institute for Clinical Excellence (Table 1) which resemble the NIH guidelines of 1991, now complemented by the European Association for Endoscopic Surgery (EAES) guidelines from December 2004.[7]

The first step in the selection process is to ask if the patient is likely to benefit from weight loss. Is compliance realistic and is the patient fit enough to tolerate the procedure (and any complications that may result)? Is the surgeon, the team (Table 2) and the institution sufficiently experienced and equipped to provide the procedure? As the short-term risks of obesity surgery clearly exceed that of conservative treatment, all patients should have tried other ways of weight loss prior to surgery.

Table 1 Current selection criteria for bariatric surgery

- Age 18–55 years
- BMI 35 kg/m^2 with a co-morbidity or > 40 kg/m^2 or over
- No alcohol or drug dependence
- No delusional or psychotic illness
- Agreement to life-long follow-up

Table 2 The multidisciplinary team

Metabolic physician
Dietician
Psychologist or psychiatrist
Surgeon
Anaesthetist
Physiotherapist
Hospital management

Absolute contra-indications to bariatric surgery are a lack of capacity to comply with a follow-up programme such as in patients with severe cognitive or mental retardation, malignant hyperphagia unresponsive to psychotherapy and pharmacological treatment, and medical conditions such as autoimmune disorders or oesophageal varices.[7]

PATIENT CO-MORBIDITIES

Sufficient evidence is now available that most obesity-related morbidities respond to weight loss. In a recent meta-analysis that included 9 series of LGB, there was complete resolution of diabetes in 76.8% of patients after bariatric procedures overall, with 84% resolving after GBP and 48% after LGB.[5] Even 20% excess weight loss can lead to a halving of diabetic risk, while hypertension, progression and risk of ischaemic heart disease and musculoskeletal pain with limitation of activity are all reduced in severity and prevalence.[8–10] Depression, which is often a consequence of obesity, responds to weight loss and quality of life is improved,[8,9] while there is resolution of sleep apnoea in 87% of affected patients after weight loss.[5,8]

Prediction of outcome remains a major challenge and in an investigation from Adelaide which studied factors that motivated patients to seek surgery, including patients' concerns regarding appearance, embarrassment, medical conditions, health concerns, physical fitness and physical limitation, none were found to correlate with long-term weight loss.[11] Some behavioural patterns predict a better outcome. A past history of success at weight loss is a good sign of motivation and is associated with a greater likelihood of success, while patients who have lost weight in the immediate pre-operative period are more likely to have a better long-term weight loss. Peri-operative psychological counselling and, in particular, identification and treatment of binge eating disorders improves the outcome of surgery[12] while pre-existing depression does not lead to a worse outcome and is not an exclusion criteria.

Other negative predictors, but not exclusion criteria, include, increasing body mass index (BMI), insulin resistance and type II diabetes, and poor physical activity.[5,8,13]

AGE

In selected patients over 55 years of age, LGB seems to be as effective as in younger age groups.[7,14] However, obesity-related morbidities are often well established and less reversible in the older patient, and the benefits of improvement in morbidities are for a shorter period of time. Surgery for adolescents (12–19 years) is controversial: 80% of obese adolescents go on to become obese adults and many of the body image and psychological problems of obesity become established in youth. Although the outcome after LGB in adolescence in terms of weight loss is comparable to that in adults,[15] it is difficult to be sure the patients are fully informed and understand the long-term implications of surgery. The EAES has deferred recommendations on surgery in this group pending further research and surgery in this age group should be limited to patients who have a BMI greater than 40 kg/m^2, have reached musculoskeletal maturity and probably should only be performed by high volume centres.[7]

PROCEDURE SELECTION

Sweet eaters, binge eaters, patients with oesophageal dysmotility, and those who are super-obese (> 50 kg/m^2) may benefit from a bypass procedure. However, despite a common assumption that sweet eating is a contra-indication to LGB, results from two recent series demonstrate that sweet eaters have outcomes as good as other patients after LGB.[16,17] With regard to the super-obese population, outcomes in patients with BMI > 60 kg/m^2 appear to be almost as good as those with lesser degrees of obesity.[18] An Italian multicentre study reported on 239 super-obese patients with a mean BMI of 54 kg/m^2; although the conversion rate was higher and many remained obese with BMI greater than 35 kg/m^2, there was significant reduction of obesity-related morbidities with an excess weight loss of 38.9% at 3 years.[19]

Key point 1

- Adherence to selection guidelines helps to ensure better outcomes. Obesity-related morbidities are improved or reversed following weight loss. Sweet eating and binge eating are not contra-indications to laparoscopic gastric banding but eating disorders require identification and treatment before surgery. Depression responds to weight loss. Super-obesity is not a contra-indication for laparoscopic gastric banding.

SURGICAL TECHNIQUE DEVELOPMENTS

Correct placement of the ports determines the subsequent progress of the operation, taking into account subsequent downward displacement of the abdominal wall mass with the reverse Trendelenberg position (Fig. 2). The band is placed just below the gastro-oesophageal junction. After preparing the angle of His on the left of the gastro-oesophageal junction, the initial dissection is close to the right pillar of the crus, creating a very limited retro-oesophageal tunnel: the lesser sac should not be entered as this increases the likelihood of prolapse of the posterior portion of the stomach. The pars flaccida technique which has superseded the perigastric approach includes the fat and neurovascular bundle of the upper lesser curvature within the band.[1,13,20–23] The greatest obstacle to access to the hiatus is the congested, swollen liver of

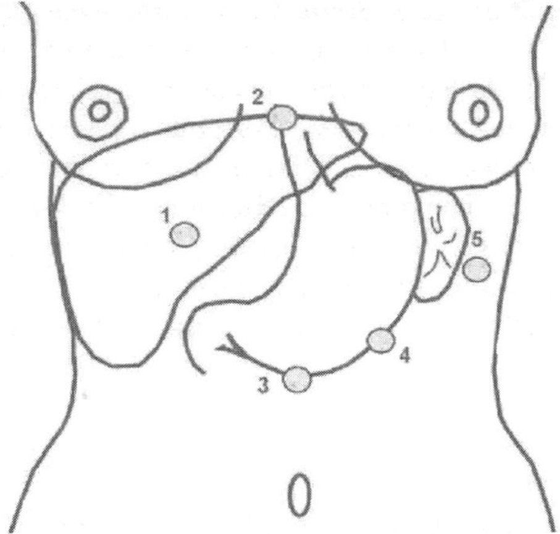

Fig. 2 Position of trocars for LGB: 1, liver retractor; 2, left hand working port; 3, laparoscope; 4, right hand working port (12/15 mm); 5, retraction and working port.

steatosis. A low energy diet or a 'milk' diet in the 2 weeks preceding surgery[24] and avoidance of a 'good-bye party', where patients overeat in anticipation of surgery, may help achieve some shrinkage of liver bulk.

THEORY BEHIND MECHANISM OF ACTION

The varieties of band all observe the same general principles: a soft, flexible, and adjustable balloon or cushion against the stomach, connected by a tube to a reservoir port system which is accessible from outside (Fig. 3). The band

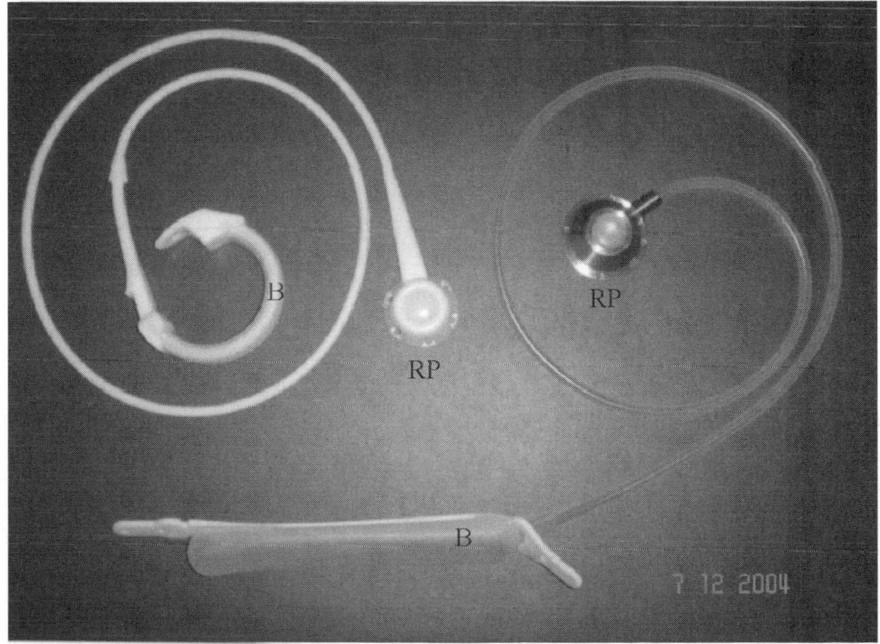

Fig. 3 Two types of commonly used band showing reservoir port (RP), tubing, balloon (B) (SAGB®, Obtech, Ethicon Endo-Surgery and the Lap-Band®, Inamed, USA)

probably acts by inducing satiety. Dixon *et al.*[25] describe an elaborate study during which subjects were given a meal after fasting, with the band deflated in one study arm, and inflated and restrictive in the other. The sensation of fullness and satiety is maintained for the duration of a meal but also for up to 14 h of fasting after a meal in the restricted group. In the unrestricted group, within 2 days of loss of the restrictive effect of the band, there was a cessation of satiety. Gut hormones which drive hunger do not immediately alter after LGB and it is only as a secondary consequence of starvation and alteration of eating behaviour that there is a drop in levels of ghrelin, the hunger-stimulating hormone. Thus, a new eating habit is adopted.

The pouch size may be a determinant of the degree of satiety, and band inflation pressures which can be estimated by manometry through the reservoir port may be a more accurate guide to efficacy than band volume.[26] Wider, softer bands may lessen the risk of slippage and high band-pressures are thought to be one of the factors leading to erosion.

AFTERCARE

Patients eat immediately upon recovery from the anaesthetic. Super-obese patients, particularly those of android type (male pattern) obesity who have a very large amount of perigastric fat may suffer from dysphagia immediately after surgery. Provided there is no prolapse of the stomach above the band, nor any suspicion of incarceration, these patients are able to tolerate oral fluids after 24–48 h of support with intravenous fluid maintenance. ITU admission following bariatric procedures is rare but should ideally be planned. Those most likely to require admission are older, heavier patients, those undergoing re-do procedures and those suffering from ventilation-dependant sleep apnoea.[27] De Waele *et al.*[28] report on the feasibility of day-case LGB, although with an average of 9 h from the end of surgery to discharge this may not be practical in many UK units.

FOLLOW-UP

Adjustability is a key feature of the band systems and knowing when and how much to adjust requires careful judgement. A properly placed and adjusted band produces prolonged satiety after a small meal. Depending on the type of band, an injection of between 5–9 ml is the maximum tolerated and adjustments are easily carried out in the out-patient department without the routine use of local anaesthetic or video fluoroscopy. This represents a considerable out-patient workload. In a series from Switzerland, a median number of 8 out-patient consultations, including 1 deflating and 4 filling adjustments, were required in the first year of follow-up.[29] Adoption of a single 'bolus' fill at 4 weeks with a follow-up at 5 months may be a cost-saving strategy in reducing out-patient attendances.[30]

Dynamic radio-isotope scintigraphy using [^{99m}Tc]-labelled yoghurt for gastric band adjustment provides real-time and representative imaging of the degree of hold up at the band and leads to a significant reduction of need for subsequent re-adjustments.[31] The EAES has recommended a range of follow-up intervals with a higher intensity one: 1, 2, 3, 4, 6, 8, 10, 12, 15, 18, 21, 24, then 6 monthly thereafter and a low intensity programme of minimum frequency: 1, 3, 6, 12, 24 monthly.[7]

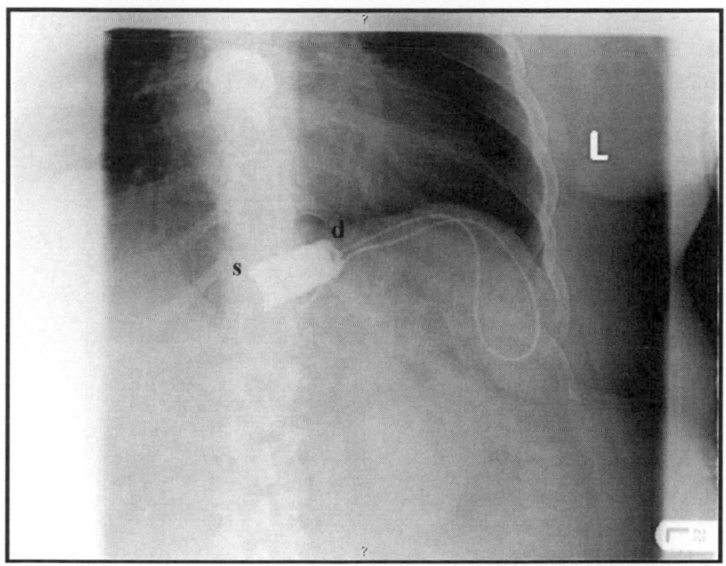

Fig. 4 Band position. Plain radiograph showing correct oblique position of band, with spine (s) and diaphragm (d) landmarks at either 'end'.

Cholelithiasis and its sequelae are associated with obesity, this risk increasing with any period of rapid weight loss.[32] Prophylactic cholecystectomy, although commonly performed during bypass procedures, has no place in the asymptomatic patient undergoing LGB but treatment with ursodeoxycholic acid for 6 months can help reduce the risk of gallstone formation.[33]

IMAGING

Plain radiography in the antero-posterior position provides sufficient information on the placement of the band (Fig. 4). A correctly positioned band lies at an oblique angle with one tip near the spine and the other near the diaphragm. Movement of the band away from either of these points, with a downward and lateral displacement may indicate slippage or erosion.[34] Barium swallow after band inflation should show an oesophageal 'vestibule' but no gastric pouch (Fig. 5). It is relatively simple to measure the pouch size in an antero-posterior projection provided the diameter of the band is known and the projection taken into account, and this can help determine the volume needed for band adjustments: narrowing of the oesophageal outlet, oesophageal dilatation or atony, reflux, or pouch dilatation with insufficient emptying are all indications for removing fluid from the band system. An oesophageal outlet of over 8 mm or immediate passage of barium with a single peristaltic wave, suggest the need for filling.[34,35]

REFLUX AND OESOPHAGEAL MOTILITY

Motility disorders are detected in as many as 30% of cases by pre-operative manometry but nearly all are sub-clinical and routine testing is not indicated. Achalasia is a contra-indication to band placement and, if discovered

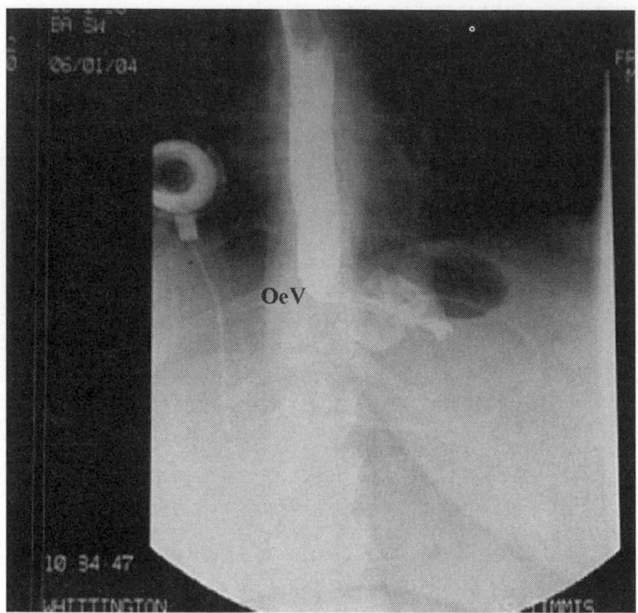

Fig. 5 Satisfactory barium swallow after initial band inflation, demonstrating central concentric narrowing of oesophageal outlet, with an oesophageal vestibule (OeV) and no gastric pouch.

postoperatively, necessitates prompt removal of the band. Secondary achalasia resulting from over-inflation of the band and excessive restriction of the outlet of the oesophagus responds to deflation of the band. Gross dilatation of the oesophagus can also be exacerbated by over-eating and is sometimes seen in association with pouch dilatation; deflating the band will allow return to normal calibre with recovery of peristaltic function.[16] The band is placed just below the oesophago-gastric junction and not surprisingly increases the resting lower oesophageal sphincter pressure and decreases sphincter relaxation.[36] There is a decrease in the acid exposure of the distal oesophagus and a lowered DeMeester score when compared to pre-operative values,[36] although reflux symptoms may not always improve after LGB.[37] Oesophagitis that occurs after band placement is often due to stasis in the oesophagus associated with slower clearance. Hiatus hernia is not a contra-indication to LGB and patients with a hiatus hernia can have a crural repair at the same time as the LGB procedure.[38]

OUTCOME

When considering efficacy, one should consider not only weight loss but also the effects on co-morbidities and quality of life of the patients.[8,39] Diabetes, insulin resistance and sensitivity are sufficiently influenced by weight loss to allow monitoring of progress. Fat mass which can be calculated from bio-impedance assessment has a linear relationship with mortality and is probably a more accurate, though harder to gauge, outcome measure. Abdominal girth and waist/hip ratio give an indication of the fat distribution and are relevant with respect to risks of co-morbidities.[40] A high waist/hip ratio or android-pattern obesity is associated with a greater severity of the components of

Table 3 Results of laparoscopic gastric banding (LGB)

First author	*n*	Mean BMI pre	Mean BMI post	% EWL at 3 yrs	Mean f/u months	% pouch dilatation slippage or malpositioning	% erosion	% re-op
Dargent[16]	500	43	30 at 5 yrs	57	21	8.8	1.8	12.7
Favretti[23]	830	46	36	–	–	2.7	0.5	13.3
Forsell[37]	326	44	30	68	28	–	4.6	7
Mittermair[45]	454	47	33	72	30	2	3.1	7.9
		median	median					
Miller[42]	158	44	28	–	28	1.3	0.6	7
Zehetner[10]	190	45	36	52	39	2.6	2.1	7.4
Ceelen[21]	625	40	32	47	19.5	5.6	–	
		median	median		median			1.6
Zinzindohoue[13]	500	44	31.9	55	13	8.5	-	10.4

EWL, excess weight loss
re-op, re-operation
f/u, follow-up

metabolic syndrome, namely ischaemic heart disease, hypertension, diabetes, and dyslipidaemia and this is linked to larger adipocytes, greater insulin resistance and higher circulating free fatty acid levels. At present, the simplest and commonest expression of outcome is as a percentage change in total weight or BMI, and percentage of excess weight that is lost (excess weight loss). Outcomes of LGB from several large series are shown in Table 3.

SURGICAL FAILURE

In an established programme where the practitioners are beyond the early learning curve, failure of the patient to lose weight remains the greatest source of disappointment. A patient can be regarded as failed if they have lost less than 30% excess weight loss or still have a BMI greater than 35 kg/m^2. The time cut-off for declaring a failure is arbitrary but since weight loss is underway by 1 year and established by 15 months to 2 years, the patient's status at 24 months gives a good indication of outcome. An algorithm for an approach to this problem is given in Figure 6. However, even an excess weight loss of 20% can lead to a benefit and reduction of co-morbidity.[8–10]

It is often retrospectively that patients who have failed are discovered to have eating disorders that were not detected by pre-operative psychological screening.[13] In some series, these failures are converted to bypass procedures and these authors tend to support tailoring the procedure based on eating habits.

COMPLICATIONS

There is a steep learning curve for any bariatric procedure and DeMaria[41] reported a 72% dysphagia and 41% removal rate in a small study of 37 patients. The European experience has been more encouraging and although a 30% re-operation was seen in the first 50 patients in some early series,[10,42] this

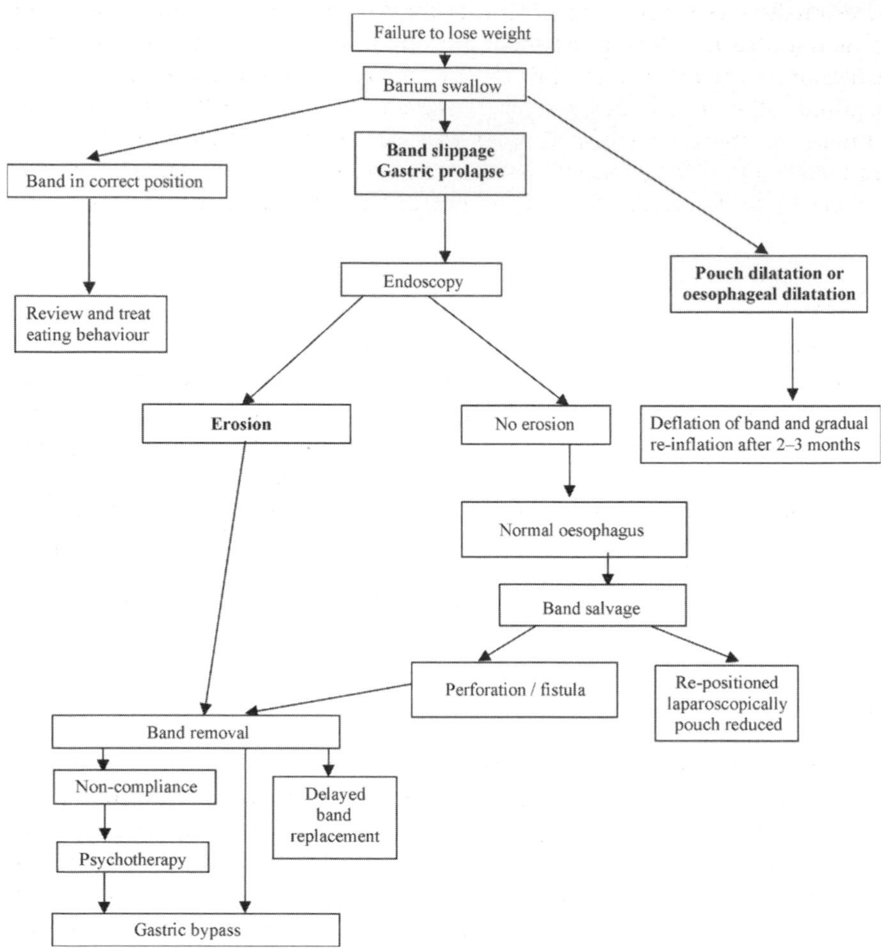

Fig. 6 The management of band failure[10,16,47]

now appears to be historical with re-operation rates of 7–12% (Table 3).[13,16,21]

Pulmonary embolus remains the most frequent cause of death after bariatric surgery.[43] The pro-thrombotic tendency of obesity, stasis and venous dilatation in the leg veins associated with pneumoperitoneum and the reverse Trendelenberg position all contribute to the risk of deep venous thrombosis. Compression boots and stockings in combination with correctly dosed heparin are essential.

EROSION OR MIGRATION

Erosion of the band into the oesophagus or stomach occurs in 0–4.6% of cases.[13,23,37,44,45] Early erosion is often associated with an oesophageal or gastric perforation undetected at the time of surgery and can present with peritonitis requiring urgent removal of the band by laparoscopy or laparotomy. More commonly, erosion presents late with failure to lose weight, or pain, and occasionally dysphagia. The diagnosis can be confirmed at endoscopy and sometimes treated during the same procedure by endoscopic band retrieval. Adhesions may make this difficult and usually a laparoscopic approach is required: after removal of the band, the gastric wall can be repaired with sutures and placement of a drain allows conservative management of any residual fistula. Tubing infection and port infection are often related to erosion and gastric perforations and their frequency falls with greater experience.[21,23]

POUCH DILATATION

An interruption to progress along the weight loss curve is usually the first sign of pouch dilatation. The pouch of stomach above the band expands in volume to form a reservoir and the patient loses the restrictive effect of the band. Once again, however, the complex interplay between eating behaviours and mechanical consequences is evident with past or current binge eating and emotionally triggered eating behaviours likelier in those with dilatations.[13] In a series of 157 LGB, 5 patients had pouch dilatations and on psychological assessment they all had binge eating behaviour.[46] Resumption of bulky foods and inflating the band too soon after surgery (within the first 2 weeks) may contribute to the development of a pouch.[47]

BAND SLIPPAGE

Band slippage, with prolapse of the stomach upwards through the band, is probably exacerbated by overeating and vomiting as well as being influenced by mechanical characteristics of the band itself. It is more likely if the band is too tight or inflated before 4 weeks postoperatively. In about 90% of patients with slippage, the presentation is with new onset reflux regurgitation and dysphagia.[21,47] Modifications of surgical technique can reduce the rate of slippage: in a series of 500 patients the perigastric approach was associated with a slippage rate in 8.5% of cases, detected at a median of 13 months, and after adopting the pars flaccida technique there were none.[13] Anterior gastro-gastric sutures reduce the risk of anterior prolapse and limiting the posterior dissection to avoid breaching and entering the lesser sac limits any shifts and movements posterior. Placement of additional sutures between the lesser curve of the stomach and the right pillar of the crus, beneath the band, may help prevent downward displacement.

Reservoir port complications, usually due to displacement, are surprisingly common, occurring in up to 11% of patients,[23] although most can be treated under local anaesthetic.[13,47]

BAND LEAKAGE

Band leakage is rarer with experience and is probably due to instrumental injury to the balloon and tubing. Suspicion of a leaking balloon is raised by failure to lose weight or the lack of any hold up of barium on a swallow despite an apparent correctly positioned band. In a series of 566 patients, Mitterrmair *et al.*[48] were able to confirm all of their 25 leakages using [^{99m}Tc]-colloid

> **Key point 2**
>
> - Close and structured follow-up is essential to identify non-compliance and late complications. Most reservoir port complications can be dealt with under local anaesthetic. The significant complications of band slippage and pouch distension occur late, often after the first year.

RE-DO AND REPLACEMENT

Most forms of re-intervention can be completed laparoscopically. A prolapse or slippage can be corrected with local re-adjustment, and the adhesions may actually help support the corrected position.[49] Balloon leakage and damage requires a replacement as do most cases of erosions. The replacement can be inserted at the same operation and does not have to be staged at an interval unless there is evidence of on-going contamination.[16] Some favour LGB for all re-do procedures, even in patients whose primary procedure was a VBG, and report a weight loss after replacement and re-positioning comparable to that achieved after a primary LGB.[17] The decision to convert to a RYGBP is harder: if there is failure in the face of an unequivocally correctly positioned and functioning band, this may well be due to abnormal eating patterns, unmasked during the follow-up of the first procedure, and a conversion RYGBP after psychotherapy may achieve better results.

> **Key point 3**
>
> - Treatment of complications requires a multidisciplinary team. Laparoscopic gastric banding in a re-do setting seems to be efficacious with a low morbidity.

CONCLUSIONS

LGB can be carried out in about 1 h, has a mortality of about 0.1% and can be performed in the ambulatory setting. The early efficacy and safety of LGB are now well established. Follow-up data are very limited and with most late complications occurring after the first year, longer term results are essential to confirm its durability.

> **Key points for clinical practice**
>
> - Adherence to selection guidelines helps to ensure better outcomes. Obesity-related morbidities are improved or reversed following weight loss. Sweet eating and binge eating are not contra-indications to laparoscopic gastric banding but eating disorders require identification and treatment before surgery. Depression responds to weight loss. Super-obesity is not a contra-indication for laparoscopic gastric banding.

> **Key points for clinical practice** (continued)
>
> - Close and structured follow-up is essential to identify non-compliance and late complications. Most reservoir port complications can be dealt with under local anaesthetic . The significant complications of band slippage and pouch distension occur late, often after the first year.
> - Treatment of complications requires a multidisciplinary team. Laparoscopic gastric banding in a re-do setting seems to be efficacious with a low morbidity.

References

1. Belachew M *et al*. Laparoscopic placement of adjustable silicone gastric band in the treatment of morbid obesity: how to do it. *Obes Surg* 1995; **5**: 66–70.
2. Morino M, Toppino M, Bonnet G, del Genio G. Laparoscopic adjustable silicone gastric banding versus vertical banded gastroplasty in morbidly obese patients: a prospective randomized controlled clinical trial. *Ann Surg* 2003; **238**: 835–841.
3. Lee WJ, Wang W, Huang MT. Laparoscopic adjustable silicone gastric banding versus vertical banded gastroplasty in morbidly obese patients. *Ann Surg* 2004; **240**: 391–392.
4. Weber M *et al*. Laparoscopic gastric bypass is superior to laparoscopic gastric banding for treatment of morbid obesity. *Ann Surg* 2004; **240**: 975–983.
5. Buchwald H *et al*. Bariatric surgery: a systematic review and meta-analysis. *JAMA* 2004; **292**: 1724–1737.
6. Biertho L *et al*. Laparoscopic gastric bypass versus laparoscopic adjustable gastric banding: a comparative study of 1,200 cases. *J Am Coll Surg* 2003; **197**: 536–544.
7. Sauerland S *et al*. Obesity surgery: evidence-based guidelines of the European Association for Endoscopic Surgery (EAES). *Surg Endosc* 2005; In press.
8. O'Brien PE, Dixon JB. Lap-band: outcomes and results. *J Laparoendosc Adv Surg Tech A* 2003; **13**: 265–270.
9. Torgerson JS, Sjostrom L. The Swedish Obese Subjects (SOS) study – rationale and results. *Int J Obes Relat Metab Disord* 2001; **25 (Suppl 1)**: S2–S4.
10. Zehetner J, Holzinger F, Triaca H, Klaiber C. A 6-year experience with the Swedish adjustable gastric band. Prospective long-term audit of laparoscopic gastric banding. *Surg Endosc* 2005; In press.
11. Libeton M, Dixon JB, Laurie C, O'Brien PE. Patient motivation for bariatric surgery: characteristics and impact on outcomes. *Obes Surg* 2004; **14**: 392–398.
12. Larsen JK *et al*. Binge eating and its relationship to outcome after laparoscopic adjustable gastric banding. *Obes Surg* 2004; **14**: 1111–1117.
13. Zinzindohoue F *et al*. Laparoscopic gastric banding: a minimally invasive surgical treatment for morbid obesity: prospective study of 500 consecutive patients. *Ann Surg* 2003; **237**: 1–9.
14. Silechia G, Greco F, Perrota N *et al*. Laparoscopic gastric banding in patients over 55 years. Abstract presented at the *9th Congress of the International Federation for the Surgery of Obesity* (IFSO), *Obes Surg* 2004; May (Suppl).
15. Dolan K, Fielding G. A comparison of laparoscopic adjustable gastric banding in adolescents and adults. *Surg Endosc* 2004; **18**: 45–47.
16. Dargent J. Surgical treatment of morbid obesity by adjustable gastric band: the case for a conservative strategy in the case of failure – a 9-year series. *Obes Surg* 2004; **14**: 986–990.
17. Dixon JB, O'Brien PE. Selecting the optimal patient for LAP-BAND placement. *Am J Surg* 2002; **184**: 17S–20S.
18. Fielding GA. Laparoscopic adjustable gastric banding for massive superobesity (> 60 body mass index kg/m^2). *Surg Endosc* 2003; **17**: 1541–1545.

19. Angrisani L *et al*. Results of the Italian multicenter study on 239 super-obese patients treated by adjustable gastric banding. *Obes Surg* 2002; **12**: 846–850.
20. Belachew M, Zimmermann JM. Evolution of a paradigm for laparoscopic adjustable gastric banding. *Am J Surg* 2002; **184**: 21S–25S.
21. Ceelen W *et al*. Surgical treatment of severe obesity with a low-pressure adjustable gastric band: experimental data and clinical results in 625 patients. *Ann Surg* 2003; **237**: 10–16.
22. Ren CJ, Fielding GA. Laparoscopic adjustable gastric banding: surgical technique. *J Laparoendosc Adv Surg Tech A* 2003; **13**: 257–263.
23. Favretti F *et al*. Laparoscopic banding: selection and technique in 830 patients. *Obes Surg* 2002; **12**: 385–390.
24. Fris RJ. Preoperative low energy diet diminishes liver size. *Obes Surg* 2004; **14**: 1165–1170.
25. Dixon AF, Dixon JB, O'Brien PE. Laparoscopic adjustable gastric banding induces prolonged satiety: a randomised blind crossover study. *J Clin Endocrinol Metab* 2004; **90**: 813–9.
26. Fried M, Lechner W, Kormanova K. Physical principles of available adjustable gastric bands: how they work. *Obes Surg* 2004; **14**: 1118–1122.
27. Helling TS, Willoughby TL, Maxfield DM, Ryan P. Determinants of the need for intensive care and prolonged mechanical ventilation in patients undergoing bariatric surgery. *Obes Surg* 2004; **14**: 1036–1041.
28. De Waele B, Lauwers M, Van Nieuwenhove Y, Delvaux G. Outpatient laparoscopic gastric banding: initial experience. *Obes Surg* 2004; **14**: 1108–1110.
29. Hauri P *et al*. Treatment of morbid obesity with the Swedish adjustable gastric band (SAGB): complication rate during a 12-month follow-up period. *Surgery* 2000; **127**: 484–488.
30. Kirchmayr W *et al*. Adjustable gastric banding: assessment of safety and efficacy of bolus-filling during follow-up. *Obes Surg* 2004; **14**: 387–391.
31. Susmallian S, Ezri T, Elis M, Charuzi I. Access-port complications after laparoscopic gastric banding. *Obes Surg* 2003; **13**: 128–131.
32. Torgerson JS, Lindroos AK, Naslund I, Peltonen M. Gallstones, gallbladder disease, and pancreatitis: cross-sectional and 2-year data from the Swedish Obese Subjects (SOS) and SOS reference studies. *Am J Gastroenterol* 2003; **98**: 1032–1041.
33. Miller K, Hell E, Lang B, Lengauer E. Gallstone formation prophylaxis after gastric restrictive procedures for weight loss: a randomized double-blind placebo-controlled trial. *Ann Surg* 2003; **238**: 697–702.
34. Pomerri F, De Marchi F, Barbiero G, Di Maggio A, Zavarella C. Radiology for laparoscopic adjustable gastric banding: a simplified follow-up examination method. *Obes Surg* 2003; **13**: 901–908.
35. Favretti F, O'Brien PE, Dixon JB. Patient management after LAP-BAND placement. *Am J Surg* 2002; **184**: 38S–41S.
36. Weiss HG *et al*. Adjustable gastric and esophagogastric banding: a randomized clinical trial. *Obes Surg* 2002; **12**: 573–578.
37. Forsell P, Hallerback B, Glise H, Hellers G. Complications following Swedish adjustable gastric banding: a long-term follow-up. *Obes Surg* 1999; **9**: 11–16.
38. Dolan K, Finch R, Fielding G. Laparoscopic gastric banding and crural repair in the obese patient with a hiatal hernia. *Obes Surg* 2003; **13**: 772–775.
39. Tolonen P, Victorzon M. Quality of life following laparoscopic adjustable gastric banding – the Swedish band and the Moorehead-Ardelt questionnaire. *Obes Surg* 2003; **13**: 424–426.
40. Ballantyne GH. Measuring outcomes following bariatric surgery: weight loss parameters, improvement in co-morbid conditions, change in quality of life and patient satisfaction. *Obes Surg* 2003; **13**: 954–964.
41. DeMaria EJ. Laparoscopic adjustable silicone gastric banding: complications. *J Laparoendosc Adv Surg Tech A* 2003; **13**: 271–277.
42. Miller K, Hell E. Laparoscopic adjustable gastric banding: a prospective 4-year follow-up study. *Obes Surg* 1999; **9**: 183–187.
43. Melinek J, Livingston E, Cortina G, Fishbein MC. Autopsy findings following gastric bypass surgery for morbid obesity. *Arch Pathol Lab Med* 2002; **126**: 1091–1095.

44. Ceelen WP, Cardon A, Pattyn P. Gastric banding for clinically severe obesity: results with the Swedish band. *Surg Technol Int* 2004; **12**: 103–109.
45. Mittermair RP, Weiss H, Nehoda H, Kirchmayr W, Aigner F. Laparoscopic Swedish adjustable gastric banding: 6-year follow-up and comparison to other laparoscopic bariatric procedures. *Obes Surg* 2003; **13**: 412–417.
46. Poole N *et al*. Pouch dilatation following laparoscopic adjustable gastric banding: psychobehavioral factors (can psychiatrists predict pouch dilatation?). *Obes Surg* 2004; **14**: 798–801.
47. Keidar A, Szold A, Carmon E, Blanc A, Abu-Abeid S. Band slippage after laparoscopic adjustable gastric banding: etiology and treatment. *Surg Endosc* 2005; In press.
48. Mittermair RP *et al*. Band leakage after laparoscopic adjustable gastric banding. *Obes Surg* 2003; **13**: 913–917.
49. Vertruyen M. Repositioning the Lap-Band for proximal pouch dilatation. *Obes Surg* 2003; **13**: 285–288.

Dinesh Singhal Orf R.C. Busch
Willem A. Bemelman Dirk J. Gouma

10

Diagnostic laparoscopy in staging gastrointestinal malignancies

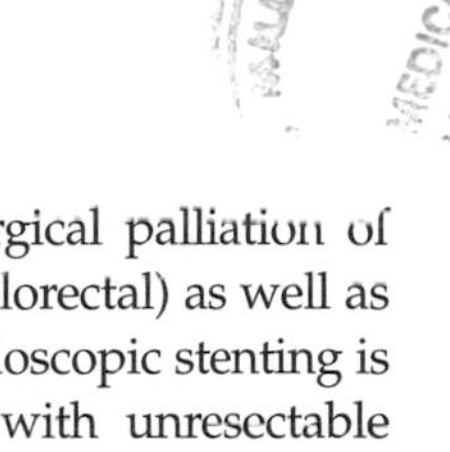

Recent studies demonstrate increasing feasibility for non-surgical palliation of unresectable gastrointestinal (GI) cancers (oesophageal and colorectal) as well as gastric outlet obstruction due to peri-ampullary cancers.[1–4] Endoscopic stenting is currently the preferred modality for palliation of patients with unresectable malignant biliary obstruction on pre-operative staging.[5,6] Adequate pre-operative staging is, therefore, of increasing importance.

Diagnostic laparoscopy was introduced as the final staging investigation in GI cancer patients who do not have advanced disease after radiological staging and therefore seem candidates for surgical resection. The aim of diagnostic laparoscopy is to detect peritoneal, superficial liver or lymph node metastases and locally advanced disease that may be missed on radiological staging and thus could avoid a non-therapeutic laparotomy.[7,8] The prerequisite for the use of laparoscopic staging is the availability, as well as the acceptance, of non-operative palliative treatment for unresectable tumours.

Early data showed substantial benefit for laparoscopic staging in several GI cancers. However, more recent data on diagnostic laparoscopy are disappointing.

Dinesh Singhal MS, DNB
Consultant, Department of Surgical Gastroenterology, Max Healthcare Group of Hospitals, Panchsteel, Patarganj and Saket, New Delhi, India

Orf R.C. Busch MD
Academic Medical Center, Department of Surgery, Meibergdreef 9, 1105 AZ Amsterdam, The Netherlands

Willem A. Bemelman MD
Academic Medical Center, Department of Surgery, Meibergdreef 9, 1105 AZ Amsterdam, The Netherlands

Dirk J. Gouma MD
Professor, Academic Medical Center, Department of Surgery, Meibergdreef 9, 1105 AZ Amsterdam, The Netherlands E-mail: d.j.gouma@amc.uva.nl (for correspondence)

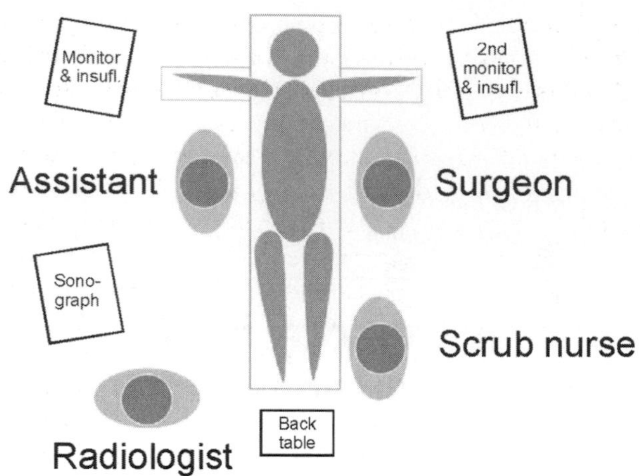

Fig. 1 Organisation of the operating room for diagnostic laparoscopy.

The introduction of helical CT scan and MRI are important factors in the refinement of the established indications for diagnostic laparoscopy.[9] In addition, the long-term benefit of non-surgical palliation for peri-ampullary cancers has recently been questioned.[10]

This review summarises the current role of diagnostic laparoscopy in GI cancers.

TECHNICAL ASPECTS

Diagnostic laparoscopy involves a laparoscopic evaluation of the abdominal cavity for metastatic disease. The technical details of the procedure have been previously described.[11–13] The organisation of the operation room, placement of ports and the conduct of the procedure are shown in Figures 1 and 2. Briefly, a CO_2 pneumoperitoneum is created by an 'open' technique or a Verress needle and using three 10 or 11 mm ports (umbilical, left and right subcostal), the

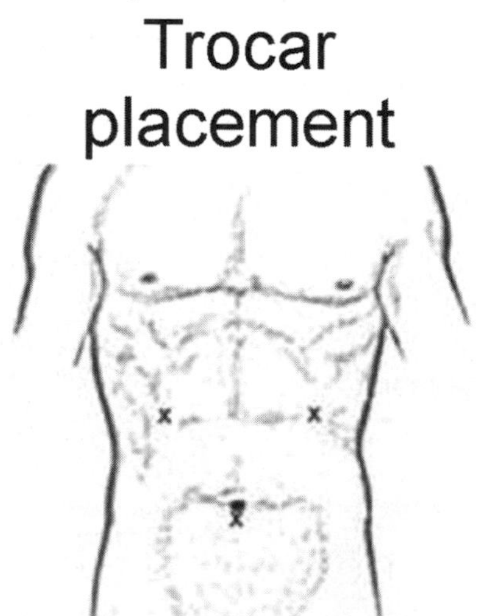

Fig. 2 Placement of ports for diagnostic laparoscopy of GI cancers.

abdomen is explored and biopsy samples taken from all suspicious lesions that would preclude resection. If no suspicious lesions are found, laparoscopic ultrasound (LUS) is performed using a 7.5 MHz probe to detect liver or lymph node metastases. Invasion into the neighbouring major vascular structures is subsequently assessed. However, after the introduction of thin slice (2 mm) helical CT scan, only 3% of patients with peri-ampullary tumours are shown to have additional lesions at LUS. Thus, a more selective use of LUS may be indicated in the staging of GI tumours.

Peritoneal cytology has also been used frequently. A study from the Amsterdam Medical Center revealed that in only 3% (7/236) of patients with peri-ampullary cancers did the peritoneal lavage show malignant cells. Also, in the entire patient population (n = 449), additional information was obtained in only 6 patients (1.3%). There was a relationship between positive cytology and obvious advanced disease shown by diagnostic laparoscopy. On multivariate analysis, survival was not affected by the findings on peritoneal lavage but by metastatic or local advanced disease.[13] In a recent experimental model, intraperitoneally applied 5-aminolevulinic acid resulted in an increased detection of occult peritoneal metastases involving colonic and ovarian carcinomatosis.[14,15]

SCORING SYSTEMS

The benefit of diagnostic laparoscopy has been reported in many different ways, including: (i) detection of additional new findings; (ii) a change of the diagnosis and/or stage, change in treatment strategy (bypass instead of resection); or (iii) avoidance of unnecessary laparotomy (detection of metastases followed by non-surgical palliation). Besides these end-points, the success rate of diagnostic laparoscopy also depends on several other factors:

1. Patient related factors – presence of intra-abdominal adhesions, obesity.
2. Tumour-related factors:

   Location – pancreatic tumours (head, body and tail) are more likely to be unresectable as compared to ampullary tumours.[16–18]

   Pre-laparoscopic stage – advanced tumours are more likely to have a higher yield at laparoscopy.

   Surgical-related factors – the use of LUS and surgical skill to detect metastases, *e.g.* to explore the lesser sac or coeliac nodes and take biopsies.

   Philosophy – to accept lesions as being metastatic without histological conformation.

3. The place of diagnostic laparoscopy in the diagnostic algorithm as well as the quality of pre-operative imaging – diagnostic laparoscopy is usually performed as the final staging investigation. The yield is, therefore, inversely related to the quality of pre-laparoscopy imaging techniques.

COMPLICATIONS

Diagnostic laparoscopy has been shown to be a safe procedure with a complication rate of 0.15–3% and a mortality of 0.05%.[19] The most dangerous part of the procedure is the introduction of the Verress needle or the first trocar. The introduction of the first trocar by an 'open' method increases the safety of the procedure especially in patients with adhesions.[20] A randomised trial at our institution demonstrated that an open technique can be performed safely without being more time consuming than the closed technique.[21]

The incidence of major vascular injuries during laparoscopy is extremely low (0.001–0.005%) but they constitute the single most common (15%) cause of mortality from the procedure.[22] In a recent review, the incidence of bowel perforation due to laparoscopic surgery was reported to be 0.22% with a mortality of 3.6%.[23]

Of the late complications, port site metastases have been discussed extensively. The incidence of this complication ranges between 0.8–2% but it occurs mostly in patients with advanced disease, generally with peritoneal metastases.[24,25] Careful tissue handling and protection of the port sites for the delivery of tissue specimens may avoid this complication.

TUMOURS OF THE OESOPHAGUS AND GASTRO-OESOPHAGEAL JUNCTION

An effective palliation for unresectable oesophageal cancer is available, *e.g.* endoscopic stenting or radiotherapy.[1] Diagnostic laparoscopy could prevent a 'non-therapeutic' laparotomy in patients with metastatic oesophageal cancer. Recent studies are summarised in Table 1.

A substantial benefit ranging between 9–25% has been shown in patients with distal oesophageal adenocarcinoma and tumours of the gastro-oesophageal junction. In an early study from our institution, only 6% patients with oesophageal carcinoma benefited from diagnostic laparoscopy compared to 20% in a later study.[24,26] This is mainly due to a change in the indication for diagnostic laparoscopy and an increase of gastro-oesophageal junction tumours in this study. The yield of diagnostic laparoscopy in patients with (squamous cell) carcinoma of the middle and the upper part of the oesophagus is too limited (3–9%) to justify its routine use.[26]

Key point 1

- Diagnostic laparoscopy is indicated only for staging of tumours of the gastro-oesophageal junction and cardia. The benefit for (squamous cell) carcinoma in the thoracic oesophagus is limited.

GASTRIC CANCER

Patients who might benefit from diagnostic laparoscopy in gastric cancer are fairly limited. Most patients will present with bleeding and/or obstruction and a resection (in particular a subtotal gastrectomy) is generally accepted as palliative treatment. The mortality is currently around 2–4%. There might be an indication for patients without severe bleeding/obstruction and with advanced T4 tumours with invasion of the pancreas or other structures (a relative contra-indication to an extensive palliative procedure).

Table 1 Diagnostic laparoscopy for carcinoma of oesophagus and gastro-oesophageal junction

	Adeno-carcinoma		Squamous cell carcinoma		
Study	*n*	Upstaged *n* (%)/laparotomy avoided	*n*	Upstaged *n*(%)	Remarks
Romijn *et al.*[48]	25	1 (4)	15	0	Additional lesions detected at LUS in 2 patients in each group but could not be biopsied. Metastases detected in 20% of the patients with lesions at the cardia
Bemelman *et al.*[49]	18[a]	2 (11)	38[b]	1 (3)[b] 2 (6)	Diagnostic laparoscopy for middle and lower oesophageal tumours not recommended
Van Dijkum *et al.*[24]	35[a]	8(20)	–	–	Laparoscopy beneficial in gastro-oesophageal junction tumours
Luketich *et al.*[50]	48	–	5	–	7 (15%) of patients had tumour up-staged
Smith *et al.*[51]	36	9 (25)	5	1	LUS led to the up-staging of 33% patients
Hulscher *et al.*[52]	48[c]	11(23)	–	–	Pre-operative staging by abdominal ultrasound and EUS. LUS led to up staging in 33% patients
Clements *et al.*[53]	45[a]	4 (9)	22	2 (9)	–

[a]Gastro-oesophageal junction tumours; [b]middle and lower third/oesophageal tumours; [c]carcinoma of gastric cardia.

In a few centres, patients with advanced disease are candidates for (pre-operative) chemo-radiotherapy and diagnostic laparoscopy might be used to confirm the staging obtained by non-invasive radiological techniques such as CT scan or EUS.

The main limitations of EUS are that it cannot adequately evaluate metastases to the (right lobe of) the liver and the lymph nodes along the celiac axis. Diagnostic laparoscopy with LUS compliments EUS for the evaluation of metastases, lymph node involvement around the celiac axis and extent of invasion of T4 tumours. Recent series of diagnostic laparoscopy for the staging of gastric cancers and changes in management after diagnostic laparoscopy are summarised in Table 2. Diagnostic laparoscopy leads to a change in the management of 29–40% of gastric cancers in these series. The benefit mainly occurs because of the detection of peritoneal and liver metastases which might also be due to selection criteria.

Key point 2

- Gastric cancer patients who do not need palliative surgery for obstruction or bleeding may benefit from laparoscopic staging.

Table 2 Diagnostic laparoscopy for gastric cancer

Study	Pre-op. staging	*n*	Change in management/ upstaged (%)	Remarks
Burke *et al.*[54]	CT scan	103	32 (31)	Only 103 patients who underwent diagnostic laparoscopy and laparotomy included here
Hunerbein *et al.*[55]	EUS + USG + CT scan + MRI	131	45 (36)	Spiral CT scan used selectively
Feussner *et al.*[56]	USG + CT scan + EUS	111	45 (40)	Only T3 and T4 tumours. Peritoneal metastases 25%. Additional value of LUS 15%. 69% of T4 lesions down-staged to T3
Smith *et al.*[51]	USG + CT scan	52	15(29)	LUS detected 4 (26%) additional lesions in addition to 11 by diagnostic laparoscopy

PRIMARY AND SECONDARY LIVER TUMOURS

Only 10–30% of malignant liver tumours are resectable.[27–29] As there are virtually no indications for palliative resection of liver tumours, diagnostic laparoscopy (with LUS) may reduce the incidence of negative exploration.

Table 3 Occult metastasis detected at diagnostic laparoscopy and LUS in patients with liver secondaries due to colorectal carcinoma

Study	Year	No	AML detected at DL and LUS (%)/laparotomy prevented	Pre-operative staging
Van Dijkum *et al.*[24]	1999	33	33	Spiral CT scan
Rahusen *et al.*[31]	1999	50	38	CT scan – 10 mm slices for the liver. Other details not stated. At diagnostic laparoscopy 13% and at LUS 25% additional lesions detected
Foroutani *et al.*[57a]	2000	55	20	Triphasic CT scan with 7 mm slices
Angelica *et al.*[32]	2003	199	10	Various combinations of CT, ultrasound, MRI, CT portography, PET scan used; 87% patients had ≥ 2 studies
de Castro *et al.*[12]	2004	43	12[b]	Multiphasic spiral CT scan (3–5 mm slices) for pre-operative staging

[a]Only LUS compared with CT scan; [b]in the entire cohort of 51 patients.
AML, additional metastatic lesions
DL, diagnostic laparoscopy

DIAGNOSTIC LAPAROSCOPY FOR LIVER SECONDARIES DUE TO COLORECTAL CARCINOMA

In the early studies of diagnostic laparoscopy with LUS, occult metastases were detected in up to 33–46% of patients, thereby precluding resection of the liver.[24,30,31] The clinical relevance of these studies for today's practice is questionable due to pre-operative imaging protocols and that the histopathological validation on LUS was not always obtained. In recent studies where standard, modern radiological imaging was used for staging, diagnostic laparoscopy revealed occult lesions in only 10% of patients.[12,32] The results of these studies are summarised in Table 3.

In view of the more limited benefit of diagnostic laparoscopy with LUS in recent studies, a selective application of this staging modality for potentially resectable liver metastases has been proposed.[33] A clinical risk score comprising five factors (lymph node positive primary tumour, disease-free interval, number of liver lesions, carcinoembryonic antigen level and size of the largest liver lesion) has been reported to predict prognosis in patients with colorectal cancers.[33] A retrospective analysis from the Memorial Sloan Kettering Hospital reported that patients with more than two risk factors are more likely to have occult metastases compared to those with a score of < 2 (42% versus 12%; $P = 0.001$). The authors proposed that diagnostic laparoscopy should be restricted to patients with more than 2 risk factors according to the scoring system in an attempt to improve utilisation of available resources.[34]

Key point 3

- Only 10–12% of patients with potentially resectable metastases from colorectal tumours have occult metastases. A selective use of diagnostic laparoscopy is, therefore, recommended.

DIAGNOSTIC LAPAROSCOPY FOR HEPATOCELLULAR CARCINOMA

Diagnostic laparoscopy with LUS for hepatocellular carcinoma (HCC) has theoretical advantage:

1. Detection of small intrahepatic metastases or multicentric tumours.
2. Safe biopsy of the primary and additional lesions.
3. Assessment of liver remnant and severity of cirrhosis (biopsy).
4. Detection of extrahepatic disease such as extension of tumour thrombi into major vessels and assessment of local invasion into adjacent structures.

According to recent published series, diagnostic laparoscopy with LUS leads to up-staging in 16–39% of patients of HCC as summarised in Table 4.

To increase the yield of diagnostic laparoscopy further, a more selective use of diagnostic laparoscopy has been proposed. Patients without cirrhosis, major vascular invasion, or bilobar tumours are less likely to benefit from diagnostic laparoscopy.[35] However, diagnostic laparoscopy and biopsy may be helpful for the differentiation of dysplastic nodules and HCC. In a recent study, diagnostic laparoscopy resulted in an up- or down-staging in 12 of 18 patients with equivocal liver lesions (AFP < 100 ng/ml) evaluated for liver transplantation.[36]

Table 4 Occult metastasis detected at diagnostic laparoscopy and LUS in patients with hepatocellular carcinoma

Study	Laparotomy prevented (%)	Pre-operative staging
Lo *et al.*[58]	16	Selected patients after Child-Pugh grading, ICG retention test, USG and CT scan and hepatic angiogram
Van Dijkum *et al.*[24]	40	Triple phase spiral CT scan
Montorsi *et al.*[59]	20	Combinations of ultrasound, CT scans after lipiodol arteriography and spiral CT scan
Angelica *et al.*[32]	20	Various combinations of CT, ultrasound, MRI, CT portography, PET scan used; 87% patients had ≥ 2 studies
de Castro *et al.*[12]	39	Multiphasic spiral CT scan (3–5 mm slices) for pre-operative staging
Lang *et al.*[60a]	36	Selected patients after Child-Pugh grading, ICG retention test, USG and CT scan and hepatic angiogram

[a]Selected patients with ruptured hepatocellular carcinoma.

LUS has been used successfully to detect additional lesions. However, improved MRI might in the future reduce the need for diagnostic laparoscopy.

Key point 4

- Diagnostic laparoscopy detects unresectable disease in 16–39% of potentially resectable hepatocellular carcinoma patients and hence is still recommended for pre-operative staging. It also

PROXIMAL BILE DUCT (KLATSKIN'S TUMOUR) AND GALL BLADDER CANCER

There is a high likelihood of unresectability (up to 80%) in patients with proximal bile duct tumours and gallbladder carcinoma due to metastases or locally advanced disease. The median survival in these patients is 6–9 months and 6 months, respectively. As the majority of these patients can be palliated non-operatively, by endoscopic or percutaneous stenting, laparoscopic staging might prevent a non-therapeutic laparotomy and result in a better quality of life.

Diagnostic laparoscopy may also be helpful to differentiate between proximal bile duct and gall bladder cancers extending into the hepato-duodenal ligament which are usually irresectable.[37]

The few studies evaluating diagnostic laparoscopy and LUS in patients with proximal bile duct cancer are summarised in Table 5. While these studies demonstrate a substantial benefit of diagnostic laparoscopy, the routine use of

Table 5 Occult metastasis detected at diagnostic laparoscopy and LUS in patients with proximal biliary tract carcinoma

Study	Hilar cholangio-carcinoma (%)	Gall bladder carcinoma (%)	Remarks
Van Dijkum *et al.*[24]	40	–	–
Weber *et al.*[38]	25	48	LUS was not done. 45% of hilar cholangiocarcinoma (52% due to advanced local disease) and 65% of gall bladder carcinoma (60% due to advanced local disease) were unresectable at laparotomy
Vollmer *et al.*[16]	–	55	Of the 11 patients, 7 were unresect-able – 6 due to metastases at diag-nostic laparoscopy. LUS revealed major vascular invasion in 1 patient
Tilleman *et al.*[37]	41	–	LUS revealed histologically proven disease in only additional 1% of patients. Not recommended

LUS remains undetermined. In one study, where it was not used, diagnostic laparoscopy revealed a high rate of unresectability due to locally advanced tumours at exploration. In contrast, in another study where LUS was used routinely, additional lesions with proven pathology were only identified in 1% of the patients.[37,38]

The difference in outcome might also be due to different staging procedures and indications for resection (with or without vascular reconstruction, *etc.*).

Key point 5

- Diagnostic laparoscopy detects unresectable disease in 25–55% of patients with potentially resectable proximal bile duct and gall bladder cancer and is recommended for routine pre-operative staging. The additional role of LUS remains doubtful.

PANCREATIC AND PERI-AMPULLARY CANCERS

The early studies of diagnostic laparoscopy for peri-ampullary tumours reported metastases in between 18–82% of the patients as summarised in Table 6. The introduction of newer staging modalities like helical CT scan (especially with 2–3 mm sections) has meant that fewer metastatic lesions are missed during the pre-laparoscopic imaging.[39] Thus a reduced benefit of between 4–13% has been reported in more recent studies (Table 7). This fact is emphasised in a review by Pisters *et al.*,[9] who stated that if occult metastatic disease is detected in more than 20% of patients during diagnostic laparoscopy, the quality of prediagnostic imaging should be considered as inadequate.

Table 6 Early studies on diagnostic laparoscopy for peri-ampullary carcinoma

Study	Year	*n*	Metastases at diagnostic laparoscopy (%)
Warshaw *et al.*[7]	1986	40	14 (35)
Cuschieri *et al.*[8]	1988	51	42 (82)
Fernandez de Castillo *et al.*[61]	1995	89	16 (18)
John *et al.*[62]	1995	40	14 (35)
Conlon *et al.*[63]	1996	108	39 (39)

Table 7 Peritoneal and/or liver metastases detected during laparotomy after high quality spiral CT scan

Study	Patients considered resectable	Resection rate (%)	Patients with metastases	Preventable laparotomy (%)
Steinberg *et al.*[64]	32	75	4	13
Friess *et al.*[65]	159	75	16	10
Rumstadt *et al.*[66]	194	89	9	5
Holzman *et al.*[67]	23	78	1	4
Spitz *et al.*[68]	118	80	18	15
Saldinger *et al.*[69]	68	76	3	4

Adapted from Pisters *et al.*[9]

In most studies, the end-point for the benefit of diagnostic laparoscopy was avoidance of a non-therapeutic laparotomy. We have shown that during follow-up a substantial percentage of patients still needed a laparotomy because of subsequent gastric outlet obstruction.[26] The benefit of diagnostic laparoscopy in terms of prevention of laparotomy in these patients is reduced from 15% to 11%. It is well known that 10–20% of patients with an unresectable peri-ampullary cancer managed by biliary drainage alone develop subsequent gastric outlet obstruction and need a surgical bypass.[40,41]

Therefore, a randomised study was performed not only to analyse the benefit of diagnostic laparoscopy in terms of detection of metastases but also to analyse whether patients with metastases should be treated by endoprosthesis or bypass surgery.

Key point 6

- Diagnostic laparoscopy detects unresectable disease in only 4–13% of patients with potentially resectable peri-ampullary carcinoma. Also, there is no substantial gain in hospital-free survival with subsequent endoscopic biliary stenting compared to surgical bypass. Therefore, diagnostic laparoscopy is not recommended for routine pre-operative staging.

This randomised trial demonstrated that endoscopic biliary stenting after diagnostic laparoscopy was not associated with a longer hospital-free survival compared with bypass surgery (Fig. 3) and there was no difference in morbidity and mortality.[10] In view of relative limited benefit observed in the first study and the negative results from the above mentioned trial, we eliminated routine laparoscopic staging for peri-ampullary cancers at the Amsterdam Medical Center in 1998.

All patients with metastatic disease detected during surgery undergo a surgical bypass.[18] This principle, however, might change after adequate palliation of duodenal obstruction with new stent devices.

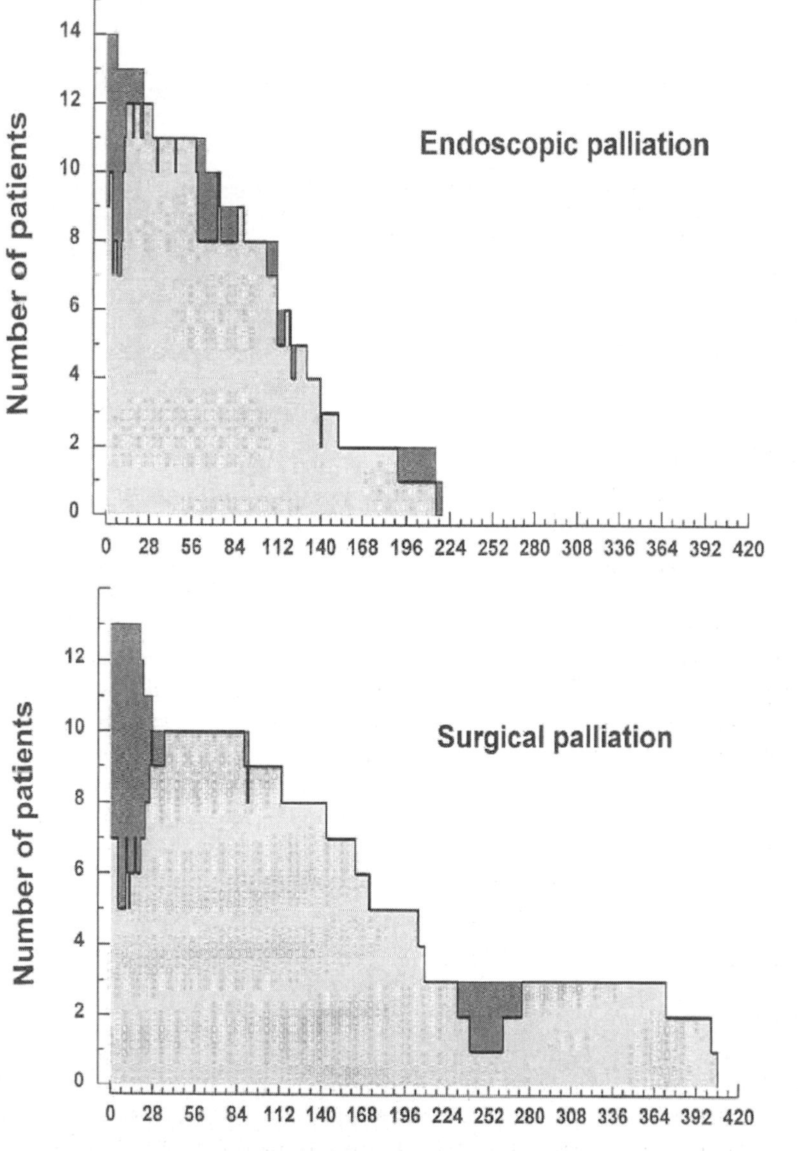

Fig. 3 Survival of patients with resectable peripancreatic carcinoma (metastasis) allocated to endoscopic and surgical palliation. Dark grey area is time spent in hospital.

Table 8 Influence of radiological imaging and time period on the yield of diagnostic laparoscopy for peri-ampullary cancer at the Amsterdam Medical Center

Study	Period	Radiological modality & technique	Laparotomy prevented by DL (%)	Evolution of DL for periampullary cancers
Bemelman *et al.*[11]	1993–1994	Ultrasonography	19	High yield of diagnostic laparoscopy
Van Dijkum *et al.*[26]	1992–1995	Ultrasonography + conventional CT scan	15	Decreasing benefit
Van Dijkum *et al.*[10]	1995–1998	5 mm sliced spiral CT scan	13	Randomised study on late outcome – substantial gain in hospital-free survival unlikely with stenting as compared to surgical bypass. Stop DL
Tilleman *et al.*[18]	1999–2001	3 mm sliced spiral CT scan	9.5[a]	Policy validated. Recommendation: routine use of DL no longer justified

[a]Actual benefit of diagnostic laparoscopy (DL).

The evolution of diagnostic laparoscopy for patients with peri-ampullary tumours at the Amsterdam Medical Center is summarised in Table 8.

DIAGNOSTIC LAPAROSCOPY AND LAPAROSCOPIC ULTRASOUND IN PANCREATIC TUMOURS

LUS is reported in many studies to increase the prediction of resectability of pancreatic head tumours.[42,43] However, there are a few limitations of these studies. First, the pre-operative CT scan quality was not always up to the currently acceptable standards, and second, locally advanced tumours are also included but full details are not always provided regarding pre-operative imaging.[9] In one study, in 8 of the 13 patients reported to have advanced lesions during LUS, lesions were already detected at pre-operative external ultrasound.[44]

The principle that vascular invasion during external ultrasound/Doppler or CT scan are doubtful and confirmation is needed by laparoscopy or laparotomy while the same findings at LUS are accepted as solid criteria for unresectability, even in the absence of histopathological validation, is remarkable.

Key point 7

- Routine additional laparoscopic ultrasound does not significantly improve the detection of pathology proven local invasion in the mesenteric vessels after standard laparoscopic evaluation. A selective use is, therefore, recommended.

COLORECTAL CANCER

The indications of routine laparoscopic staging for colorectal cancer are limited. In contrast to upper GI tract cancers, the generally accepted palliative management for patients with metastatic disease is resection or a surgical bypass. Also, the currently available imaging modalities provide accurate information for patient management in the majority of patients.

The main indication for diagnostic laparoscopy with LUS for colorectal cancers used to be the assessment of occult metastatic disease in patients with otherwise resectable liver metastases. However, with the availability of thin-slice helical CT scan, a more selective use in high-risk patients is suggested.

The potential use of diagnostic laparoscopy in these tumours might, however, change in the near future since colonic stenting has become available and accepted as palliative treatment but more recently also as a 'bridge to surgery' in patients with acute intestinal obstruction.[4,45–47]

The indication for diagnostic laparoscopy in patients with colorectal cancer may also change because of the acceptance of laparoscopic colorectal surgery for malignant lesions as well as the benefit of laparoscopic stoma formation in patients with extensive stage 4 disease. Effective palliation may be achieved by avoiding a laparotomy in selected patients.[46,47]

SUMMARY

Diagnostic laparoscopy should be considered as the final staging procedure in patients with GI tumours if non-surgical palliation is feasible. The main objective of diagnostic laparoscopy is to avoid a non-therapeutic laparotomy by the detection of metastatic lesions likely to be missed during pre-operative radiological staging. Hence, the place of diagnostic laparoscopy in the staging algorithms is determined by the accuracy of the present imaging modalities.

Diagnostic laparoscopy may be considered as a routine pre-operative staging procedure for patients with oesophageal adenocarcinoma of the GI junction, hepatocellular carcinoma, proximal bile duct, gallbladder cancer and pancreatic body and tail cancers. A relatively high number of patients with these tumours have peritoneal and superficial liver metastases that are likely to be missed by the currently available imaging techniques.

With the increasing availability and accuracy of the imaging modalities, the benefits of diagnostic laparoscopy for peri-ampullary cancers and liver secondaries due to colorectal cancer has decreased substantially.

Key points for clinical practice

- Diagnostic laparoscopy is indicated only for staging of tumours of the gastro-oesophageal junction and cardia. The benefit for (squamous cell) carcinoma in the thoracic oesophagus is limited.
- Gastric cancer patients who do not need palliative surgery for obstruction or bleeding may benefit from laparoscopic staging.

(*continued on next page*)

Key points for clinical practice *(continued)*

- Only 10–12% of patients with potentially resectable metastases from colorectal tumours have occult metastases. A selective use of diagnostic laparoscopy is, therefore, recommended.
- Diagnostic laparoscopy detects unresectable disease in 16–39% of potentially resectable hepatocellular carcinoma patients and hence is still recommended for pre-operative staging. It also improves staging of cirrhosis.
- Diagnostic laparoscopy detects unresectable disease in 25–55% of patients with potentially resectable proximal bile duct and gall bladder cancer and is recommended for routine pre-operative staging. The additional role of LUS remains doubtful.
- Diagnostic laparoscopy detects unresectable disease in only 4–13% of patients with potentially resectable peri-ampullary carcinoma. Also, there is no substantial gain in hospital-free survival with subsequent endoscopic biliary stenting compared to surgical bypass. Therefore, diagnostic laparoscopy is not recommended for routine pre-operative staging.
- Routine additional laparoscopic ultrasound does not significantly improve the detection of pathology proven local invasion in the mesenteric vessels after standard laparoscopic evaluation. A selective use is, therefore, recommended.

References

1. Homs MY, Steyerberg EW, Eijkenboom WM *et al*. Single-dose brachytherapy versus metal stent placement for the palliation of dysphagia from oesophageal cancer: multicentre randomised trial. *Lancet* 2004; **364**: 1497–1504.
2. Nassif T, Prat F, Meduri B *et al*. Endoscopic palliation of malignant gastric outlet obstruction using self-expandable metallic stents: results of a multicenter study. *Endoscopy* 2003; **35**: 483–489.
3. Mittal A, Windsor J, Woodfield J *et al*. Matched study of three methods for palliation of malignant pyloroduodenal obstruction. *Br J Surg* 2004; **91**: 205–209.
4. Law WL, Choi HK, Lee YM *et al*. Palliation for advanced malignant colorectal obstruction by self-expanding metallic stents: prospective evaluation of outcomes. *Dis Colon Rectum* 2004; **47**: 39–43.
5. Shepherd HA, Royle G, Ross AP *et al*. Endoscopic biliary endoprosthesis in the palliation of malignant obstruction of the distal common bile duct: a randomized trial. *Br J Surg* 1988; **75**: 1166–1168.
6. Smith AC, Dowsett JF, Russell RC *et al*. Randomised trial of endoscopic stenting versus surgical bypass in malignant low bile duct obstruction. *Lancet* 1994; **344**: 1655–1660.
7. Warshaw AL, Tepper JE, Shipley WU. Laparoscopy in the staging and planning of therapy for pancreatic cancer. *Am J Surg* 1986; **151**: 76–80.
8. Cuschieri A. Laparoscopy for pancreatic cancer: does it benefit the patient? *Eur J Surg Oncol* 1988; **14**: 41–44.
9. Pisters PW, Lee JE, Vauthey JN *et al*. Laparoscopy in the staging of pancreatic cancer. *Br J Surg* 2001; **88**: 325–337.
10. Nieveen van Dijkum EJ, Romijn MG, Terwee CB *et al*. Laparoscopic staging and subsequent palliation in patients with peripancreatic carcinoma. *Ann Surg* 2003; **237**: 66–73.

11. Bemelman WA, de Wit LT, van Delden OM *et al*. Diagnostic laparoscopy combined with laparoscopic ultrasonography in staging of cancer of the pancreatic head region. *Br J Surg* 1995; **82**: 820–824.
12. de Castro SM, Tilleman EH, Busch OR *et al*. Diagnostic laparoscopy for primary and secondary liver malignancies: impact of improved imaging and changed criteria for resection. *Ann Surg Oncol* 2004; **11**: 522–529.
13. van Dijkum EJ, Sturm PD, de Wit LT *et al*. Cytology of peritoneal lavage performed during staging laparoscopy for gastrointestinal malignancies: is it useful? *Ann Surg* 1998; **228**: 728–733.
14. Gahlen J, Prosst RL, Pietschmann M *et al*. Laparoscopic fluorescence diagnosis for intraabdominal fluorescence targeting of peritoneal carcinosis experimental studies. *Ann Surg* 2002; **235**: 252–260.
15. Loning M, Diddens H, Kupker W *et al*. Laparoscopic fluorescence detection of ovarian carcinoma metastases using 5-aminolevulinic acid-induced protoporphyrin IX. *Cancer* 2004; **100**: 1650–1656.
16. Vollmer CM, Drebin JA, Middleton WD *et al*. Utility of staging laparoscopy in subsets of peripancreatic and biliary malignancies. *Ann Surg* 2002; **235**: 1–7.
17. Barreiro CJ, Lillemoe KD, Koniaris LG *et al*. Diagnostic laparoscopy for periampullary and pancreatic cancer: what is the true benefit? *J Gastrointest Surg* 2002; **6**: 75–81.
18. Tilleman EH, Kuiken BW, Phoa SS *et al*. Limitation of diagnostic laparoscopy for patients with a periampullary carcinoma. *Eur J Surg Oncol* 2004; **30**: 658–662.
19. Boyd Jr WP, Nord HJ. Diagnostic laparoscopy. *Endoscopy* 2000; **32**: 153–158.
20. Bonjer HJ, Hazebroek EJ, Kazemier G *et al*. Open versus closed establishment of pneumoperitoneum in laparoscopic surgery. *Br J Surg* 1997; **84**: 599–602.
21. Bemelman WA, De Wit LT, Busch OR *et al*. Establishment of pneumoperitoneum with a modified blunt trocar. *J Laparoendosc Adv Surg Tech A* 2000; **10**: 217–218.
22. Philips PA, Amaral JF. Abdominal access complications in laparoscopic surgery. *J Am Coll Surg* 2001; **192**: 525–536.
23. van der Voort N, Heijnsdijk EA, Gouma DJ. Bowel injury as a complication of laparoscopy. *Br J Surg* 2004; **91**: 1253–1258.
24. van Dijkum EJ, de Wit LT, van Delden OM *et al*. Staging laparoscopy and laparoscopic ultrasonography in more than 400 patients with upper gastrointestinal carcinoma. *J Am Coll Surg* 1999; **189**: 459–465.
25. Shoup M, Brennan MF, Karpeh MS *et al*. Port site metastasis after diagnostic laparoscopy for upper gastrointestinal tract malignancies: an uncommon entity. *Ann Surg Oncol* 2002; **9**: 632–636.
26. van Dijkum EJ, de Wit LT, van Delden OM *et al*. The efficacy of laparoscopic staging in patients with upper gastrointestinal tumors. *Cancer* 1997; **79**: 1315–1319.
27. Scheele J, Stang R, Altendorf-Hofmann A *et al*. Resection of colorectal liver metastases. *World J Surg* 1995; **19**: 59–71.
28. Bismuth H, Adam R, Levi F *et al*. Resection of nonresectable liver metastases from colorectal cancer after neoadjuvant chemotherapy. *Ann Surg* 1996; **224**: 509–520.
29. Llovet JM, Burroughs A, Bruix J. Hepatocellular carcinoma. *Lancet* 2003; **362**: 1907–1917.
30. John TG, Greig JD, Crosbie JL *et al*. Superior staging of liver tumors with laparoscopy and laparoscopic ultrasound. *Ann Surg* 1994; **220**: 711–719.
31. Rahusen FD, Cuesta MA, Borgstein PJ *et al*. Selection of patients for resection of colorectal metastases to the liver using diagnostic laparoscopy and laparoscopic ultrasonography. *Ann Surg* 1999; **230**: 31–37.
32. D'Angelica M, Fong Y, Weber S *et al*. The role of staging laparoscopy in hepatobiliary malignancy: prospective analysis of 401 cases. *Ann Surg Oncol* 2003; **10**: 183–189.
33. Fong Y, Fortner J, Sun RL *et al*. Clinical score for predicting recurrence after hepatic resection for metastatic colorectal cancer: analysis of 1001 consecutive cases. *Ann Surg* 1999; **230**: 309–318.
34. Jarnagin WR, Conlon K, Bodniewicz J *et al*. A clinical scoring system predicts the yield of diagnostic laparoscopy in patients with potentially resectable hepatic colorectal metastases. *Cancer* 2001; **91**: 1121–1128.
35. Weitz J, D'Angelica M, Jarnagin W *et al*. Selective use of diagnostic laparoscopy prior to planned hepatectomy for patients with hepatocellular carcinoma. *Surgery* 2004; **135**: 273–281.

36. Kim RD, Nazarey P, Katz E *et al*. Laparoscopic staging and tumor ablation for hepatocellular carcinoma in Child C cirrhotics evaluated for orthotopic liver transplantation. *Surg Endosc* 2004; **18**: 39–44.
37. Tilleman EH, de Castro SM, Busch OR *et al*. Diagnostic laparoscopy and laparoscopic ultrasound for staging of patients with malignant proximal bile duct obstruction. *J Gastrointest Surg* 2002; **6**: 426–430.
38. Weber SM, DeMatteo RP, Fong Y *et al*. Staging laparoscopy in patients with extrahepatic biliary carcinoma. Analysis of 100 patients. *Ann Surg* 2002; **235**: 392–399.
39. Freeny PC, Traverso LW, Ryan JA. Diagnosis and staging of pancreatic adenocarcinoma with dynamic computed tomography. *Am J Surg* 1993; **165**: 600–606.
40. Lillemoe KD, Cameron JL, Hardacre JM *et al*. Is prophylactic gastrojejunostomy indicated for unresectable periampullary cancer? A prospective randomized trial. *Ann Surg* 1999; **230**: 322–328.
41. Van Heek NT, de Castro SM, van Eijck CH *et al*. The need for a prophylactic gastrojejunostomy for unresectable periampullary cancer: a prospective randomized multicenter trial with special focus on assessment of quality of life. *Ann Surg* 2003; **238**: 894–902.
42. John TG, Wright A, Allan PL *et al*. Laparoscopy with laparoscopic ultrasonography in the TNM staging of pancreatic carcinoma. *World J Surg* 1999; **23**: 870–881.
43. Taylor AM, Roberts SA, Manson JM. Experience with laparoscopic ultrasonography for defining tumour resectability in carcinoma of the pancreatic head and periampullary region. *Br J Surg* 2001; **88**: 1077–1083.
44. Minnard EA, Conlon KC, Hoos A *et al*. Laparoscopic ultrasound enhances standard laparoscopy in the staging of pancreatic cancer. *Ann Surg* 1998; **228**: 182–187.
45. Carne PW, Frye JN, Robertson GM *et al*. Stents or open operation for palliation of colorectal cancer: a retrospective, cohort study of perioperative outcome and long-term survival. *Dis Colon Rectum* 2004; **47**: 1455–1461.
46. Milsom JW, Kim SH, Hammerhofer KA *et al*. Laparoscopic colorectal cancer surgery for palliation. *Dis Colon Rectum* 2000; **43**: 1512–1516.
47. Hartley JE, Monson JR. The role of laparoscopy in the multimodality treatment of colorectal cancer. *Surg Clin North Am* 2002; **82**: 1019–1033.
48. Romijn MG, van Overhagen H, Spillenaar Bilgen EJ *et al*. Laparoscopy and laparoscopic ultrasonography in staging of oesophageal and cardial carcinoma. *Br J Surg* 1998; **85**: 1010–1012.
49. Bemelman WA, van Delden OM, van Lanschot JJ *et al*. Laparoscopy and laparoscopic ultrasonography in staging of carcinoma of the esophagus and gastric cardia. *J Am Coll Surg* 1995; **181**: 421–425.
50. Luketich JD, Meehan M, Nguyen NT *et al*. Minimally invasive surgical staging for esophageal cancer. *Surg Endosc* 2000; **14**: 700–702.
51. Smith A, Finch MD, John TG *et al*. Role of laparoscopic ultrasonography in the management of patients with oesophagogastric cancer. *Br J Surg* 1999; **86**: 1083–1087.
52. Hulscher JB, Nieveen van Dijkum EJ, de Wit LT *et al*. Laparoscopy and laparoscopic ultrasonography in staging carcinoma of the gastric cardia. *Eur J Surg* 2000; **166**: 862–865.
53. Clements DM, Bowrey DJ, Havard TJ. The role of staging investigations for oesophago-gastric carcinoma. *Eur J Surg Oncol* 2004; **30**: 309–312.
54. Burke EC, Karpeh MS, Conlon KC *et al*. Laparoscopy in the management of gastric adenocarcinoma. *Ann Surg* 1997; **225**: 262–267.
55. Hunerbein M, Rau B, Hohenberger P *et al*. The role of staging laparoscopy for multimodal therapy of gastrointestinal cancer. *Surg Endosc* 1998; **12**: 921–925.
56. Feussner H, Omote K, Fink U *et al*. Pretherapeutic laparoscopic staging in advanced gastric carcinoma. *Endoscopy* 1999; **31**: 342–347.
57. Foroutani A, Garland AM, Berber E *et al*. Laparoscopic ultrasound vs triphasic computed tomography for detecting liver tumors. *Arch Surg* 2000; **135**: 933–938.
58. Lo CM, Lai EC, Liu CL *et al*. Laparoscopy and laparoscopic ultrasonography avoid exploratory laparotomy in patients with hepatocellular carcinoma. *Ann Surg* 1998; **227**: 527–532.
59. Montorsi M, Santambrogio R, Bianchi P *et al*. Laparoscopy with laparoscopic ultrasound for pretreatment staging of hepatocellular carcinoma: a prospective study. *J Gastrointest Surg* 2001; **5**: 312–315.

60. Lang BH, Poon RT, Fan ST *et al*. Influence of laparoscopy on postoperative recurrence and survival in patients with ruptured hepatocellular carcinoma undergoing hepatic resection. *Br J Surg* 2004; **91**: 444–449.
61. Fernandez-del Castillo C, Rattner DW, Warshaw AL. Further experience with laparoscopy and peritoneal cytology in the staging of pancreatic cancer. *Br J Surg* 1995; **82**: 1127–1129.
62. John TG, Greig JD, Carter DC *et al*. Carcinoma of the pancreatic head and periampullary region. Tumor staging with laparoscopy and laparoscopic ultrasonography. *Ann Surg* 1995; **221**: 156–164.
63. Conlon KC, Dougherty E, Klimstra DS *et al*. The value of minimal access surgery in the staging of patients with potentially resectable peripancreatic malignancy. *Ann Surg* 1996; **223**: 134–140.
64. Steinberg WM, Barkin J, Bradley III EL *et al*. Workup of a patient with a mass in the head of the pancreas. *Pancreas* 1998; **17**: 24–30.
65. Friess H, Kleeff J, Silva JC *et al*. The role of diagnostic laparoscopy in pancreatic and periampullary malignancies. *J Am Coll Surg* 1998; **186**: 675–682.
66. Rumstadt B, Schwab M, Schuster K *et al*. The role of laparoscopy in the preoperative staging of pancreatic carcinoma. *J Gastrointest Surg* 1997; **1**: 245–250.
67. Holzman MD, Reintgen KL, Tyler DS *et al*. The role of laparoscopy in the management of suspected pancreatic and periampullary malignancies. *J Gastrointest Surg* 1997; **1**: 236–244.
68. Spitz FR, Abbruzzese JL, Lee JE *et al*. Preoperative and postoperative chemoradiation strategies in patients treated with pancreaticoduodenectomy for adenocarcinoma of the pancreas. *J Clin Oncol* 1997; **15**: 928–937.
69. Saldinger PF, Reilly M, Reynolds K *et al*. Is CT angiography sufficient for prediction of resectability of periampullary neoplasms? *J Gastrointest Surg* 2000; **4**: 233–237.

Talvinder Singh Gill John H. Scholefield

11

Update on adjuvant therapy in colorectal cancer

Colorectal cancer is the second most common malignancy in Western societies and the second commonest cause of death from cancer.[1] About 150,000 colorectal cancers are diagnosed in Europe each year. Surgery remains the primary treatment for this disease. About two-thirds of patients undergo resection with curative intent, but 30–50% of these patients will relapse and die of their disease.[2]

Adjuvant therapy is treatment given after the primary treatment to increase the chances of a cure. In colorectal cancer, it is administered in addition to surgical treatment of the primary tumour before (neo-adjuvant) or after resection of all macroscopic disease. The options include (i) chemotherapy; (ii) radiotherapy; and (iii) immunotherapy.

The pattern of recurrence in colon and rectal cancers is different. Colonic cancers usually recur in the form of disseminated disease and so systemic adjuvant treatment in the absence of distant metastatic disease is the main requirement. Local recurrence following curative resection of rectal cancer is a major problem and adjuvant treatment for locoregional control is also required in addition to systemic therapy.

CHEMOTHERAPY

5-Fluorouracil has remained the mainstay of chemotherapy for colorectal cancer over the last 40 years. In 1990, adjuvant chemotherapy using fluorouracil with

Talvinder Singh Gill MBBS MS FRCS(Glas)
Specialist Registrar, Department of Surgery, Queen's Medical Centre, University Hospital NHS Trust, Nottingham NG7 2UH, UK

John H. Scholefield MB ChB FRCS ChM
Professor of Surgery, Queen's Medical Centre, University Hospital NHS Trust, Nottingham NG7 2UH, UK (for correspondence)

levamisole was reported to improve disease-free and overall survival in Dukes' C (stage III) colon cancer.[3] Subsequent studies have shown that fluorouracil with folinic acid confers similar benefit but is less toxic and optimal duration of treatment is 6 months rather than a year.[4,5]

When given as adjuvant therapy after the complete resection of a Dukes' C colon cancer, fluorouracil and folinic acid treatment increases the disease-free survival at 5 years from about 42% to 58% and the overall 5-year survival from about 51% to 64%.[6] Fluorouracil and folinic acid have now become widely accepted as first-line adjuvant therapy for lymph node positive tumours.

Key point 1

- Adjuvant chemotherapy using 5-fluorouracil and folinic acid is standard adjuvant treatment after curative resection of colorectal cancer in patients with lymph node positive disease.

The use of adjuvant fluorouracil and folinic acid in patients with Dukes' B cancer is more controversial. For this group of patients, the probability of 5-year disease-free survival increases from 72% to 76% after treatment ($P = 0.049$), but the likelihood of overall survival increases from 80% to 81% only ($P = 0.113$).[6]

QUASAR was one of the largest single trials of adjuvant chemotherapy in colorectal cancer recruiting patients. Patients with surgically curative resections of colon or rectal cancer were randomised following surgery to adjuvant chemotherapy or observation. Chemotherapy consisted of either six 5-day, 4-weekly or 30 once-weekly courses of intravenous fluorouracil (370 mg/m^2) with either high-dose (175 mg) or low-dose (25 mg) L-folinic acid, and with either levamisole or placebo. A total of 3238 patients were randomised (91% Dukes' B, 71% colon cancer, median age 63 years). Direct randomised comparisons found no benefit for high-dose compared with low-dose folinic acid or levamisole.[7] With a median follow-up of 4.2 years, risk of death with chemotherapy versus control was 0.88 (95% CI 0.75–1.05; $P = 0.15$) and recurrence 0.82 (95% CI 0.70–0.97; $P = 0.02$). Adjuvant chemotherapy was equally effective in patients with rectal cancer.[5]

Chemotherapy produces a small (1–6%) survival benefit for stage B patients, sufficient to outweigh the inconvenience and cost for high-risk and younger patients. Longer follow-up and meta-analysis of all trials is needed to clarify the balance of benefits and side-effects for older patients. Dukes' B colorectal cancers are a heterogeneous group, patients with 'bad-B' disease should be identified and treated differently to 'good-B' disease. Low-risk cancer can be defined as well-differentiated tumours not involving serosa, with no vascular or perineural invasion and complete circumferential resection margin. Adjuvant chemotherapy for patients with low-risk Dukes' B colon cancer is unlikely to be of benefit. The decision to offer adjuvant therapy for Dukes' B disease needs to be individualised to the circumstances of each specific patient (*e.g.* poorly differentiated, vascular invasion, perineural invasion) and should be balanced against the possible risks of treatment-related toxicity and the cost of treatment.

Key point 2

- The data on the role of adjuvant chemotherapy for patients with Dukes' B (stage II) disease have been inconsistent. Chemotherapy should be offered as an adjuvant treatment to the younger and high-risk patients with Duke's B cancer.

Oral adjuvant chemotherapy regimens have clear advantages for healthcare providers over intravenous infusion in terms of compliance, convenience and cost of administration.

Capecitabine is an oral prodrug converted within the cell to 5-fluorouracil. Some trials in advanced colorectal cancer have shown an improved response rate over an infusional regimen with acceptable toxicity. The X-ACT study randomised a total of 1987 patients from 164 centres between 1998 and 2001. Patients with resected Dukes' C colon cancer were randomised to oral capecitabine (1250 mg/m^2 twice daily days 1–14, every 3 weeks) or intravenous fluorouracil and folinic acid (Mayo Clinic regimen: folinic acid 20 mg/m^2 + 5-fluorouracil 425 mg/m^2 days 1–5, every 4 weeks) for 24 weeks' treatment. The primary end-point was at least equivalence in disease-free survival. Median follow-up was 3.8 years. Capecitabine was at least equivalent to fluorouracil and folinic acid with regard to disease-free survival in the per protocol population (HR 0.89 [95% CI 0.76–1.04]). In this study, an 'intention to treat' analysis showed a strong trend towards superior disease-free survival for capecitabine versus fluorouracil and folinic acid, and a trend to superiority for overall survival.[8] Capecitabine may replace fluorouracil and folinic acid in the adjuvant therapy of colon cancer as it is likely to be more cost-effective to use an oral adjuvant regimen compared with an intravenous regimen.

Uracil/Tegafur is another oral option. This has shown similar median survival in metastatic colorectal cancer as with fluorouracil and folinic acid.[9] Tegafur is converted to 5-fluorouracil *in vivo* and uracil enhances the concentration of fluorouracil in tumours.

Key point 3

- Oral adjuvant chemotherapy with capecitabine is becoming more popular and may replace intravenous therapy.

During the past 5 years, various new treatments for advanced colorectal cancer have emerged. The treatment of advanced colorectal cancer was disappointing, with fluorouracil and folinic acid yielding response rates of 10–25% with little effect on survival. Several phase III trials have now shown that adding irinotecan or oxaliplatin doubles the response rates to around 50% and increases progression-free survival.[10,11] New treatments traditionally trialled in advanced disease first may be expected to have a much greater effect on survival if used as adjuvant treatment for earlier stages of disease. The adjuvant trials looking at the addition of these new modalities to fluorouracil and folinic acid are therefore awaited with great interest.

OXALIPLATIN

Oxaliplatin distorts DNA into adducts and reduces thymidylate synthase levels. Oxaliplatin has been shown to down-size liver metastases, to enable potentially curative resection to be performed in several patients whose tumour would previously have been considered inoperable. Survival rates of 34% at 5 years and 20% at 10 years for patients undergoing liver resection after neo-adjuvant chemotherapy (fluorouracil, folinic acid, and oxaliplatin) are similar to those of patients undergoing primary resection.[12]

The results of the MOSAIC study suggest a role for oxaliplatin in the adjuvant treatment of colorectal cancer. This large, international, phase III study recruited 2246 patients with Dukes' B (stage II) and Dukes' C (stage III) colon cancer. The trial looked at the addition of oxaliplatin to standard postoperative adjuvant chemotherapy with fluorouracil and folinic acid and showed that adding oxaliplatin resulted in a reduction in relapse rates of 23% ($P = 0.0002$). The increase in disease-free survival (78.2% versus 72.9%) was also significant ($P = 0.002$). This difference was far more evident among patients with Dukes' C cancer (72.2% versus 65.3%) than among those with Dukes' B cancer (87.0% versus 84.3%). There was no significant difference in estimated overall survival at 3 years between the two groups (87.7% versus 86.6%). Peripheral neuropathy was the main side effect of adding oxaliplatin, occurring in 92.1% of patients and classified as grade 3 in 12.4% of the patients receiving this treatment.[13] Grade 3 neuropathy is severe paresthesias and/or disabling objective sensory loss interfering with function.

With only 3 years' follow-up, it is too early to say whether this will translate into a 'gold standard' survival advantage at 5 years, but 3-year, disease-free survival has been shown to be a good predictor of 5-year overall survival in trials of adjuvant treatment of colon cancer.[14] If these outcomes are confirmed, this regimen offers the opportunity of nearly doubling the benefit of adjuvant fluorouracil and folinic acid in colon cancer and may save many thousands of lives. However, the costs of these drugs are several times those of the present agents and this may create new problems for healthcare providers.

IRINOTECAN

Irinotecan is a potent inhibitor of topoisomerase I, an enzyme involved in DNA repair. Irinotecan used in advanced colorectal cancer increases median overall survival by about 3 months.[15] The main toxicities observed with irinotecan are: acute cholinergic syndrome, neutropenia, delayed onset diarrhoea, nausea and vomiting, fatigue and alopecia.

The Intergroup trial CALGB C89803 randomised 1264 patients of Dukes' C colon cancer, to receive either fluorouracil and folinic acid or irinotecan plus fluorouracil and folinic acid after potentially curative resection. Median follow-up was 2.6 years. The addition of irinotecan showed no improvement in terms of either overall survival ($P = 0.88$) or disease-free survival ($P = 0.84$), but was associated with greater degree of neutropenia, neutropenic fever and death on treatment.[16]

QUASAR 2 and several other phase III trials are currently ongoing to assess the potential benefits of combining irinotecan with chemotherapy in the adjuvant setting.

> **Key point 4**
>
> - Addition of irinotecan to chemotherapeutic regimens has shown promising results in advanced colorectal cancer but its use as an adjuvant therapy is not established yet.

RADIOTHERAPY

Radiotherapy is only occasionally used for colon cancer in the adjuvant setting, where circumferential resection margins are involved after potentially curative resection. Fears about irradiating the small bowel limit the use of radiotherapy in treating colon cancer.

Adjuvant radiotherapy for rectal cancer is a rapidly evolving area. A meta-analysis of 22 randomised trials of adjuvant radiotherapy for rectal cancer considered 8507 patients and concluded that radiotherapy had neither survival benefit (62%) nor improvement in resectability rate (85%) over surgery alone (63% and 86%, respectively). Yearly risk of local recurrence was 46% lower in those who had pre-operative radiotherapy and 37% lower in patients who had postoperative radiotherapy. Pre-operative radiotherapy reduced the risk of local recurrence and death from rectal cancer, but early deaths from other causes increased (8% versus 4% died, $P < 0.0001$).[17]

Traditionally, there are widely differing approaches to adjuvant radiotherapy between the US and Europe. In the US, radiotherapy for rectal cancer is normally given postoperatively, whereas in Europe pre-operative radiotherapy is generally preferred.

POSTOPERATIVE RADIOTHERAPY: US APPROACH

Postoperative combination therapy is standard practice for resectable rectal cancer in the US. The National Institutes of Health (NIH) Consensus Conference[18] made a clinical announcement on adjuvant therapy for rectal cancer in 1990 and concluded: 'combined postoperative chemotherapy and radiation therapy improves local control and survival in stage II and III patients and is recommended'. The advantage of postoperative adjuvant radiotherapy is that accurate histopathological staging makes appropriate treatment selection easier.

In the National Surgical Adjuvant Breast and Bowel Project (NSABP) R-02 study, 694 patients with stage II and III rectal cancer were randomly assigned to receive adjuvant chemotherapy with or without radiotherapy. The addition of postoperative radiotherapy did not improve disease-free or overall survival, but it significantly reduced the cumulative incidence of locoregional relapse from 13% to 8% at 5 years.[19]

PRE-OPERATIVE RADIOTHERAPY: EUROPEAN APPROACH

The European approach to adjuvant radiotherapy for rectal cancer favours pre-operative radiotherapy. This view has developed from a meta-analysis of the results of studies showing reduced rates of local failure with pre-operative radiotherapy.[17,20,21]

The Swedish Rectal Cancer Trial in 1997 showed a short-term regimen of high-dose pre-operative radiotherapy reduces rates of local recurrence and improves survival among patients with resectable rectal cancer.[22] After 5 years of follow-up, the rate of local recurrence was 11% in the group that received radiotherapy before surgery and 27% in the group treated with surgery alone. The overall 5-year survival rate was 58% in the radiotherapy-plus-surgery group and 48% in the surgery-alone group. This trial also confirmed that multiple (three or four) field radiation technique reduces the toxicity of intensive, short-course radiation.

Key point 5

- A short-term regimen of high-dose pre-operative radiotherapy reduces rates of local recurrence and improves survival among patients with resectable rectal cancer.

The improvement in surgical techniques and the use of total mesorectal excision (TME) has also reduced the number of local recurrences. The best TME surgeons already have local recurrence rates of less than 10%, and some < 5%.[23] These surgeons used adjuvant radiotherapy more sparingly, but probably only a few surgeons can achieve these standards and will need to use adjuvant radiotherapy more frequently.

A randomised, prospective, multicentre trial was conducted by the Dutch Colorectal Cancer Group to compare the effect of pre-operative radiotherapy combined with total mesorectal excision surgery with total mesorectal excision surgery alone. They found the rate of local recurrence at 2 years was 5.3%. The local recurrence rate at 2 years was 2.4% in the radiotherapy-plus-surgery group and 8.2% in the surgery-only group ($P < 0.001$). The beneficial effect of pre-operative radiotherapy was more significant for tumours in mid-rectum (5.1–10.0 cm from anal verge). The overall survival at 2 years was same (82%) in both groups. There was not much difference in proportion of patients with metastatic disease at 2 years (14.8% versus 16.8%).[24] Five-year follow-up results are awaited.

Key point 6

- Pre-operative radiotherapy does reduce the rate of local recurrence even when it was given before total mesorectal excision. The beneficial effect of pre-operative radiotherapy was more significant for tumours in mid-rectum.

Pre-operative radiotherapy is better tolerated by the patient and seems to have greater efficacy but the potential for toxicity is significant. Long-term complications of short-course radiotherapy remain uncertain and more follow-up is required. The difficulty with pre-operative radiotherapy is case selection.

The role of MRI is increasingly important in this selection. Selective use of postoperative radiotherapy based on more efficient predictors of local recurrence could be a more cost-effective strategy than indiscriminate use of pre-operative radiotherapy. The present UK MRC CR-07 trial should address some of these issues and initial results are expected in 2005.

CHEMO-RADIOTHERAPY

The literature on the efficacy of adjuvant chemo-radiotherapy for colorectal cancer is conflicting.[25]

The German CAO/ARO/AIO-94 study recruited more than 800 patients to compare pre-operative fluorouracil-based chemo-radiotherapy versus postoperative combined modality treatment for stage II and III resectable rectal cancer. The results have not shown much difference in distant metastasis (32%) or overall survival (74%). The rate of local recurrence was 6% in the pre-operative treatment arm and 12% in the postoperative treatment ($P = 0.006$). The disease-free survival and sphincter preservation rate was 65% and 39%, respectively, in the pre-operative group compared to 61% and 19% in the postoperative group.[26]

The European Organisation for Research and Treatment of Cancer (EORTC) 22921 study is a major European trial, randomised for pre-operative radiotherapy alone versus chemo-radiotherapy. This trial closed in April 2003 and has accrued 1011 patients. Preliminary results have shown that the addition of fluorouracil and folinic acid to pre-operative radiotherapy significantly reduced tumour size, pTN stage, and significantly decreased lymphatic, venous and perineural invasion rates.[27]

The French Foundation of Digestive Cancerology (FFCD) 9203 study is a very similar French trial. Preliminary analysis was performed on 685 eligible patients. Surgery was performed 3–10 weeks after the treatment. Pre-operative chemo-radiotherapy significantly increased toxicity and tumour sterilisation as compared to radiotherapy alone. The postoperative mortality and sphincter preservation rate was unaltered.[28]

The Polish Sphincter Preservation Study randomised 316 patients between pre-operative long fractionation chemo-radiotherapy and the short five-fraction radiotherapy only. The results of this study have shown that pre-operative chemo-radiotherapy with surgery after an interval of 4–6 weeks offers no advantage in sphincter preservation in comparison to short fractionation radiotherapy and immediate surgery (58% versus 61%).[29]

Long-term results of these trials are awaited; of particular interest will be any change in the rate of local recurrence and disease-free or overall survival with the addition of chemotherapy to pre-operative radiotherapy.

PATIENT SELECTION AND ROLE OF MRI

High-resolution magnetic resonance imaging (MRI) has recently been reported to be a reliable tool for the pre-operative identification of the circumferential resection margin. MRI is superior to CT for the pre-operative assessment of potential circumferential resection margin and lymph node involvement. MRI is becoming a requirement in the pre-operative work-up of patients with rectal cancer. Tumour involvement of the circumferential resection margin is a strong predictor of local recurrence, likelihood of distant metastasis and survival after resection of rectal cancer.[30,31] MRI can provide reliable pre-operative information on the distance between the tumour and the proposed surgical resection margin and identify patients at high risk of circumferential resection margin involvement to select patients for neo-adjuvant therapy. Several studies[32] including the recent MERCURY trial[33] have shown that MRI is a reliable tool for selecting patients for neo-adjuvant therapy.

Key point 7

- Pre-operative MRI is mandatory for the evaluation of rectal cancer to assess the potential circumferential resection margin and to select the appropriate treatment option.

IMMUNOTHERAPY

Immunotherapy for cancer is not a new concept, but there have been several false dawns in its development. Nevertheless, interest in immunotherapy as adjuvant therapy in colorectal cancer is again increasing, as more is understood about the molecular biology of the immune response. Various tumour vaccines including against carcinoembryonic antigen (CEA) have been tried. Phase I/II trials are currently underway to assess the efficacy of tumour vaccines. Several monoclonal antibodies have shown promising results in advanced colorectal cancer. New treatment options are currently being evaluated as adjuvant treatment in colorectal cancer. The results of these trials are awaited with interest.

CETUXIMAB

Cetuximab is a monoclonal antibody against the epidermal growth factor receptor (EGFR). EGFR/HER1 is a member of the human epidermal growth factor receptor (HER) family of tyrosine kinase cell-surface receptors that are dysregulated in many types of tumour; its expression has been associated with poor prognosis in colon cancer.[34]

Cituximab has activity and little toxicity in colon cancers that are resistant to chemotherapy, both as a single agent and in combination with chemotherapy. It appears to be synergistic with irinotecan, even in irinotecan-resistant tumours. Experience with cetuximab in the treatment of colorectal cancer is presently limited to patients with advanced disease resistant to irinotecan. In this subgroup, the objective response rate with cetuximab alone is 10%, whereas the combination of cetuximab and irinotecan causes disease regression in about 22% of patients.[35]

BEVACIZUMAB (AVASTIN)

Bevacizumab is a recombinant, humanised monoclonal antibody against vascular endothelial growth factor (VEGF). Angiogenesis is critical for tumour growth and is also important for invasion and metastasis. VEGF, a diffusible glycoprotein produced by normal and neoplastic cells is an important regulator of physiological and pathological angiogenesis and is over-expressed in 48–53% of colorectal cancers.[36] In addition to its direct anti-angiogenic effects, bevacizumab may also improve the delivery of chemotherapy by altering tumour vasculature and decreasing the elevated interstitial pressure in tumours.[37,38]

In a large trial, 813 patients (who had received no previous therapy for metastatic colorectal cancer) were randomised to receive irinotecan, fluorouracil and folinic acid with either bevacizumab or a placebo. This trial demonstrated the superiority of the arm with bevacizumab in terms of median overall survival (20.3 months versus 15.6 months; $P < 0.001$), the objective response rate (44.8% versus 34.8%; $P = 0.004$), and median progression-free survival (10.6 months versus 6.2 months, $P < 0.001$). The main side effect of bevacizumab was grade III hypertension, reported in 11.0% of patients.[39] The US Food and Drug Administration has licensed bevacizumab for first-line treatment of metastatic colon cancer.

The use of bevacizumab and of cituximab in combination with adjuvant chemotherapy will now be explored in the adjuvant setting and holds out the promise of further incremental benefits. QUASAR 2 is a multicentre international study that will assess the role of bevacizumab as adjuvant treatment of colorectal cancer.

Key point 8

- Monoclonal antibodies in addition to chemotherapy have shown a 6-month increase in overall survival for metastatic colorectal cancer. Phase III trials are currently evaluating their role in adjuvant treatment.

Immunohistochemical studies and pharmacogenetics will probably play a bigger role in the future in identifying the markers predictive of response to different adjuvant treatments and the detection of gene abnormalities responsible for susceptibility to severe side effects in a particular patient.

CONCLUSIONS

Adjuvant chemotherapy has been standard treatment after curative resection of colorectal cancer in patients with lymph node positive disease. It also helps younger patients with poor prognostic variables even in the absence of disease in lymph nodes. 5-Fluorouracil and folinic acid are currently used as first-line chemotherapy. Newer agents are showing promise of improved outcomes and are likely to change practice in the years to come.

The role of adjuvant radiotherapy for rectal cancer is still evolving. MRI scan has become increasingly important to select patients for neo-adjuvant therapy. Pre-operative chemo-radiotherapy should be considered for patients with locally advanced rectal cancer or when circumferential resection margin is involved on MRI scan.

Monoclonal antibodies have shown promising results in advanced disease and are being evaluated in the adjuvant setting.

Key points for clinical practice

- Adjuvant chemotherapy using 5-fluorouracil and folinic acid is standard adjuvant treatment after curative resection of colorectal cancer in patients with lymph node positive disease.
- The data on the role of adjuvant chemotherapy for patients with Dukes' B (stage II) disease have been inconsistent. Chemotherapy should be offered as an adjuvant treatment to the younger and high-risk patients with Duke's B cancer.
- Oral adjuvant chemotherapy with capecitabine is becoming more popular and may replace intravenous therapy.
- Addition of irinotecan to chemotherapeutic regimens has shown promising results in advanced colorectal cancer but its use as an adjuvant therapy is not established yet.
- A short-term regimen of high-dose pre-operative radiotherapy reduces rates of local recurrence and improves survival among patients with resectable rectal cancer.
- Pre-operative radiotherapy does reduce the rate of local recurrence even when it was given before total mesorectal excision. The beneficial effect of pre-operative radiotherapy was more significant for tumours in mid-rectum.
- Pre-operative MRI is mandatory for the evaluation of rectal cancer to assess the potential circumferential resection margin and to select the appropriate treatment option.
- Monoclonal antibodies in addition to chemotherapy have shown a 6-month increase in overall survival for metastatic colorectal cancer. Phase III trials are currently evaluating their role in adjuvant treatment.

References

1. Pisani P, Parkin DM, Bray F, Ferlay J. Estimates of the worldwide mortality from 25 cancers in 1990. *Int J Cancer* 1999; **83**: 18–29.
2. Abulafi AM, Williams NS. Local recurrence of colorectal cancer: the problem, mechanisms, management and adjuvant therapy. *Br J Surg* 1994; **81**: 7–19.
3. Moertel CG, Fleming TR, Macdonald JS *et al.* Levamisole and fluorouracil for adjuvant therapy of resected colon carcinoma. *N Engl J Med* 1990; **322**: 352–358.
4. International Multicentre Pooled Analysis of Colon Cancer Trials (IMPACT) Investigators. Efficacy of adjuvant fluorouracil and folinic acid in colon cancer. *Lancet* 1995; **345**: 939–944.
5. Gray RG, Barnwell J, Hills R, McConkey C, Williams N, Kerr D, for the QUASAR Collaborative Group. QUASAR: a randomized study of adjuvant chemotherapy (CT) vs. observation including 3238 colorectal cancer patients [abstract]. *Proc Am Soc Clin Oncol* 2004; **23**: 3501.

6. Gill S, Loprinzi CL, Sargent DJ *et al*. Pooled analysis of fluorouracil-based adjuvant therapy for stage II and III colon cancer: who benefits and by how much? *J Clin Oncol* 2004; **22**: 1797–1806.
7. QUASAR Collaborative Group. Comparison of fluorouracil with additional levamisole, higher-dose folinic acid, or both, as adjuvant chemotherapy for colorectal cancer: a randomized trial. *Lancet* 2000; **355**: 1588–1596.
8. Cassidy J, Scheithauer W, McKendrick J *et al*. Capecitabine (X) vs. bolus 5-FU/LV as adjuvant therapy for colon cancer (the X-ACT study): positive efficacy results of a phase III trial [abstract]. *Proc Am Soc Clin Oncol* 2004; **23**: 3509.
9. Douillard J, Hoff PM, Skillings JR *et al*. Multicenter phase III study of uracil/Tegafur and oral leucovorin versus fluorouracil and leucovorin in patients with previously untreated metastatic colorectal cancer. *J Clin Oncol* 2002; **20**: 3605–3616.
10. De Gramont A, Figer A, Seymour M *et al*. Leucovorin and fluorouracil with or without oxaliplatin as first line treatment in advanced colorectal cancer. *J Clin Oncol* 2000; **18**: 2938–2947.
11. Giacchetti S, Perpoint B, Zidani R *et al*. Phase III multicentre randomized trial of oxaliplatin added to chronomodulated fluorouracil-leucovorin as first line treatment of metastatic colorectal cancer. *J Clin Oncol* 2000; **18**: 136–147.
12. Adam R. Chemotherapy and surgery: new perspectives on the treatment of unresectable liver metastases. *Ann Oncol* 2003; **ii (Suppl 2)**: 13–16.
13. Andre T, Boni C, Mounedji-Boudiaf L *et al*. Oxaliplatin, fluorouracil, and leucovorin as adjuvant treatment for colon cancer. The Multicenter International Study of Oxaliplatin/5-Fluorouracil/Leucovorin in the Adjuvant Treatment of Colon Cancer (MOSAIC) Investigators. *N Engl J Med* 2004; **350**: 2343–2351.
14. Sargent D, Wieand S, Goldberg R *et al*. *3 year DFS vs. 5 year OS as an endpoint for adjuvant colon cancer studies: data from randomized trials*. Rockville, MD: Food and Drug Administration, 2003.
15. Douillard JY, Cunningham D, Roth AD *et al*. Irinotecan combined with fluorouracil compared with fluorouracil alone as first line treatment for metastatic colorectal cancer: a multicentre randomised trial. *Lancet* 2000; **355**: 1041–1047.
16. Saltz LB, Niedzwiecki D, Hollis D *et al*. Irinotecan plus fluorouracil/leucovorin (IFL) versus fluorouracil/leucovorin alone (FL) in stage III colon cancer (Intergroup trial CALGB C89803) [abstract]. *Proc Am Soc Clin Oncol* 2004; **23**: 3500.
17. Colorectal Cancer Collaborative Group. Adjuvant radiotherapy for rectal cancer: a systematic overview of 8507 patients from 22 randomised trials. *Lancet* 2001; **358**: 1291–1304.
18. NIH Consensus Conference. Adjuvant therapy for patients with colon and rectal cancer. *JAMA* 1990; **264**: 1444–1450.
19. Wolmark N, Wieand HS, Hyamns DM *et al*. Randomised trial of post-operative adjuvant chemotherapy with or without radiotherapy for carcinoma of the rectum. National Surgical Adjuvant Breast and Bowel Project Protocol R-02. *J Natl Cancer Inst* 2000; **92**: 388–396.
20. Glimelius B, Isacsson U, Jung B, Pahlman L. Radiotherapy in addition to radical surgery in rectal cancer: evidence for a dose-response effect favouring preoperative treatment. *Int J Radiat Oncol Biol Phys* 1997; **37**: 281–287.
21. Goldberg PA, Nicholls RJ, Porter NH, Love S, Grimsey JE. Long-term results of a randomized trial of short-course low-dose adjuvant preoperative radiotherapy for rectal cancer: reduction in local treatment failure. *Eur J Cancer* 1994; **30A**: 1602–1606.
22. Swedish Rectal Cancer Trial. Improved survival with preoperative radiotherapy in resectable rectal cancer. *N Engl J Med* 1997; **336**: 980–987.
23. MacFarlane JK, Ryall RDH, Heald RJ. Mesorectal excision for rectal cancer. *Lancet* 1993; **341**: 457–460.
24. Kapiteijn E, Marijnen CA, Nagtegaal ID *et al*. Preoperative radiotherapy combined with total mesorectal excision for resectable rectal cancer. *N Engl J Med* 2001; **345**: 638–646.
25. Glimelius B. Chemoradiotherapy for rectal cancer – is there an optimal combination? *Ann Oncol* 2001; **12**: 1039–1045.
26. Sauer R, Fietkau R, Wittekind C *et al*. Adjuvant versus neoadjuvant combined modality treatment for locally advanced rectal cancer: first results of the German rectal cancer

study (CAO/ARO/AIO-94). *Int J Radiat Oncol Biol Phys* 2003; **57**: s124–s125.
27. Bosset JF, Calais G, Mineur L *et al*. Does the addition of chemotherapy (CT) to preoperative radiotherapy (preopRT) increase the pathological response in patients with resected rectal cancer? Report of the 22921 EORTC phase III trial [abstract]. *Proc Am Soc Clin Oncol* 2004; **23**: 3504.
28. Conroy T, Bonnetain F, Chapet O *et al*. Preoperative (preop) radiotherapy (RT) + 5FU/folinic acid (FA) in T3,4 rectal cancers: Preliminary results of the FFCD 9203 randomized trial [abstract]. *Proc Am Soc Clin Oncol* 2004; **23**: 3626.
29. Bujko K, Nowacki MP, Nasierowska-Guttmejer A *et al*. Sphincter preservation following preoperative radiotherapy for rectal cancer: report of a randomised trial comparing short-term radiotherapy vs. conventionally fractionated radio-chemotherapy. *Radiother Oncol* 2004; **72**: 15–24.
30. Birbeck KF, Macklin CP, Tiffin NJ *et al*. Rates of circumferential resection margin involvement vary between surgeons and predict outcomes in rectal cancer surgery. *Ann Surg* 2002; **235**: 449–457.
31. Wibe A, Rendedal PR, Svensson E *et al*. Prognostic significance of the circumferential resection margin following total mesorectal excision for rectal cancer. *Br J Surg* 2002; **89**: 327–334.
32. Beets-Tan RG, Beets GL, Vliegen RF *et al*. Accuracy of magnetic resonance imaging in prediction of tumour-free resection margin in rectal cancer surgery. *Lancet* 2001; **357**: 497–504.
33. Burton S, Daniels I, Stellakis M *et al*. Evaluation of the role of MRI in staging rectal cancer within the multidisciplinary team setting. *Colorectal Dis* 2004; **6 (Suppl. I)**: 34.
34. Grunwald V, Hidalgo M. Developing inhibitors of the epidermal growth factor receptor for cancer treatment. *J Natl Cancer Inst* 2003; **95**: 851–867.
35. Cunningham D, Humblet Y, Siena M *et al*. Cetuximab (C225) alone or in combination with irinotecan (CPT-11) in patients with epidermal growth factor receptor (EGFR)-positive, irinotecan-refractory metastatic colorectal cancer (MCRC) [abstract]. *Proc Am Soc Clin Oncol* 2003; **22**: 252.
36. Lee JC, Chow NH, Wang ST *et al*. Prognostic value of vascular endothelial growth factor expression in colorectal patients. *Eur J Cancer* 2000; **36**: 748–753.
37. Jain RK. Normalizing tumour vasculature with anti-angiogenic therapy: a new paradigm for combination therapy. *Nat Med* 2001; **7**: 987–989.
38. Willett CG, Boucher Y, di-Tomaso E *et al*. Direct evidence that the VEGF-specific antibody bevacizumab has antivascular effects in human rectal cancer. *Nat Med* 2004; **10**: 145–147.
39. Hurwitz H, Fehrenbacher L, Novotny W *et al*. Bevacizumab plus irinotecan, fluorouracil, and leucovorin for metastatic colorectal cancer. *N Engl J Med* 2004; **350**: 2335–2342.

Stella Vig Alison Halliday

12

Carotid endarterectomy

The suggestion that stroke might be caused by carotid atherosclerosis was made as early as 1856.[1] At post mortem, atherosclerotic plaque was found at the carotid bifurcation of patients dying of a stroke.[2] The first pre-mortem diagnostic cerebral angiogram was performed in 1927,[3] and in 1954, Eastcott *et al.*[4] first reported benefit from carotid artery resection in a patient with repeated transient ischaemic events.

INDICATIONS

Carotid endarterectomy is only worthwhile if the risks are less than the benefits. Patients with tight carotid stenosis may have symptoms but many have none, and recent large randomised controlled trials have now provided reliable data identifying who should undergo surgery.

SYMPTOMATIC

Amaurosis fugax, transient ischaemic attacks and mild strokes affecting the carotid territory are, when associated with tight ipsilateral carotid stenosis, symptoms that may be appropriately treated by carotid endarterectomy.

The North American Symptomatic Carotid Endarterectomy Trial (NASCET) and the European Carotid Surgery Trial (ECST) reported benefits of carotid endarterectomy in several thousand patients randomised to surgery with

Stella Vig MCh.FRCS(Gen Surg)
Consultant Vascular Surgeon, Mayday Hospital, Croydon, Surrey, UK
E-mail: svig@doctors.org.uk

Alison Halliday MS FRCS
Consultant Vascular Surgeon and Reader in Cardiovascular Sciences, St George's Hospital, Blackshaw Road, London SW17 0QT, UK (for correspondence)
E-mail: alison.halliday@stgeorges.nhs.uk

appropriate medical therapy or medical therapy alone.[5,6] NASCET reported that carotid endarterectomy was beneficial for patients who, within the previous 6 months had focal transient ischaemic attacks or non-disabling stroke, and who had carotid stenosis of 70–99% (but not occlusion). At follow-up, the 2-year risk of ipsilateral stroke was reduced by carotid endarterectomy from 26% to 9% ($P < 0.001$). The 30-day peri-operative stroke and death rate was 5.8%. Six patients with tight stenosis needed carotid endarterectomy to prevent 1 ipsilateral stroke in 2 years. The study was tightly controlled excluding patients with disabling stroke, uncontrolled hypertension, diabetes mellitus, unstable angina, myocardial infarction within the previous 6 months and those who had progressive neurological dysfunction, such as dementia.

The European Carotid Surgery Trial (ECST) mirrored NASCET's findings. Carotid endarterectomy reduced the risk of stroke and death over 3 years from 21.9% to 12.3% in patients who underwent carotid endarterectomy ($P < 0.01$). The ECST 30-day peri-operative stroke and death rate was 7.5%. The on-going US Veterans Administration trial was then stopped because ECST and NASCET data showed clear benefit with carotid endarterectomy for high-grade symptomatic stenoses.[7]

Benefit, however, was not clear for patients with lesser stenoses. In ECST, surgery for more moderate stenoses (30–69%) was of no benefit, as the surgical morbidity and mortality outweighed the gain in stroke-free survival.

Some apparent differences in NASCET and ECST results were explained by the use of alternative methods of measuring angiographic stenosis. In NASCET, maximal luminal diameter stenosis was compared with the diameter of the normal internal carotid artery past the bulb. The ECST method of measurement differed and an ECST stenosis of 70% was equivalent to a NASCET stenosis of 40%. When angiograms were re-measured using the NASCET method, the results of both trials were the same. For severe stenosis (ECST > 82%, NASCET > 70%), there was equal benefit from surgery and the relative risk of disabling stroke or death was halved.

For patients with less severe stenoses (ECST 70–79% = NASCET 50–69%), carotid endarterectomy reduced the relative risk of disabling stroke or death by 27% (95% CI, 15–44%).

Recent analysis by Rothwell *et al.*[8] has shown that benefit from endarterectomy depends not only on the severity of carotid stenosis but also on minimising delay to surgery after the presenting event. For maximum benefit, carotid endarterectomy should be done within 2 weeks of relevant hemispheric symptoms.

Key point 1

- Symptomatic patients with a > 70% carotid artery stenosis benefit from carotid endarterectomy.

ASYMPTOMATIC (NO FOCAL SYMPTOMS WITHIN 6 MONTHS)

The first evidence supporting prophylactic carotid endarterectomy was reported in 1993 by the US Veterans Administration hospitals' trial.[9] Four years after carotid endarterectomy, patients with carotid stenosis of 50% or greater (measured according to the NASCET method) had significantly fewer transient ischaemic attacks and strokes than controls (8% versus 20.6%; $P < 0.001$). In the surgical groups, the 30-day stroke and death rate was 4.3%.

A larger randomised trial, the Asymptomatic Carotid Atherosclerosis Study (ACAS), recruited patients with 60–99% stenosis (NASCET method).[10] The 5-year rate of ipsilateral stroke and death (including a very low rate of peri-operative stroke and death) was twice as high in the control group (11% versus 5.1% for carotid endarterectomy patients). Sixty-seven patients needed to have carotid endarterectomy to prevent one disabling stroke or death in 2 years.

The largest trial to date is the Asymptomatic Carotid Surgery Trial (ACST).[11] Patients were allocated to immediate versus delayed carotid endarterectomy (operation only if clearly needed). The non-peri-operative results favoured immediate carotid endarterectomy (stroke risks 3.8% versus 11%; gain 7.2%; 95% CI, 5.0–9.4; $P < 0.0001$). The overall 30-day stroke or death rate was 3.1% (95% CI, 2.3–4.1).

In asymptomatic patients younger than 75 years of age, with carotid stenosis of 70% or greater, immediate carotid endarterectomy halved the net 5-year stroke risk from about 12% to about 6% (including the 3% peri-operative hazard). The trialists cautioned that outside trials inappropriate selection of patients or poor surgery could obviate any benefit.

A recent Cochrane review cautions readers, suggesting that although there is significant evidence favouring carotid endarterectomy for asymptomatic carotid stenosis, the effect is small in terms of absolute risk reduction.[12]

Key point 2

- In asymptomatic patients younger than 75 years of age, with at least 70% carotid stenosis, immediate carotid endarterectomy halved the net 5-year stroke risk from about 12% to about 6% (this included 3% peri-operative hazard). Surgery should be considered in these patients providing results are comparable to those in trials. Carotid endarterectomy in appropriate asymptomatic patients should be considered beneficial as a long-term (5 or more years) strategy.

PRE-OPERATIVE ASSESSMENT

In the past, carotid angiography was routinely used to measure carotid stenosis and to investigate completeness of the circle of Willis. It was found to be unnecessarily hazardous and carotid duplex has now become the standard non-invasive tool for investigating carotid disease. Conventional angiography is now rarely used and may be replaced by safer magnetic resonance (MR) and CT angiography.[13] In symptomatic patients, a pre-operative CT or MRI is important because < 2% of patients have other significant brain pathology including malignant tumours, and operation may be inappropriate and dangerous.

Key point 3

- Pre-operative assessment should include up-to-date (< 2 weeks) carotid duplex and patients with stroke or hemispheric transient ischaemic attacks should have brain imaging. Before general or local anaesthesia, patients should have appropriate management of co-morbidity; half of deaths are due to cardiac disease.

ANAESTHESIA

Locoregional anaesthesia allows the surgeon and anaesthetist to assess cognitive and motor function during endarterectomy but it may be inappropriate for technically demanding carotid endarterectomies or anxious patients. A Cochrane review of local versus general anaesthesia for carotid endarterectomy reported data from seven randomised and 41 non-randomised studies.[14] Meta-analysis of non-randomised studies showed that local anaesthetic was associated with significant reductions in odds of death (35 studies), stroke (31 studies), stroke or death (26 studies), myocardial infarction (22 studies), and pulmonary complications (7 studies), within 30 days of operation. Meta-analysis of randomised studies showed that with local anaesthetic there was a significant reduction in postoperative haematoma within 30 days of operation, but no evidence of reduction in peri-operative stroke. Better evidence may come from an on-going large randomised control trial (GALA), which plans to randomise up to 5000 patients between general and local anaesthesia.

Key point 4

- Carotid endarterectomy may be safely performed under local or general anaesthetic.

OPERATIVE

INTRA-OPERATIVE TECHNIQUE

A conventional longitudinal carotid endarterectomy is described. The patient is positioned on the table with a head ring allowing extension of the neck and rotation of the head away from the operating side. The patient is placed slightly head up. If a patch is to be used, prophylactic antibiotics are given. Local anaesthetic with adrenaline may be infiltrated prior to the skin incision to decrease skin edge bleeding. A skin incision is made along the anteromedial border of sternocleidomastoid. After ligation of the common facial vein, the internal jugular vein is retracted laterally exposing the carotid sheath (Fig. 1). Heparin is given and the common, external and internal carotid arteries are exposed. Care is taken to identify and preserve the vagus and hypoglossal

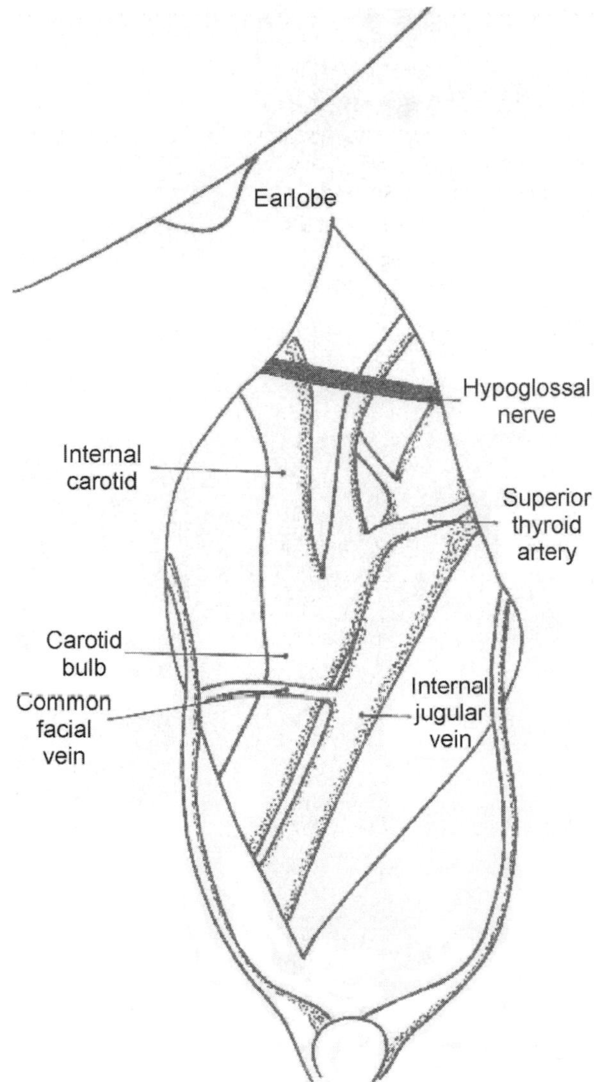

Fig. 1 Schematic representation of carotid exposure.

nerves; occasionally, the glossopharyngeal nerve is seen. The internal carotid artery is clamped first to prevent embolisation; after clamping an arteriotomy is made from common to normal distal internal carotid artery. A Javid or Pruitt-Inahara shunt may be placed to improve cerebral perfusion (Fig. 2).[15,16] A plane is developed with a Watson-Cheyne dissector ensuring that sufficient media in the artery wall is preserved. The plaque is carefully removed from common, external and involved internal carotid artery and the distal intima is tacked down with a 7/O prolene. This ensures that restored flow will not cause arterial dissection. After adequate flushing with heparin, the arteriotomy is closed primarily or using a patch. The external and common clamps are released allowing any potential emboli to be flushed into the external carotid

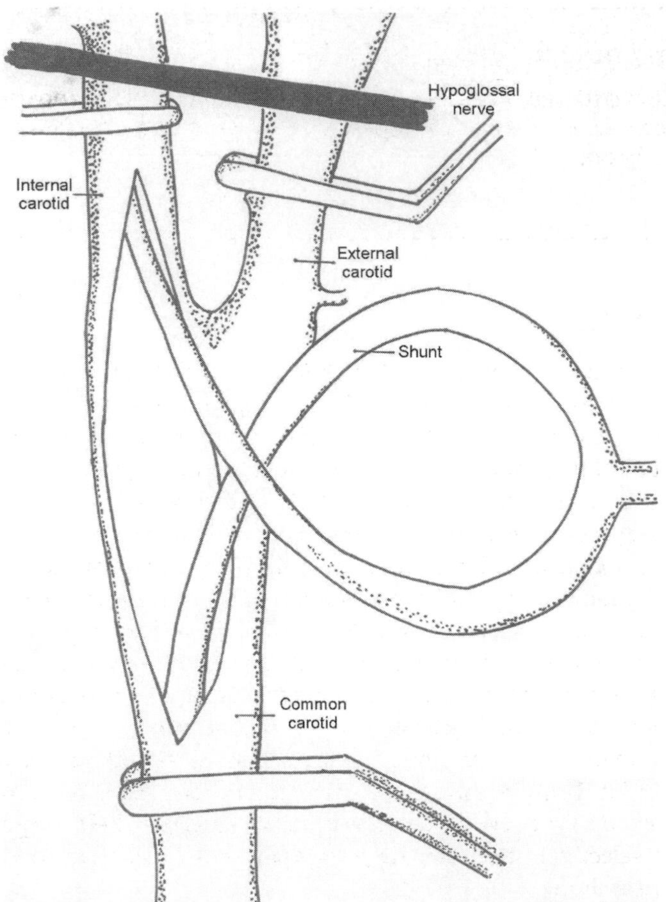

Fig. 2 Schematic representation of carotid with Pruitt-Inahara shunt *in situ*.

circulation. The internal clamp is then released restoring flow. After ensuring there is no bleeding, the neck is closed in layers over a suction drain, which is removed the next day. The patient is closely observed in recovery or high dependency unit for a few hours, and usually discharged within 2–3 days.

In conventional carotid endarterectomy, a longitudinal arteriotomy is used and the atherosclerotic plaque removed under direct vision. Eversion carotid endarterectomy (Ecarotid endarterectomy) technique uses transverse arteriotomy, 'blind' plaque removal and re-implantation of the carotid artery. A Cochrane review reported no significant differences in the rates of peri-operative stroke and/or death (1.7% versus 2.6%; odds ratio, 0.44; 95% CI, 0.10–1.82) and stroke during follow-up (1.4% versus 1.7%; OR, 0.84; 95% CI, 0.43–1.64) between eversion and conventional carotid endarterectomy techniques.[17] Ecarotid endarterectomy was associated with a significantly lower rate of re-stenosis > 50% during follow-up (2.5% versus 5.2%; OR, 0.48;, 95% CI, 0.32–0.72). There was no evidence that Ecarotid endarterectomy was safer than conventional carotid endarterectomy, and no differences in local complications between either techniques.

Key point 5

- Conventional and eversion techniques are both safe endarterectomy techniques and choice depends on experience of the individual surgeon.

MONITORING

The best direct test of cerebral function in awake patients is when carotid endarterectomy is carried out under locoregional anaesthesia. Clamping the internal carotid may cause focal or global hypoperfusion and an intraluminal shunt should be available for insertion if shunting is not a routine procedure. Although EEG may be accurate in detecting cerebral ischaemia, it is not widely used.[18] Indirect measurements of cerebral perfusion include stump pressure and transcranial Doppler. Stump pressure is measured by inserting a needle into the carotid artery and then clamping the external and common carotid arteries to detect internal carotid arterial backflow. Stump pressures below 25 mmHg are associated with increased likelihood of cerebral ischaemia.[19] Non-invasive transcranial Doppler monitoring is a direct measure of blood velocity in the middle cerebral artery. This cannot be used in 10–20% of patients because their temporal bone is too thick to detect intracranial flow.[20] Transcranial Doppler provides cerebral blood velocity throughout the operation and for a few hours after in recovery. It may help surgeons to shunt patients selectively and can help monitor shunt function and detect intra-operative emboli.

CEREBRAL PROTECTION – CAROTID SHUNT

Carotid artery clamping may reduce cerebral blood flow. If the circle of Willis is complete or nearly complete, the ipsilateral cerebral perfusion may be normal or adequate but an intraluminal carotid shunt may be required to restore flow. There are two types of shunt in common use – Javid and Pruitt-Inahara. The Pruitt-Inahara shunt is T-shaped, held in place with inflatable cuffs in common and internal carotid arteries (Fig. 3). The Javid shunt is tapered with bulbous proximal and distal ends that are held in place by clamps (Fig. 4). Shunts may be inserted selectively or routinely. There is no significant difference in peri-operative rates of all stroke, ipsilateral stroke or death in patients routinely or selectively shunted.[21]

PATCH OR NO PATCH

Patch angioplasty might reduce risk of postoperative stroke and carotid re-stenosis. A Cochrane review assessed safety and efficacy of routine or selective carotid patching compared with primary arterial closure.[22] Meta-analysis showed that carotid patch angioplasty was associated with reduction in risk of stroke (any type; OR, 0.33; P = 0.004), ipsilateral stroke (OR, 0.31; P = 0.0008),

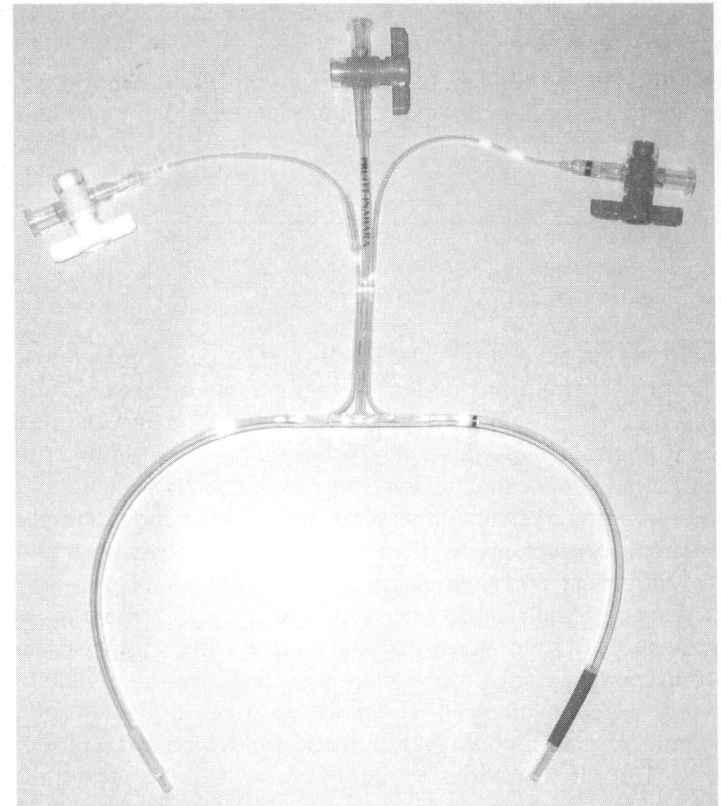

Fig. 3 A Pruitt-Inahara shunt.

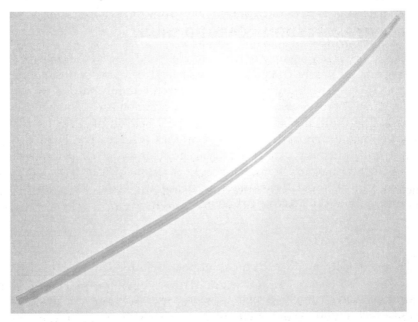

Fig. 4 A Javid shunt.

and stroke or death, both during the peri-operative period (OR, 0.39; $P = 0.007$) and during long-term follow-up (OR, 0.59; $P = 0.004$). There was also a reduced risk of peri-operative arterial occlusion (OR, 0.15; $P = 0.00004$) and decreased re-stenosis during long-term follow-up (OR, 0.20; $P < 0.00001$). Patch angioplasty may be carried out with vein, Dacron or PTFE. A further Cochrane review reported reduced peri-operative stroke risk and re-stenosis when PTFE patches were compared with collagen-impregnated Dacron grafts.[23] One possible long-term complication after patch angioplasty is development of carotid pseudo-aneurysms. Synthetic patches produced significantly fewer pseudo-aneurysms compared with vein (OR, 0.09).

Key point 6

- Patch angioplasty reduces risk of postoperative stroke and long-term re-stenosis.

QUALITY ASSURANCE

Strokes after carotid endarterectomy have a poor outlook. Apart from shunting and patching techniques, other intra-operative 'quality controls' have been used to try to minimise complications.

INTRA-OPERATIVE ANGIOSCOPY

Intra-operative completion angioscopy allows visualisation of the endarterectomised artery and distal internal carotid artery prior to release of the internal clamp. The use of angioscopy in 500 patients enabled intimal flaps to be repaired in 3% and luminal thrombus to be removed in 4% of patients.[24] This non-randomised series had an intra-operative stroke rate of 0.2%, ipsilateral embolic stroke occurred in 0.8% of patients, and the 30-day death/stroke rate was 2.2%.

INTRA-OPERATIVE DUPLEX

Duplex ultrasonography may be used after clamp removal to identify correctable abnormalities; in one series, 2.3% of patients had intimal flaps, free-floating clots, ICA stenoses, ICA pseudo-aneurysms or retrograde CCA dissection.[25] The overall stroke and death rate was 0.8%, but the study was uncontrolled. Comparison of intra-arterial angiography with duplex suggests that duplex has a higher sensitivity for detecting minor defects missed by angiography.[26]

POSTOPERATIVE CARE

Peri-operative complications of carotid endarterectomy include myocardial infarction, stroke, and death. Hypotension may lead to carotid thrombosis. Hypertension may cause haemorrhagic stroke, wound haematoma or hyperperfusion syndrome.

In the postoperative phase, Dextran 40 has been shown to reduce embolic signals thereby reducing the risk of postoperative stroke.[27]

COMPLICATIONS

STROKE

Postoperative stroke risk depends on case selection, anaesthetic and surgical technique. Data from the NASCET and ECST trials reported 30-day peri-operative stroke and death rates between 5.8% and 7.3%; in asymptomatic patients this was lower (2–4%).[5–7,9–11]

CRANIAL NERVE INJURY

Intra-operative risk of cranial nerve injury is 5% with 4% persisting beyond hospital discharge and 1% present after 1 year.[28] The commonest injury is to the hypoglossal nerve followed by the marginal branch of the mandibular, then the recurrent laryngeal nerve.

BLEEDING/HAEMATOMA FORMATION

Large or rapidly expanding haematomas require urgent re-exploration, as there is a risk of airway obstruction.

HYPERPERFUSION SYNDROME

This is uncommon but dangerous. Hyperaemic cerebral perfusion can cause cerebral oedema and haemorrhagic stroke. Patients may complain of severe headache that improves with blood pressure control. Postoperative hyper-perfusion may be rapidly detected and treatment monitored using transcranial Doppler.

RECURRENT STENOSIS

Clinically significant recurrent stenoses are uncommon and patients are not routinely followed beyond 6 weeks after operation. Late occlusion and recurrent stenosis may be as low as 0.6% and 0.5%, respectively.[29] Re-stenoses may often occur at the site of a residual anatomical defect or stenosis.[30] Patch angioplasty may decrease the risk of long-term re-stenosis especially in females who appear at an increased risk.

SUMMARY

Carotid endarterectomy has now been proven to prevent fatal and disabling stroke in patients with symptomatic and asymptomatic carotid disease. Benefit from carotid endarterectomy only occurs if the complication rate of the procedure is low. Low complications rates are achievable with meticulous surgical technique, monitoring and quality assurance.

Key points for clinical practice

- Symptomatic patients with a > 70% carotid artery stenosis benefit from carotid endarterectomy.
- In asymptomatic patients younger than 75 years of age, with at least 70% carotid stenosis, immediate carotid endarterectomy halved the net 5-year stroke risk from about 12% to about 6% (this included 3% peri-operative hazard). Surgery should be considered in these patients providing results are comparable to those in trials. Carotid endarterectomy in appropriate asymptomatic patients should be considered beneficial as a long-term (5 or more years) strategy.
- Pre-operative assessment should include up-to-date (< 2 weeks) carotid duplex and patients with stroke or hemispheric transient ischaemic attacks should have brain imaging. Before general or local anaesthesia, patients should have appropriate management of co-morbidity; half of deaths are due to cardiac disease.
- Carotid endarterectomy may be safely performed under local or general anaesthetic.
- Conventional and eversion techniques are both safe endarterectomy techniques and choice depends on experience of the individual surgeon.
- Patch angioplasty reduces risk of postoperative stroke and long-term re-stenosis.

References

1. Savory WS. Case of a young woman in whom the main arteries of both upper extremities and of the left side of the neck were completely obliterated. *Med Chir Trans Lond* 1856; **39**: 205–219.
2. Fisher M. Occlusion of the carotid arteries: further experiences. *Arch Neurol Psychiatry* 1954; **72**: 187–204.
3. Moniz E. L'encephalographic arterielle: son importance dans la localization des tumeurs cerebrales. *Rev Neurol* 1927; **2**: 72–90.
4. Eastcott HHG, Pickering GW, Rob C. Reconstruction of internal carotid artery in a patient with intermittent hemiplegia. *Lancet* 1954; **2**: 994–996.
5. European Carotid Surgery Trialists' Collaborative Group. MRC European Carotid Surgery Trial: interim results for patients with severe (70–99%) or with mild (0–29%) carotid stenosis. *Lancet* 1991; **337**: 1235–1243.
6. North American Symptomatic Carotid Endarterectomy Trial Collaborators. Beneficial effects of carotid endarterectomy in symptomatic patients with high grade stenosis. *N Engl J Med* 1991; **325**: 445–453.
7. Mayberg MR, Wilson SE, Yatsu F *et al*. Carotid endarterectomy and prevention of cerebral ischemia in symptomatic carotid stenosis. *JAMA* 1991; **266**: 3289–3294.
8. Rothwell PM, Eliasziw M, Gutnikov SA, Warlow CP, Barnett HJ, Carotid Endarterectomy Trialists Collaboration. Endarterectomy for symptomatic carotid stenosis in relation to clinical subgroups and timing of surgery. *Lancet* 2004; **363**: 915–924.
9. Hobson RW, Weiss DG, Fields WS *et al*. Efficacy of carotid endarterectomy for asymptomatic carotid stenosis. The Veterans Affairs Cooperative Study Group. *N Engl J Med* 1993; **328**: 221–227.

10. Asymptomatic Study Executive Committee. Endarterectomy for asymptomatic carotid artery stenosis. *JAMA* 1995; **273**: 1421–1428.
11. MRC Asymptomatic Carotid Surgery Trial (ACST) Collaborative Group. Prevention of disabling and fatal strokes by successful carotid endarterectomy in patients without recent neurological symptoms: randomised controlled trial. *Lancet* 2004; **363**: 1491–1499.
12. Chambers BR, You RX, Donnan GA. Carotid endarterectomy for asymptomatic carotid stenosis (Cochrane Review). The Cochrane Library, Issue 4, 2004.
13. Griewing B, Morgensten C, Driesner F *et al*. Cerebrovascular disease assessed by color-flow and power Doppler ultrasonography. Comparison with digital subtraction angiography in internal carotid stenosis. *Stroke* 1996; **27**: 95–100.
14. Rerkasem K, Bond R, Rothwell PM. Local versus general anaesthesia for carotid endarterectomy. *Cochrane Database System Rev* 2004(2): CD000126.
15. Javid H, Julian OC, Dye WS *et al*. Seventeen-year experience with routine shunting in carotid artery surgery. *World J Surg* 1979; **3**: 167–177.
16. Pruitt C. Vascular shunting. *Contemp Surg* 1983; **23**: 1.
17. Cao PG, De Rango P, Zannetti S, Giordano G, Ricci S, Celani MG. Eversion versus conventional carotid endarterectomy for preventing stroke (Cochrane Review). The Cochrane Library, Issue 4, 2004.
18. Pistolese GR., Appolloni A, Ronchery S *et al*. Update on cerebral monitoring and protective methods. *Ann Ital Chir* 1997; **68**: 441–451.
19. Moore WS, Hall AD. Carotid artery back pressure: a test of cerebral tolerance to temporary carotid occlusion. *Arch Surg* 1969; **99**: 702–710.
20. Benichou H, Berferon P, Ferandi M *et al*. Doppler transcranien pre et peroperatoire: prevision et surveillance de la tolerance au clampage carotidien. *Ann Chir Vasc* 1991; **5**: 21–25.
21. Bond R, Rerkasem K, Counsell C *et al*. Routine or selective carotid artery shunting for carotid endarterectomy (and different methods of monitoring in selective shunting). *Cochrane Database System Rev* 2002(2): CD000190.
22. Bond R, Rerkasem K, AbuRahma AF, Naylor AR, Rothwell PM. Patch angioplasty versus primary closure for carotid endarterectomy. *Cochrane Database System Rev* 2004(2): CD000160.
23. Bond R, Rerkasem K, Naylor R, Rothwell PM. of different types for carotid patch angioplasty. *Cochrane Database System Rev* 2004(2): CD000071.
24. Naylor AR, Hayes PD, Allroggen H *et al*. Reducing the risk of carotid surgery: a 7-year audit of the role of monitoring and quality control assessment. *J Vasc Surg* 2000; **32**: 750–759.
25. Ascher E, Markevich N, Kallakuri S, Schutzer RW, Hingorani AP. Intraoperative carotid artery duplex scanning in a modern series of 650 consecutive primary endarterectomy procedures. *J Vasc Surg* 2004; **39**: 416–420.
26. Valenti D, Gaggiano A, Berardi G *et al*. Intra-operative assessment of technical defects after carotid endarterectomy: a comparison between angiography and colour duplex scan. *Cardiovasc Surg* 2003; **11**: 26–29.
27. Levi CR, Stork JL, Chambers BR *et al*. Dextran reduces embolic signals after carotid endarterectomy. *Ann Neurol* 2001; **50**: 544–547.
28. Cunningham EJ, Bond R, Mayberg MR, Warlow CP, Rothwell PM. Risk of persistent cranial nerve injury after carotid endarterectomy. *J Neurosurg* 2004; **101**: 445–448.
29. Ballotta E, Da Giau G, Piccoli A, Baracchini C. Durability of carotid endarterectomy for treatment of symptomatic and asymptomatic stenoses. *J Vasc Surg* 2004; **40**: 270–278.
30. Padayachee TS, Arnold JA, Thomas N, Aukett M, Colchester AC, Taylor PR. Correlation of intra-operative duplex findings during carotid endarterectomy with neurological events and recurrent stenosis at one year. *Eur J Vasc Endovasc Surg* 2002; **24**: 435–439.

Stephen G.E. Barker Sayed Aly
Jane Turner Richard Leigh

13

Ulceration and the diabetic foot

Diabetic patients are 4 times more likely to develop peripheral vascular disease (PVD), with a 5-times greater likelihood of developing critical limb ischaemia.[1,2] Ischaemic changes can contribute to ulceration. A diminished blood supply following stenosis or occlusion in the lower limb causes the tissues and skin to become atrophic and easily damaged. Small abrasions simply may not heal and infections may not clear.

Nerve damage in the diabetic foot may result from the direct effect of sugars on the nerve and the formation of sorbitol via the polyol pathway. This causes demyelination of large fibres, or on the vasa nervorum, causing nerve ischaemia.[3] Platelet plugging of the vasa nervorum might occur also. The resulting neuropathy contributes to ulceration in the feet in three ways:

1. *Sensory neuropathy* – loss of sensitivity to pain. Trauma can occur without the patient feeling any damage.

2. *Autonomic neuropathy* – the skin of the lower limbs become 'anhydrotic' (due to decreased sweating), losing elasticity. Subsequent cracking of the

*Colour figures (plates) referred to in this chapter are to be found in the 'Colour plates section' at the front of this volume (p1–8).

Stephen G.E. Barker MS FRCS
Senior Lecturer/Consultant, The Academic Vascular Surgery Unit, Middlesex Hospital, Mortimer Street, London W1T 3AA, UK. E-mail: stephen.barker@ucl.ac.uk. (for correspondence)

Sayed Aly PhD FRCS
Consultant Vascular & Endovascular Surgeon, Mater University Hospital, Eccles Road, Dublin 7, Ireland. E-mail: sayed@doctors.org.uk

Jane Turner BSc
Research Assistant, The Academic Vascular Surgery Unit, Middlesex Hospital, Mortimer Street, London W1T 3AA, UK

Richard Leigh BSc MChS
Chief Podiatrist, Department of Podiatry, UCLH Trust, Middlesex Hospital, Cleveland Street, London W1T 8AA, UK. E-mail: podiatry.dept@uclh.org

skin creates a portal of entry for infection. Arterio-venous shunting may help predispose Charcot's arthropathy (Plate XI, p6).

3. *Motor neuropathy* – muscle imbalance in the foot may cause deformity and clawing of the toes. These changes increase load on the metatarsals, promoting callus formation and 'cavitation' of deeper tissues. Interstitial fluid ruptures to the skin's surface, allowing bacteria to enter and infection to develop (Plate XII, p6).

Key point 1

- Diabetic foot ulcers are contributed to by: (i) sensory, motor and autonomic neuropathy; (ii) ischaemia; and (iii) infection.

IMAGING TECHNIQUES

ANKLE-BRACHIAL PRESSURE INDEX

The ankle-brachial pressure index (ABPI) is often employed as a screening tool but, in many patients with significant stenosis in the lower extremities, it would be missed with ABPI measurements alone. In a comparative study of both colour duplex ultrasound and ankle-brachial index measurements,[4] the ABPI had a low sensitivity, but a high specificity. However, the often-calcified vessels in the diabetic foot can invalidate the ratio as the vessels remain incompressible.

Key point 2

- The ankle-brachial pressure index is very often misleading.

DUPLEX ULTRASOUND

Duplex ultrasound assesses both anatomical and functional abnormality in the various arterial segments. Significant stenosis is indicated by a peak systolic velocity ratio greater than two across the arterial lesion.[5–7] Waveform analysis can give additional information about the degree of stenosis.

TRANSCUTANEOUS OXYGEN PRESSURE MAPPING

Transcutaneous oxygen pressure ($TcPO_2$) mapping can be used to determine the severity of foot ischaemia, thus aiding selection of appropriate treatment and decreasing the total cost of care. Studies show that if transmetatarsal $TcPO_2$ level is 30 mmHg or greater, treatment should be conservative comprising local wound care, debridement, or a more minor ablative procedure.[8] If the transmetatarsal $TcPO_2$ level is below 30 mmHg, it will anticipate the need for vascular reconstruction. An initial, or post-intervention transmetatarsal $TcPO_2$

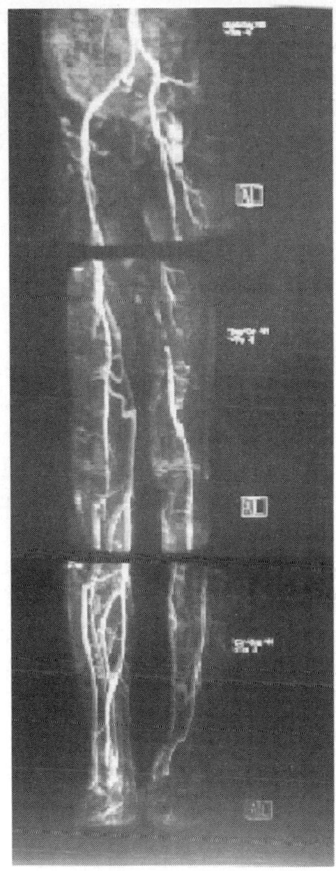

Fig. 1 MRA – femoral and distal disease of left leg.

level of 30 mmHg or greater was more accurate than a palpable pedal pulse in predicting ultimate wound healing, or resolution of rest pain.[9–11]

ANGIOGRAPHY

Angiography remains the 'gold standard' for assessment of the lower arterial system prior to any intervention. It can be performed via femoral or brachial catheterisation, with iodine-based contrast used to visualise the blood vessels. Angiography is not without complication, in particular; bleeding, dissection, embolisation, and nephrotoxicity (especially at starting blood creatinine levels of 110 mmol or more). Intravascular contrast injection is associated with an increased risk of lactic acidosis; a condition that can have a high mortality, especially in diabetics on Metformin.

MAGNETIC RESONANCE ANGIOGRAPHY

Magnetic resonance angiography (MRA) is likely to be the future investigation of choice. Current systems give clear visualisation of vessels above knee level, but tend to give rather 'fuzzy' images of crural vessels distally. Diabetic patients with poor renal function may benefit from MRA (Fig. 1). One comparative study has shown MRA to be significantly better than digital subtraction angiography (DSA) in revealing peripheral run-off vessels and patent pedal vessels suitable for distal bypass grafting.[12]

If osteomyelitis is suspected, plain radiographs remain of use. Three-phase bone scintigraphy, or infection-specific radiopharmaceuticals may aid diagnosis. MR imaging is extremely valuable to show even very early infection, with changes in bone marrow, oedema of soft tissues, cavitation and sinus formation.

INFECTION

In diabetic ulceration, granulocyte motility and activity is slowed[13–15] and the epidermis is compromised, exposing deeper structures. Due to the suppressed immune state overall, diabetic foot ulcers tend to acquire rapid, poly-microbial infection; often a mixture of Gram-positive, Gram-negative and anaerobic strains.[16] Bacteria that overcome the host defences quickly colonise the wound,[17] increasing in density until their cell signalling increases ('quorum sensing') and gene expression alters.[18] This bacterial response produces a three-dimensional polysaccharide matrix,[19] forming a 'biofilm', which increases virulence,[20] lessens the host response to bacteria[21] and increases antimicrobial resistance.[22] This 'bioburden' may be responsible for delayed wound healing[23] where bacterial numbers reach 'critical colonisation' with no overt host response,[24] or infection when the 'bioburden' reaches beyond the point of critical colonisation (10^5 bacteria/g)[25] and bacteria invade the tissues causing direct cell damage. Necrotic tissue should be debrided to reduce the 'bioburden'. Similarly, infected bone requires proper surgical debridement to enable healing.[26,27]

Key point 3

- Diabetic foot ulcers tend to acquire a poly-microbial infection including Gram-positive and Gram-negative bacteria as well as anaerobic strains.

On presentation of an infected diabetic foot ulcer, deep swabs or a tissue biopsy should be taken for microbiological culture and microscopy.[28,29] Initially, all cellulitic infections should be treated with triple agent, broad-spectrum antibiotic cover until sensitivities become available to focus treatment. Spreading cellulitis, deep sepsis, or osteomyelitis should be treated initially with intravenous antibiotics, then oral antibiotic cover for several weeks (Plate XIII, p7).

MANAGEMENT OF ARTERIAL DISEASE

Management of the diabetic foot remains a complex clinical problem and an aggressive multidisciplinary approach to diabetic foot disease involving the primary care provider, medical specialists, interventional radiology, podiatry, and plastic and vascular surgeons will provide optimal medical and surgical care. The principles of diabetic wound care include correction of systemic factors; such as blood glucose control, cardiovascular risk-factor management and smoking, and correction of local factors, such as wound debridement, pressure relief, infection control and revascularisation when indicated. Regular and careful inspection of the leg and foot becomes essential.

Early investigation becomes important when a patient presents with evidence of infection. Subsequently, adequate drainage and antibiotic therapy are mandatory. If an infected foot requires surgical debridement, or open partial forefoot amputation, observing the wound on a daily basis is important. A wound free from necrotic tissue should be maintained in a moist, warm environment to encourage the cellular division and migration of epithelium required for healing. Exudate should be managed to prevent the wound from bathing in fluid, or from completely drying out.

Key point 4

- Diabetic foot infections should be treated promptly with triple antibiotic therapy and appropriate surgery.

Once infection is eradicated, improved signs of healing, including the development of wound granulation, normally occur in a few days. If wounds are not showing signs of improved healing, arteriography is necessary. Early drainage, debridement, and local foot amputations combined with liberal use of revascularisation results in a cumulative limb salvage rate of greater than 70% at 5 years in high-risk groups.[30–33]

In 1999, the American Diabetes Association recognised several basic principles of diabetic wound healing: (i) off-loading; (ii) debridement; (iii) use of appropriate dressings; (iv) antibiotics; and (v) vascular reconstruction and amputation, or reconstructive foot surgery when necessary.

The indication for vascular reconstruction in a diabetic population is as in non-diabetics and can be in the form of either endovascular therapy, by-pass surgery, or a combination of both. Advanced 'run-off' disease to begin with is, however, associated with a high incidence of major amputation.

ENDOVASCULAR MANAGEMENT

Balloon angioplasty, with or without stent placement, is used for most inflow vessel and femoro-popliteal lesions. The outcome depends on the site, length, morphology of the lesion and the state of the distal run-off vessels. Currently, stents are metallic and permanent and may be self-expanding, or require balloon expansion.

Balloon angioplasty for distal popliteal and crural run-off vessels is achievable using a small balloon for a short stenosis. However, complications may risk losing the entire vessel and associated run-off. At present, there is no clear evidence in the literature to support routine distal balloon angioplasty.

BYPASS SURGERY

It is likely that there is no significant difference between diabetics and non-diabetics as to bypass graft patency, number of re-interventions and amputations. Diabetes *per se* is not a contraindication in attempting vascular surgical procedures in patients with critical leg ischaemia.[34]

Key point 5

- Diabetes *per se* is not a contraindication in attempting revascularisation. However, advanced arterial 'run-off' disease is associated with a high incidence of amputation.

In-flow vessel disease is common in diabetic patients. In a recent study, diabetic patients comprised a greater proportion of the total number of patients requiring inflow bypass, as well as a greater proportion of patients requiring subsequent outflow bypass for unresolved ischaemic symptoms.[35,36] In-flow reconstructions can be achieved surgically with an aorto-bifemoral, or axillo-bifemoral bypass in cases of bilateral disease. Femoro-femoral crossover, or ilio-femoral bypass can be used in unilateral disease. Femoral endartectomy, with or without a profundoplasty, remains a very useful and simple procedure.

INFRA-INGUINAL BYPASS SURGERY IN THE DIABETIC FOOT

In both diabetic and non-diabetic patients, the indications and patency rates for infra-inguinal bypass surgery necessitate good inflow alongside reasonable run-off vessels. Absence of either will lead to the failure of the graft. However, severe, circumferential calcification of patent outflow target arteries should not dissuade vascular surgeons from attempting distal bypass grafting for limb salvage.

The favoured graft material for surgeons is long saphenous vein, but arm vein can be a substitute. In the absence of vein, prosthetics can be used. Although the type of prosthetic used for above-knee femoro-popliteal bypass grafts does not seem to affect 5-year patency rates, patient age and graft size do. The risk for graft occlusion is significantly increased for those less than 65 years of age and for grafts with a diameter less than 7 mm.[37]

In a study of bypass grafts to a single crural, or pedal vessel, with critical lower limb ischaemia, it was found that the patency rate of femoro-tibial and peroneal bypass depended on the inflow state, the availability of a venous conduit, the number of calf vessels patent, the presence of straight flow to the foot and the presence of patent pedal vessels.[38] These factors can help in the selection of patients for femoro-distal reconstruction and may explain the wide variation in published results.[39,40] In the absence of a good venous conduit, a synthetic graft can be used with a distal vein cuff.

Currently, there is interest to use a 'short' bypass for infra-popliteal reconstruction, especially in diabetic patients. In a retrospective review of almost 2000 bypass grafts with distal anastomoses to infra-popliteal vessels, primary patency, secondary patency and foot salvage rates at 2 years were 60%, 65%, and 77%, respectively (for the severe calcification group), and 74%, 82%, and 93%, respectively (for the no calcification group). Good results can be achieved in the majority of diabetic patients undergoing short popliteal-distal bypasses.[41] An alternative combines intra-operative balloon angioplasty (IBA) of the superficial femoral artery with a distal bypass graft originating from the popliteal artery, as a method of lower extremity revascularisation in diabetic patients.[42]

Where failing infra-inguinal bypass grafts are identified by duplex ultrasound, diabetic patients should undergo a prompt and detailed angiographic evaluation. Despite a high recurrent stenoses rate (48%), high rates of limb salvage (93%) and assisted primary graft patency (79%) justify routine duplex surveillance, pre-operative angiography and aggressive graft revision in diabetic patients with infra-inguinal grafts.[43]

Prognostic factors for early failure of bypass to the foot in diabetic patients with critical ischaemia have been examined.[44] Vein graft of questionable quality, major wound healing problems, use of the reversed vein technique and a narrow lumen (< 1.5 mm) of the recipient artery, increased the likelihood of failed primary patency. Conversely, short vein bypass, translocated or composite veins, major postoperative oedema of the leg, or questionable quality of the wall of the recipient artery had no significant independent effect. A combination of chronic renal failure and very limited foot circulation has a significant adverse outcome; current literature indicates poor survival and limb salvage rates in diabetic patients with renal failure who present with ulcerated or gangrenous lower extremities (Plate XIV, p7). Even in those limbs that were successfully revascularised, the amputation rate was as high as 37%.[45,46] The low cost of revascularisation (average, £4320) compared with amputation (primary amputation, £12,730) justifies attempted reconstruction. However, repeated attempts to reconstruct the limbs of patients with severe distal disease who may benefit more from primary amputation, will significantly increase the cost: a failed bypass leading to amputation costing, on average, £17,066.

FREE FLAP TRANSFER

Aggressive attempts at revascularisation have extended the time limits for limb salvage. However, prior extensive tissue loss compromises the later healing process. This often results in amputation despite bypass graft patency. Microvascular free tissue transfer combined with arterial revascularisation may allow healing and, hence, limb preservation. The advantages of this technique are that it provides immediate soft-tissue coverage, limiting the amputation level and improving healing time, resulting in early ambulation. It provides extra run-off for any revascularisation as illustrated by a decrease in peripheral resistance, contributing to graft patency. The application of healthy, well-vascularised tissue limits infection and enhances neovascularisation. Thereby, the limb is preserved. This combined plastics and vascular approach is the ultimate alternative to amputation.

A pedal bypass (using autogenous vein graft) combined with a free muscle flap was performed in 13 patients with critical leg ischaemia. Patency was achieved in 11 cases 6-months' postoperatively.[47] Similar results have been reported elsewhere.[48–53] However, the combination of diabetes and chronic renal insufficiency, particularly with a need for dialysis, is a powerful predictor of failure and should be considered a strong contraindication for this procedure.[54]

AMPUTATION IN DIABETES

Limb salvage is one of the cardinal aims of vascular surgery. The incidence and indications for major limb amputations and infra-popliteal bypass during two consecutive 16-month periods were analysed.[46] There was an increase in the incidence of bypasses to the infra-popliteal arteries (and a corresponding decrease in the number of major amputations). Factors that may have contributed to this increase include the availability of DSA and a change in referral patterns within the hospital so that, with the exception of trauma, all patients considered for major amputation were initially assessed by a vascular surgeon.

Amputations of lower extremities can be classified into major limb amputation and foot amputation. Major limb amputations can be above-knee, or below-knee (with trans-femoral, Gritti-Stokes and knee disarticulation also described). Foot amputations can be a definitive treatment, or in combination with bypass surgery. These are classified as: ray amputation for toe necrosis; Chopart's mid-tarsal amputation; Lisfranc's tarso-metatarsal joint amputation; Syme's amputation, or through ankle.

Total calcanectomy is described as an alternative procedure to trans-tibial amputation in patients with chronic osteomyelitis of the calcaneus, achieving eradication of infection and the preservation of improved functional ambulation. In a review of eight patients treated with a total calcanectomy for a chronic non-healing plantar ulcer of the heel and osteomyelitis of the calcaneus, four patients maintained the same ambulation level postoperatively in a modified heel-containment orthosis.[55–57]

'OFF-LOADING' AND PRESENT APPLIANCES

Removing, or re-distributing mechanical force – 'off-loading' – from a diabetic foot is an important factor in wound care and can alter skin physiology.[58] There are several devices and techniques used for off-loading:

1. Clinical padding, such as semi-compressed felt.
2. Orthotic management, using various types of foam sponge which can be added to pre-fabricated insoles used in clinic, or layered in bespoke insoles.
3. Footwear with adjustable insoles, such as the 'DH boot'.
4. Total contact casting (TCC) is a specialist technique using felts, stockinette, plaster of Paris bandage and fibreglass plaster, to prevent movement at the ankle and transfer weight to the lower leg.
5. The Scotch cast boot is similar to the TCC, but finishes below the ankle and often contains a 'window' in the cast.
6. Pneumatic Walker (Air-cast) is a full-length plastic boot that works in a similar way to TTC, using internal balloons to achieve weight transfer.
7. Pressure Relieving Ankle Foot Orthosis (PRAFO) is a device for off-loading, utilising a metal frame with adjustable strapping and footing.
8. Charcot's Restraint Orthotic Walker (CROW) is a removable, lined, plastic full-length boot which is moulded to a cast of the patient's leg and foot. It tends to be used for patients with foot deformity (as seen in Charcot's arthropathy, sometimes with severe ulceration).
9. Crutches, Zimmer frames or wheelchairs can be used to aid off-loading, under the supervision of a physiotherapist.

> **Key point 6**
>
> - Avoiding focused pressure areas – 'off-loading' – is an essential element of prevention and treatment of diabetic foot ulcers.

HYPERBARIC OXYGEN

Reversal of hypoxia halts the progression of diabetic neuropathy, lending further support to the role of hypoxia in the pathogenesis of nerve destruction in diabetes mellitus.[59]

Patients undergoing hyperbaric oxygen therapy rest in a chamber which is pressurised to 2–3 times atmospheric pressure with 100% oxygen. Breathing the hyperbaric oxygen increases patients' haemoglobin and plasma oxygen concentrations. Hyper-oxygenated blood has several beneficial effects on damaged tissues. Poorly perfused tissues receive increased oxygen, reducing ischaemic damage and increase the fibroblast division necessary for matrix formation; microvascular angiogenesis, antimicrobial activity, phagocytosis and white cell activity are increased; vasoconstriction occurs, reducing oedema and the loss of grafted skin. Leukocyte action is suppressed, so peri-wound tissues may be preserved.

MANAGEMENT IN THE COMMUNITY

Defined care pathways between acute and community sites are essential in care of diabetic foot ulcers. Close liaison between acute and community sites should target foot health, preventive care and simple screening procedures. Also, they should ensure ease of access to podiatry clinics and specialist care when problems arise. Joint working structures should be formed so that wound care is agreed between practitioners. These strategies will enable patients to leave hospital at the earliest convenient time. Equality of service provision for minority groups may need addressing. Establishing review and audit systems will determine outcomes and facilitate efficacy of practice.

> **Key point 7**
>
> - The management of diabetic foot ulcers is multidisciplinary and necessitates close liaison with acute and community healthcare workers.

TREATING DIABETIC ULCERATION

Current treatments for diabetic foot ulceration broadly include:

1. *Removal of necrotic tissue with desloughing agents*: hydrocolloids, larvae, enzymes.
2. *Managing exudate*: polyurethane foams, capillarity dressings, Kerraboot, Vacuum Assisted Closure (VAC), alginates, cellulose composites, non-adherent dressings, film dressings.

3. *Skin grafting and replacement tissue*: autologous and heterologous skin replacements, bioengineered dermal fibroblasts.
4. *Growth factors*: platelet derived growth factor (PDGF).
5. *Reducing the bacterial bioburden*: topical antiseptics, topical antibiotics, iodine-releasing dressings/solutions/spray/ointments, honey, chlorhexadine or iodine impregnated tulle gras, charcoal-based dressings.
6. *Aiding cell motility*: Hyaluronan.

Some of the latest products available include:

Silver-impregnated dressings
With the evolution of organisms with multiresistance to antibiotics, the introduction of silver-impregnated dressings has emerged. Silver can be added to many dressing types, thereby combining the effectiveness of the dressing with antimicrobial activity.

The Kerraboot®
The Kerraboot® is a non-contact wound-care device comprising a plastic boot with a super-absorbant footpad. It maintains warmth and moisture at the wound site, necessary to promote angiogenesis and epithelialisation. Free drainage from the ulcer site prevents accumulation of growth-inhibitory exudate. Odour is virtually eliminated by use of a 'trapping' layer forming part of the boot's overall construction.

THE FUTURE

The nation has become sedentary, generally more obese and, on average, older. These are risk factors associated with an increased risk of developing diabetes. As the number of patients with diabetes rises, we are met with the challenges of detection and prevention. Type 2 diabetes is often detected very late and this group suffers similar foot pathology to those with long-term Type 1 diabetes. Routine screening of the nation for diabetes remains improbable, but the targeting of 'high-risk' groups may improve diagnosis rates and facilitate early intervention. In addition, new techniques to determine the probability of neuropathy and vascular disease and predictive measures for wound healing and infection could be invaluable. Regular exercise and a 'balanced' diet are simple steps to prevention of such pathology. However, educating and achieving life-style changes of a nation will not be a simple task.

Key point 1

- Diabetes is on the increase globally. Type 2 diabetic patients are often detected late, but this group can suffer similar foot pathology to long-term Type 1 patients.

There is no national database of foot pathology, treatments or outcomes in the UK. Such a database, linked to acute and community site IT, could be used for audit which would likely increase efficacy of treatment. This may become a more realistic proposition with UK Government initiatives to have integrated 'electronic patient record' systems in all Trusts by 2010. National collection of outcome data could provide the evidence required to move diabetic foot treatment away from 'best practice' to 'evidence-based medicine'.

Key points for clinical practice

- Diabetic foot ulcers are contributed to by: (i) sensory, motor and autonomic neuropathy; (ii) ischaemia; and (iii) infection.
- The ankle-brachial pressure index is very often misleading.
- Diabetic foot ulcers tend to acquire a poly-microbial infection including Gram-positive and Gram-negative bacteria as well as anaerobic strains.
- Diabetic foot infections should be treated promptly with triple antibiotic therapy and appropriate surgery.
- Diabetes *per se* is not a contraindication in attempting revascularisation. However, advanced arterial 'run-off' disease is associated with a high incidence of amputation.
- Avoiding focused pressure areas – 'off-loading' – is an essential element of prevention and treatment of diabetic foot ulcers.
- The management of diabetic foot ulcers is multidisciplinary and necessitates close liaison with acute and community healthcare workers.
- Diabetes is on the increase globally. Type 2 diabetic patients are often detected late, but this group can suffer similar foot pathology to long-term Type 1 patients.

References

1. Jirkovska A, Boucek P, Woskova V, Bartos V, Skibova J. Identification of patients at risk for diabetic foot: a comparison of standardized non-invasive testing with routine practice at community diabetes clinics. *J Diabetes Complications* 2001; **15**: 63–68.
2. Blot SI, Monstrey SJ. The use of laser Doppler imaging in measuring wound-healing progress. *Arch Surg* 2001; **136**: 116.
3. Linsenmeier RA, Braun RD, McRipley MA *et al*. Retinal hypoxia in long-term diabetic cats. *Ophthalmol Vis Sci* 1998; **39**: 1647–1657.
4. Suzuki E, Egawa K, Nishio Y *et al*. Prevalence and major risk factors of reduced flow volume in lower extremities with normal ankle-brachial index in Japanese patients with type 2 diabetes. *Diabetes Care* 2003; **26**: 1764–1769.
5. Mazzariol F, Ascher E, Hingorani A, Gunduz Y, Yorkovich W, Salles-Cunha S. Revascularisation without preoperative contrast arteriography in 185 cases: lessons learned with duplex ultrasound arterial mapping. *Eur J Vasc Endovasc Surg* 2000; **19**: 509–515.
6. Aly S, Jenkins MP, Zaidi FH, Coleridge Smith PD, Bishop CC. Duplex scanning and effect of multi-segmental arterial disease on its accuracy in lower limb arteries. *Eur J Vasc Endovasc Surg* 1998; **16**: 345–349.
7. Aly S, Sommerville K, Adiseshiah M, Raphael M, Coleridge Smith PD, Bishop CC. Comparison of duplex imaging and arteriography in the evaluation of lower limb arteries. *Br J Surg* 1998; **85**: 1099–1102.

8. Ballard JL, Eke CC, Bunt TJ, Killeen JD. A prospective evaluation of transcutaneous oxygen measurements in the management of diabetic foot problems. *J Vasc Surg* 1995; **22**: 485–490, discussion 490–492.
9. Urbanova R, Jirkovska A, Woskova V, Wohl P. Transcutaneous oximetry in the diagnosis of ischemic disease of the lower extremities in diabetics. *Vnitr Lek* 2001; **47**: 330–332.
10. Cavallini M, Caterino S, Murante G, Gianotti R. Efficacy of the popliteal to distal bypass in salvage of the ischemic diabetic foot. *Ann Ital Chir* 1995; **66**: 473–478.
11. Attinger C, Venturi M, Kim K, Ribiero C. Maximizing length and optimizing biomechanics in foot amputations by avoiding cookbook recipes for amputation. *Semin Vasc Surg* 2003; **16**: 44–66.
12. Kreitner KF, Kalden P, Neufang A *et al*. Diabetes and peripheral arterial occlusive disease: prospective comparison of contrast-enhanced three-dimensional MR angiography with conventional digital subtraction angiography. *Am J Roentgenol* 2000; **174**: 171–179.
13. Nolan CM, Beaty HN, Bagdade JD. Further characterization of the impaired bactericidal function of granulocytes in patients with poorly controlled diabetes. *Diabetes* 1978; **27**: 889–894.
14. MacRury SM, Gemmell CG, Paterson KR, MacCuish AC. Changes in phagocytic function with glycaemic control in diabetic patients. *Clin Pathol* 1989; **42**: 1143–1147.
15. Terranova A. The effects of diabetes mellitus on wound healing. *Plast Surg Nurs* 1991; **11**: 20–25.
16. Calvet HM, Yoshikawa TT. Infections in diabetes. *Infect Dis Clin North Am* 2001; **15**: 407–421.
17. Bowler PG, Pickworth JJ, Lilly HA. Wound microbiology – the effect of occlusion. Presented at the American Academy of Dermatology 48th Annual Meeting. 1989, December 2–7. Poster 80.
18. Davies DG, Parsek MR, Pearson JP, Iglewski BH, Costerton JW, Greenberg EP. The involvement of cell-to-cell signals in the development of a bacterial biofilm. *Science* 1998; **280**: 295–298.
19. Watnick PI, Kolter R. Steps in the development of a *Vibrio cholerae* El Tor biofilm. *Mol Microbiol* 1999; **34**: 586–595.
20. Lewis K. Riddle of biofilm resistance. *Antimicrob Agents Chemother* 2001: **45**: 999–1007.
21. Johnson GM, Lee DA, Regelmann WE, Gray ED, Peters G, Quie PG. Interference with granulocyte function by *Staphylococcus epidermidis* slime. *Immunity* 1986; **54**: 13–20.
22. Russell AD. Biocide use and antibiotic resistance: the relevance of laboratory findings to clinical and environmental situations. *Lancet Infect Dis* 2003; **3**: 794–803.
23. Serralta VW, Harrison-Balestra C, Cazzaniga AL, Davis SC, Mertz M. Lifestyles of bacteria in wounds: presence of biofilms? *Wounds* 2001; **13**: 29–34.
24. Falanga V, Grinnell F, Gilchrest B, Maddox YT, Moshell A. Workshop on the pathogenesis of chronic wounds. *J Invest Dermatol* 1994; **102**: 125–127.
25. Dow G, Browne A, Sibbald RG. Infection in chronic wounds: controversies in diagnosis and treatment. *Ostomy Wound Manage* 1999; **45**: 23–40.
26. Norden CW. Acute and chronic osteomyelitis. *Infect Dis* 1999; **2**: 43.1–43.8.
27. Bodegom ME, Jahrome AK, Raymakers JTFJ, Van Baal JG. Surgical treatment of chronic osteomyelitis of the neuropathic toe. *Surgery. The Diabetic Foot*. 2004; **7**: 51–53.
28. Bowler P, Duerden B, Armstrong D. Wound microbiology and associated approaches to wound management. *Clin Microbiol Rev* 2001; **14**: 244–269.
29. Cooper R, Lawrence JC. The isolation and identification of bacteria from wounds. *J Wound Care* 1996; **5**: 335–340.
30. Sumpio BE, Lee T, Blume PA. Vascular evaluation and arterial reconstruction of the diabetic foot. *Clin Podiatr Med Surg* 2003; **20**: 689–708.
31. Becker W. Imaging osteomyelitis and the diabetic foot. *Q J Nucl Med* 1999; **43**: 9–20.
32. Learch TJ, Gentili A. Advanced imaging of the diabetic foot and its complications. *Am J Roentgenol* 2000; **175**: 1328.
33. Tan JS, File Jr TM. Diagnosis and treatment of diabetic foot infections. *Baillières Clin Rheumatol* 1999; **13**: 149–161.
34. Raffetto JD, Chen MN, LaMorte WW *et al*. Factors that predict site of outflow target artery anastomosis in infrainguinal revascularization. *J Vasc Surg* 2002; **35**: 1093–1099.

35. Faries PL, Brophy D, LoGerfo FW *et al*. Combined iliac angioplasty and infrainguinal revascularization surgery are effective in diabetic patients with multilevel arterial disease. *Ann Vasc Surg* 2001; **15**: 67–72.
36. Faries PL, LoGerfo FW, Hook SC *et al*. The impact of diabetes on arterial reconstructions for multilevel arterial occlusive disease. *Am J Surg* 2001; **181**: 251–255.
37. Green RM, Abbott WM, Matsumoto T *et al*. Prosthetic above-knee femoro-popliteal bypass grafting: five-year results of a randomized trial. *J Vasc Surg* 2000; **31**: 417–425.
38. Schneider PA, Caps MT, Ogawa DY, Hayman ES. Intra-operative superficial femoral artery balloon angioplasty and popliteal to distal bypass graft: an option for combined open and endovascular treatment of diabetic gangrene. *J Vasc Surg* 2001; **33**: 955–962.
39. Panayiotopoulos YP, Tyrrell MR, Owen SE, Reidy JF, Taylor PR. Outcome and cost analysis after femorocrural and femoropedal grafting for critical limb ischaemia. *Br J Surg* 1997; **84**: 207–212.
40. Robinson JG, Cross MA, Brothers TE, Elliott BM. Do results justify an aggressive strategy targeting the pedal arteries for limb salvage? *J Surg Res* 1995; **59**: 450–454.
41. Hicks RC, Moss J, Higman DJ, Greenhalgh RM, Powell JT. The influence of diabetes on the vasomotor responses of saphenous vein and the development of infra-inguinal vein graft stenosis. *Diabetes* 1997; **46**: 113–118.
42. Wolfle KD, Bruijnen H, Reeps C *et al*. Tibioperoneal arterial lesions and critical foot ischaemia: successful management by the use of short vein grafts and percutaneous transluminal angioplasty. *Vasa* 2000; **29**: 207–214.
43. Toursarkissian B, D'Ayala M, Shireman PK, Schoolfield J, Sykes MT. Lower extremity bypass graft revision in diabetics. *Vasc Surg* 2001; **35**: 369–377.
44. Isaksson L, Lundgren F. Prognostic factors for failure of primary patency within a year of bypass to the foot in patients with diabetes and critical ischaemia. *Eur J Surg* 2000; **166**: 123–128.
45. Arora S, Pomposelli F, LoGerfo FW, Veves A. Cutaneous microcirculation in the neuropathic diabetic foot improves significantly but not completely after successful lower extremity revascularization. *J Vasc Surg* 2002; **35**: 501–505.
46. Quigley FG, Ling J, Avramovic J. Impact of femoro-distal bypass on major lower limb amputation rate. *Aust NZ J Surg* 1998; **68**: 35–37.
47. Lorenzetti F, Tukiainen E, Alback A, Kallio M, Asko-Seljavaara S, Lepantalo M. Blood flow in a pedal bypass combined with a free muscle flap. *Eur J Vasc Endovasc Surg* 2001; **22**: 161–164.
48. Quinones-Baldrich WJ, Kashyap VS, Taw MB *et al*. Combined revascularization and microvascular free tissue transfer for limb salvage: a six-year experience. *Ann Vasc Surg* 2000; **14**: 99–104.
49. Vermassen FE, van Landuyt K. Combined vascular reconstruction and free flap transfer in diabetic arterial disease. *Diabetes Metab Res Rev* 2000; **16 (Suppl 1)**: S33–S36.
50. McCarthy 3rd WJ, Matsumura JS, Fine NA, Dumanian GA, Pearce WH. Combined arterial reconstruction and free tissue transfer for limb salvage. *J Vasc Surg* 1999; **29**: 814–820.
51. Gooden MA, Gentile AT, Demas CP, Berman SS, Mills JL. Salvage of femoropedal bypass graft complicated by interval gangrene and vein graft blowout using a flow-through radial forearm fascio-cutaneous free flap. *J Vasc Surg* 1997; **26**: 711–714.
52. Gooden MA, Gentile AT, Mills JL *et al*. Free tissue transfer to extend the limits of limb salvage for lower extremity tissue loss. *Am J Surg* 1997; **174**: 644–648, discussion 648–649.
53. Tosenovsky P, Zalesak B, Janousek L, Koznar B. Microvascular steal syndrome in the pedal bypass and free muscle transfer? *Eur J Vasc Endovasc Surg* 2003; **26**: 562–564.
54. Attinger CE, Ducic I, Neville RF, Abbruzzese MR, Gomes M, Sidawy AN. The relative roles of aggressive wound care versus revascularization in salvage of the threatened lower extremity in the renal failure diabetic patient. *Plast Reconstr Surg* 2002; **109**: 1281–1290, discussion 1291–1292.
55. Baumhauer JF, Fraga CJ, Gould JS, Johnson JE. Total calcanectomy for the treatment of chronic calcaneal osteomyelitis. *Foot Ankle Int* 1998; **19**: 849–855.
56. Fleischli JG, Laughlin TJ. Subtotal calcanectomy for the treatment of large heel ulceration and calcaneal osteomyelitis in the diabetic patient. *J Foot Ankle Surg* 1999; **38**: 373–374.
57. Diamantopoulos EJ, Haritos D, Yfandi G *et al*. Management and outcome of severe diabetic foot infections. *Exp Clin Endocrinol Diabetes* 1998; **106**: 34.

58. Piaggesi A, Viacava P, Rizzo L *et al*. Semi-quantitative analysis of the histopathological features of the neuropathic foot ulcer: effects of pressure relief. *Diabetes Care* 2003; **26**: 3123–3128.
59. Kessler L, Bilbault P, Ortega F *et al*. Hyperbaric oxygenation accelerates the healing rate of non-ischemic chronic diabetic foot ulcers: a prospective randomized study. *Diabetes Care* 2003; **26**: 2378–2382.

Plate XI Bone scan showing unilateral increased radiolabel uptake in mid-tarsal Charcot's arthropathy.

Plate XII Diabetic neuropathic ulceration.

Plate XIII Cellulitis, gangrene and osteomyelitis in an infected 'sausage' toe.

Plate XIV Dry gangrene associated with microvascular disease.

Nicholas R. Brook Michael L. Nicholson

14

Developments in live donor renal transplantation

Live kidney donation is assuming a prominent role in renal transplant programmes because of the persistent increase in patients requiring definitive treatment for end-stage renal failure. While cadaveric transplant rates remain more or less static, live donor transplantation has increased 3-fold in the US over the past decade, where it now accounts for 43% of renal transplant activity.[1] Figures from United Kingdom Transplant indicate 24% of all renal transplants were from live donors for the year 2003–2004.[2] Superior recipient post-transplant outcome compared to cadaveric kidneys,[3] the potential for transplantation before dialysis, and the ability to plan the procedure (allowing optimisation of recipient condition) justify this growth in live donation. New techniques and novel approaches have been developed to facilitate live donation and increase transplant activity. This chapter presents some of the important recent developments and controversies in live donor renal transplantation.

Key point 1

- Greater numbers of transplants are being performed from live renal donors because the supply of cadaveric organs is increasingly unable to meet demand.

*Colour figures (plates) referred to in this chapter are to be found in the 'Colour plates section' at the front of this volume (p1–8).

Nicholas R. Brook BSc MSc BM MRCS(Ed)
Specialist Registrar in Urology, Transplant Surgery Group, Department of Cardiovascular Sciences, University Hospitals of Leicester NHS Trust, Gwendolen Road, Leicester LE5 4PW, UK
E-mail: nicholasbrook@fastmail.fm (for correspondence)

Michael L. Nicholson MD FRCS
Professor of Transplant Surgery, Transplant Surgery Group, Department of Cardiovascular Sciences, University Hospitals of Leicester NHS Trust, Gwendolen Road, Leicester LE5 4PW, UK

PRE-OPERATIVE IMAGING OF LIVE RENAL DONORS

Pre-operative imaging of live donors is mandatory for a number of reasons – it confirms the presence of two functioning kidneys, identifies their position, indicates absence of pathology that would preclude donation, and provides anatomical information necessary for planning the procedure. The ideal form of imaging is minimally invasive and provides accurate morphological information on the renal parenchyma, collecting system and vascular anatomy.[4,5] Traditionally, imaging has been performed using angiography,[4,6] but there are inherent risks with this invasive procedure. Venous imaging is limited with arterial contrast injection,[7] and separate excretion urographic studies are necessary to visualise the collecting system.[5] These disadvantages have been the driving force behind the introduction of computed tomographic angiography (CTA) for anatomical assessment of living renal donors. CTA is non-invasive and cheaper than other imaging techniques.[7] Pre-operative anatomical information is, of course, necessary for open donor nephrectomy, but it assumes paramount importance in the laparoscopic procedure because of reduced exposure, and particular difficulties in the identification of complex renal vein tributaries. Thus, the location, size and number of renal veins and tributaries need to be described accurately pre-operatively. Spiral CTA imaging compares favourably with conventional angiography in the prediction of gross renal arterial and venous anatomy[8] and is a powerful tool for identification of renal vein tributary anatomy (Fig. 1).[9]

Prior to imaging, all potential donors are assessed by physical examination, undergo blood group and HLA matching with the intended recipient, complement-dependent cytotoxicity cross-matching, and isotope GFR measurement. At the Leicester unit, CTA is performed on a spiral GE Prospeed SX scanner. Arterial and venous anatomy is evaluated using a dual phase protocol with

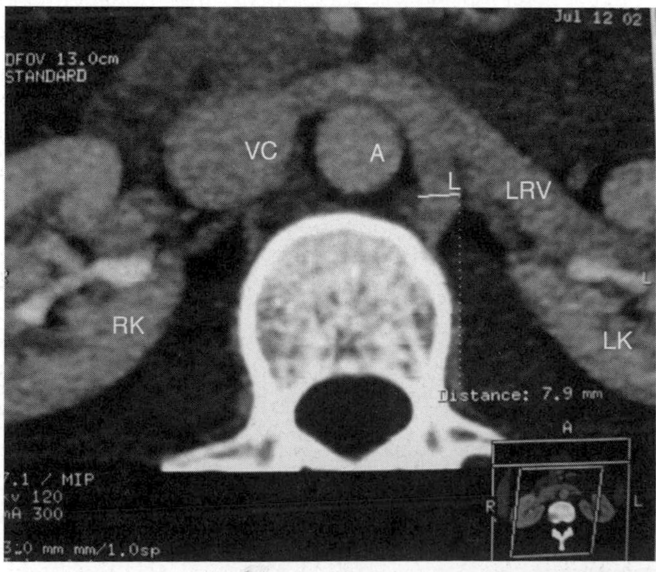

Fig. 1 CT renal angiogram demonstrating right and left kidneys (RK, LK), aorta (A), vena cava (VC), left renal vein (LRV) and a large posterior lumbar tributary (L) inserting into posterior aspect of LRV. The diameter of the lumbar vein is calculated at 7.9 mm.

venous injection of iodinated contrast media (Iopamidol®). Arterial phase imaging is performed from the level of the coeliac axis origin to include the lower renal pole. Venous phase imaging (60 s after contrast injection) includes the cephalo-caudal extent of the left renal vein and the left renal sinus.

> **Key point 2**
>
> - Spiral CT renal angiography is now the imaging modality of choice before live renal donation. It allows delineation of vascular anatomy and excludes gross donor renal pathology.

DEVELOPMENT OF MINIMAL ACCESS DONOR NEPHRECTOMY

The live donor nephrectomy operation has traditionally been performed through an open incision, necessitating a prolonged period of recovery. This, and the cosmetic implications of a large flank wound[10] may be discouragements to potential donors (Fig. 2).

To reduce such disincentives, there has been a move towards minimally invasive donor nephrectomy, first performed as a classical transperitoneal laparoscopic procedure (LapDN) by Louis Kavoussi and Lloyd Ratner in 1995.[11] Retrospective reports suggest LapDN is associated with decreased severity and duration of postoperative pain, shorter in-patient stay, quicker return to work and normal activities, and improved cosmetic result when compared to open donor nephrectomy (Fig. 3).[2,13] Furthermore, the overall societal cost of LapDN is lower and recipient quality of life scores are higher.[14]

Despite the current lack of published statistically powered randomised clinical trials, retrospective data suggest that minimal access donor nephrectomy not only

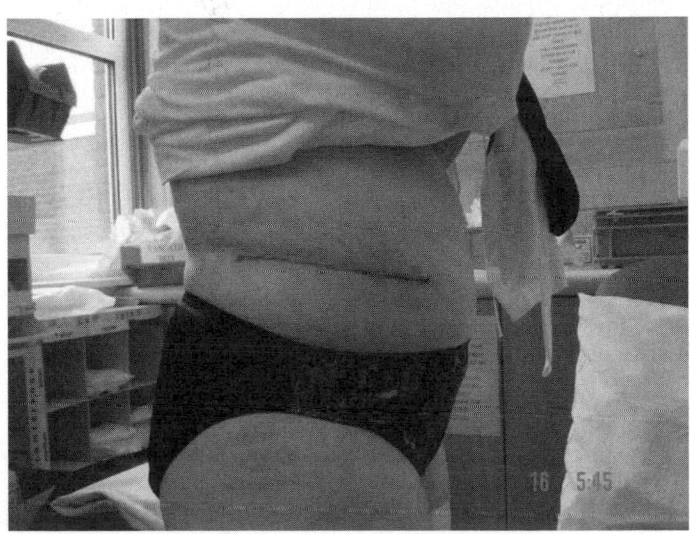

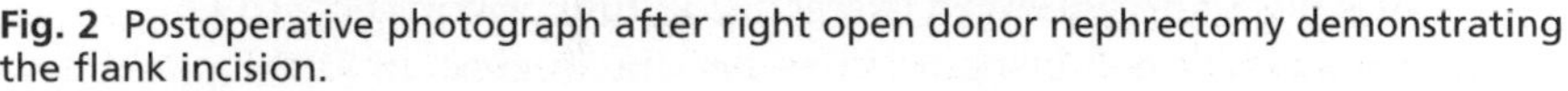

Fig. 2 Postoperative photograph after right open donor nephrectomy demonstrating the flank incision.

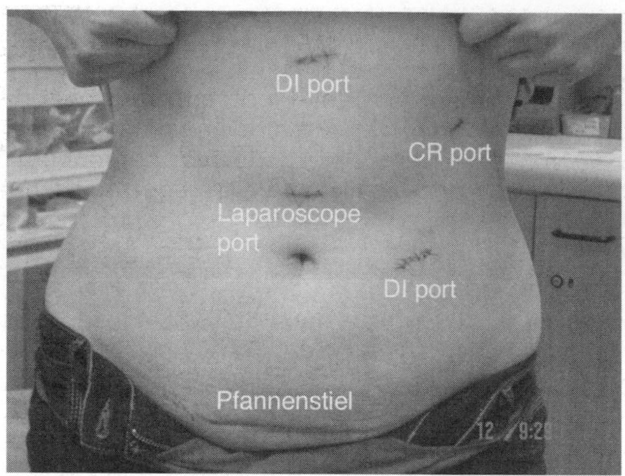

Fig. 3 Postoperative photograph of laparoscopy port sites and Pfannenstiel incision after left laparoscopic donor nephrectomy. DI, dissecting instrument; CR, colon retractor.

offers postoperative advantages to the donor but also increases the number of transplants performed by reducing donor disincentives: estimates range from a 25%[15] to a 100%[16] increase in transplant activity. In the US, 31% of live kidney donor procedures are performed laparoscopically, and 65% of centres offer the procedure.[17] Despite encouraging UK figures indicating year-on-year increases in live donor activity,[18] few centres have adopted minimally invasive techniques. With accumulating evidence that high quality grafts can be procured from laparoscopically-procured kidneys,[3,13] the main hurdle for expansion of laparoscopic donor nephrectomy is lack of operative experience of the technique amongst UK transplant surgeons. Three approaches have been described and advocated, comprising transperitoneal,[19] extraperitoneal,[20,21] and hand-assisted[22] live donor nephrectomy. The hand-assisted operation is said to be easier to learn than transperitoneal laparoscopic donor nephrectomy,[22] and can be safely and efficiently performed by surgeons with less laparoscopic experience.[23] The retroperitoneal approach avoids breaching the peritoneum, and may also have a particular application in right donor nephrectomy.[20]

Key point 3

- Traditional open donor nephrectomy requires a large incision, with associated potential for postoperative complications. Laparoscopic donor nephrectomy is a relatively new technique that may reduce some of the disincentives for live donors.

MINIMALLY INVASIVE DONOR NEPHRECTOMY TECHNIQUES

TRANSPERITONEAL LAPAROSCOPIC DONOR NEPHRECTOMY (LEFT)

The patient is placed in a modified lateral decubitus position and a CO_2 pneumoperitoneum is established using a Veress needle. In general, four laparoscopic

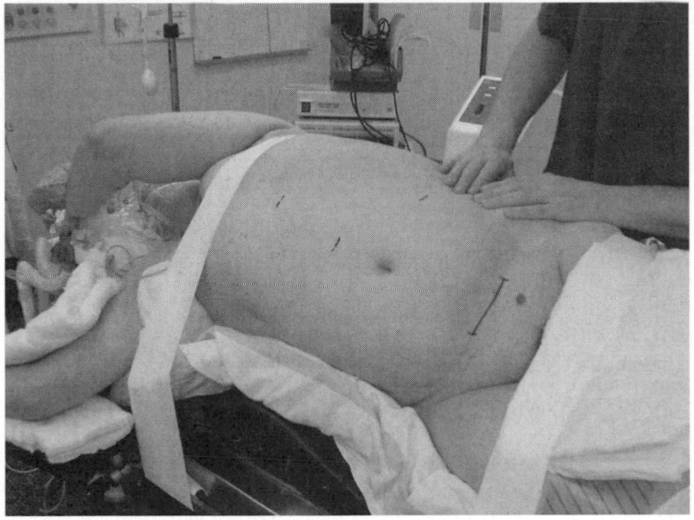

Fig. 4 Pre-operative photograph for left laparoscopic donor nephrectomy. The patient is in the modified left lateral position, and the port sites and Pfannenstiel incision are marked.

ports are required. The videolaparoscope is introduced through a 12 mm umbilical port and two further 12 mm ports are placed in the epigastrium and left iliac fossa for the main dissecting instruments (Fig. 4).

A retractor for the colon can be passed through a 5 mm port placed in the mid-axillary line. The procedure starts with scissor diathermy of the lateral peritoneal reflection of the splenic flexure and descending colon to the level of the pelvic brim; this enables the colon to be reflected medially, demonstrating the kidney within Gerota's fascia. The ureter and gonadal vessels are identified at the pelvic brim, anterior to the psoas muscle. The gonadal vein is followed superiorly to its junction with the renal vein, which is dissected to the left border of the aorta. The adrenal, gonadal, and posterior lumbar tributaries of the vein are controlled with Ligaclips® and divided. The renal artery is then identified; it is normally found just posterior to the divided adrenal vein, but is occasionally situated inferio-posterior to the renal vein. The artery is dissected back to its origin at the aorta, a manoeuvre best achieved with hook diathermy. Attention is turned back to the ureter; after dissection of the peri-ureteric tissue medial to the gonadal vein, it is clipped and divided. The remaining lateral, posterior and superior fascial attachments of the kidney are divided to leave it connected only by the vascular pedicle. A 6–8 cm Pfannenstiel incision is fashioned, and an Ethibond® purse-string suture placed in the peritoneum, which is then incised. A plastic kidney retrieval bag (Endo-catch II® retrieval system) is passed through this incision; tightening the purse-string suture allows the pneumoperitoneum to be maintained. Prior to vessel division, the kidney is placed in the retrieval bag. The renal artery and vein are clipped and divided with a vascular stapler, and the bag and kidney are removed through the incision.

For right transperitoneal donor nephrectomy, the positioning of the patient and placement of the ports is a mirror image of the left side. The dissection can commence with division of the triangular ligament of the liver, but this is unnecessary if a liver retractor is inserted through a separate port. The peritoneal reflection is cut at the border of the liver exposing the adrenal gland and the superior edge of the kidney. The duodenum is partially Kocherised, and displaced medially with the pancreas, exposing the inferior vena cava. Gerota's fascia is opened and the remainder of the dissection is as described for the left side (Plate XV, p8).

Control of the short renal vein is more difficult. This may require the use of a subcostal transverse muscle cutting incision, with control of the IVC using a Satinsky side-biting clamp. This permits harvesting of maximum vessel length, and the transverse incision is used for extraction of the allograft.

HAND-ASSISTED LAPAROSCOPIC DONOR NEPHRECTOMY

The hand-assisted technique offers certain advantages over classical laparoscopy, namely the ability to use tactile sense to facilitate dissection, retraction, and exposure.[24] It is becoming an accepted technique in the field of urology for nephrectomy and nephroureterectomy.[25] For left hand-assisted donor nephrectomy, the patient is placed in the partial lateral decubitus position with the operating table in an arch position to extend the flank. Two 12 mm trocars are used; one in the mid-clavicular line just below the umbilicus and a second in the anterior axillary line above the iliac crest. This latter port is used for the 30° videolaparoscope. In right hand-assisted nephrectomy, port placement mirrors that of the left but the ports are placed more caudally to allow improved visualisation under the right lobe of the liver.[26] The hand-assist device is applied to the abdomen in the midline, above or below the umbilicus, and an 8–10 cm incision is made within the ring. An alternative site is a limited Rutherford-Morison incision in the iliac fossa.[27] The operator fits an occlusive sleeve over his non-dominant hand and places the hand in the abdomen. The ring of the sleeve is locked to the outer ring of the device, rendering the system airtight. The order and process of the dissection are identical to the transperitoneal laparoscopic technique and the kidney is extracted through the hand-port incision.

Slight modifications of the final stages of the hand-assisted procedure have been described, and include application of topical papaverine, desufflation of the abdomen, and no manipulation of the renal artery for 5 min before its transection.[28] These manoeuvres reduce the risk of ischaemic injury to the donor kidney.

RETROPERITONEOSCOPIC OPERATIVE TECHNIQUE

The retroperitoneal approach displays the renal anatomy in a very different manner, and it may be easier to harvest the full length of the vessels on the right side. The disadvantage is that a more limited operating space is available than with the transperitoneal or hand-assisted laparoscopic techniques. The patient is placed in a standard full-flank position with the table flexed. A three-port technique is used and retroperitoneal access is gained just below the tip of the 12th rib. After digital dissection and balloon dilatation of the retroperitoneal space (with laparoscopic confirmation), a 12 mm port is inserted and the retroperitoneal space is filled with CO_2. A further 12 mm port is placed under laparoscopic vision, 2–3 fingers breath above the anterior superior iliac spine, and a 5 mm port is placed lateral to the paraspinal muscles.[29] An alternative is to use five trocars, and a gasless technique:[30] a mini-lumbotomy is fashioned under the 12th rib, and the retroperitoneal space is developed by blunt dissection. The peritoneum is pushed forwards, allowing insertion of four trocars under digital guidance; the fifth trocar is inserted through the initial incision. The retroperitoneal space is maintained by the use of a lifting retractor. Regardless of whether gas is used or not, the dissection is similar; the renal hilum is identified and the artery is dissected circumferentially from the hilum up to its retrocaval position. The renal vein is then mobilised. The ureter and peri-ureteric tissue are dissected to the pelvis, then clipped and divided.[20] Once the kidney is freed from its attachments, the artery is double-clipped and divided. The vein is secured with an Endo-GIA® stapler. If a lumbotomy has been fashioned,[30] it can be extended to allow extraction of the kidney. Alternatives are extraction through an iliac fossa[31] or pararectal[29] incision.

Key point 4

- The most common minimal access technique is a classical transperitoneal laparoscopic operation. The hand-assisted laparoscopic and retroperitoneal approaches may have advantages in certain settings.

ADDRESSING CONCERNS IN MINIMALLY INVASIVE DONOR NEPHRECTOMY

Some concerns surround the application of minimal access surgery for kidney donation. The procedure is technically demanding, and there is potential for damage to the renal vessels and ureter during dissection. It takes longer than open nephrectomy, and exposes the allograft to a short period of warm ischaemic damage. There is also the potential for reduced graft perfusion before extraction in the presence of a pneumoperitoneum. The technique will only gain acceptance if morbidity is not transferred from the donor to the recipient.

CONTRA-INDICATIONS

There are no absolute contra-indications to minimal access donor nephrectomy other than those applying to the open operation. The relative contra-indications are dictated by donor factors and the experience of the surgeon and centre. The donor must be anaesthetically fit, with special consideration given to the physiological stress of pneumoperitoneum or pneumoretroperitoneum. Obesity is a relative contra-indication for both open and laparoscopic surgery, but the hand-assisted approach may be better suited in such patients.[32] Previous abdominal surgery is a further relative contra-indication because of the potential for adhesions. Multiplicity of renal vessels should not hinder

LapDN: if the left kidney has multiple vessels, it can still be taken unless there is a clear advantage to the donor to leave the left,[33] or recipient implantation would be technically difficult.

EFFECT OF PNEUMOPERITONEUM

Transient intra-operative oliguria secondary to decreased renal blood flow is a frequent occurrence during laparoscopic procedures. Proposed mechanisms include decreased cardiac output, renal vein compression, ureteral obstruction, renal parenchymal compression and systemic hormonal effects.[34] Intracranial pressure rises during pneumoperitoneum, with release of vasoconstrictor agents that may decrease renal blood flow.[35] Use of a lower pressure reduces the adverse effects of pneumoperitoneum on renal perfusion parameters.[35] In donor nephrectomy, impaired renal blood flow may compromise allograft function, and compound the injurious effects of warm and cold ischaemia and operative manipulation of the kidney. Laparoscopically-derived donor kidneys display higher serum creatinine up to 1 month post-transplant compared to OpenDN,[16,36] but thereafter graft function is equivalent in the two groups.[16,36,37] There is a single report of increased requirement for postoperative dialysis after LapDN; Norgueria *et al.*[38] reported that 5.3% of laparoscopically derived kidneys needed dialysis in the first post-transplant week, compared to 0% of kidneys from open donors.

Intravascular volume expansion has been used to counteract alterations in renal haemodynamics in a porcine model of CO_2 pneumoperitoneum.[39] Although volume expansion reversed decreases in renal blood flow and urine output, it did not attenuate the changes in creatinine clearance induced by pneumoperitoneum. The pioneers of LapDN report using 8–10 l of crystalloid pre- and intra-operatively[3] to maintain renal perfusion at satisfactory levels in the presence of pneumoperitoneum. At the Leicester unit, two episodes of marked unilateral pulmonary oedema in the dependent lung have led us to change this practice (we now volume-load the donor with 2 l of crystalloid the night before surgery, and use replacement fluids only during surgery) with no apparent detriment to renal function.

RECIPIENT SERUM CREATININE

In a comparison of open, laparoscopic and hand-assisted donor nephrectomy,[40] recipient serum creatinine was statistically equal in all three groups up to 1 year. Wolf and colleagues' randomised trial of OpenDN versus hand-assisted DN[28] demonstrated equal graft function up to 3 months post-transplant. In a retrospective study of recipients of kidneys from LapDN (n = 132) versus OpenDN (n = 99), mean serum creatinine was statistically higher in the LapDN group at 1 week and 1 month after transplant.[38] By 6 months, there were no differences and by 1 year, the LapDN group had lower serum creatinine. The rate of delayed graft function was higher in the LapDN group than the OpenDN group (7.6 versus 2%). In a more recent report by Ratner and colleagues[16] of LapDN (n = 110) and OpenDN recipients (n = 48), the rate of decline of serum creatinine was faster in the open group for the first four days but there were no significant differences thereafter.

ACUTE REJECTION AND EARLY AND LATE GRAFT LOSS

Pretransplant ischaemia may render the donor kidney more immunogenic, by inducing major histocompatibility complex (MHC) class II expression.[41,42] However, acute rejection rates and severity of rejection do not seem to be higher in laparoscopic (despite the longer warm time) than in open live donor kidneys.[16,33,43,44] In Wolf's randomised trial of open and hand-assisted procedures, the number of treated rejection episodes in the first 3 months was similar in the two groups.[28] Allograft survival was statistically equal in the two groups, although it should be stated that allograft loss in the hand-assisted group was 3/23 (13%) and 1/27(3%) in the open group. One graft loss was due to medically supervised withdrawal of immunosuppression, and the other two to pathologically proven ischaemic necrosis not due to renal vein thrombosis or acute rejection. Herein lies the importance in the modification of their technique, with topical papaverine applied to the artery, desufflation of the abdomen and cessation of manipulation of the kidney for at least 5 min before transection of the artery to maximise blood flow. Since the introduction of this triad of adaptations, no allograft losses have occurred.

Key point 5

- Concerns over allograft damage during minimal access donation do not seem to be founded, as long as certain operative principles are adhered to.

URETERIC COMPLICATIONS

Post-transplant complications associated with ureteric ischaemia were more common in some groups' initial experience of the LapDN.[45,46] Philosophe *et al.*[47] described a ureteric complication rate (necessitating operative repair) of 7.7% in LapDN compared to 0.6% for OpenDN. The problem is related to stripping of the delicate ureteric blood supply originating from the renal artery and travelling parallel to the ureter. Modifications of technique, such as ensuring sufficient peri-ureteral tissue is taken, and that the dissection does not occur too close to the renal pelvis[3] (dissect no further laterally than the medial border of the gonadal vein[46]) have reduced the complication rate. A further technique is to take the gonadal vein and ureter together in a clip or stapling device.[45] Similar rates of ureteric complications were observed in open versus hand-assisted donation (1/27 and 2/23, respectively).[28] The group performing this study used the technique of taking the ureter and gonadal vein together since the inception of the hand-assisted technique.

MULTIPLE RENAL VESSELS

The presence of multiple arteries is not a barrier to successful use of grafts from laparoscopic donors. In a series of 320 LapDN procedures,[48] multiple renal arteries were demonstrated in 64 cases (20%), with bench arterial reconstruction in 14 and multiple arterial implantation in the other 50 (16%). Brown *et al.*[12] reported multiple renal arteries in 26% of their 50 laparoscopic donors, with no effect on

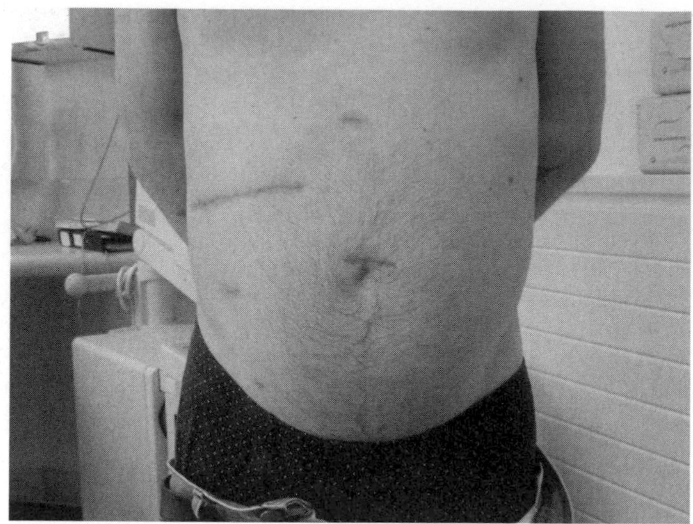

Fig. 5 Postoperative photograph after right laparoscopic donor nephrectomy with right upper quadrant incision for insertion of a Satinsky clamp, allowing control of the vena cava and harvesting of the full length of the renal vein. The incision is also used for allograft extraction.

subsequent graft function or survival. Hsu *et al.*[49] reviewed their experience of 353 laparoscopic donor nephrectomies, finding one renal artery in 277 cases (78.5%), two arteries in 71 cases (20.1%) and three in 5 cases (1.4%). Despite evidence that warm ischaemic time is increased in the presence of multiple renal arteries, there was no association with intra-operative blood loss, postoperative hospital stay, graft function or complication rate for the donor.

RIGHT DONOR NEPHRECTOMY

Historic reviews of open donor nephrectomy indicate use of right donor kidneys in 20–30% of cases, but the literature regarding laparoscopic donor nephrectomy suggests the right side is used in less than 10% of cases.[46,50,51] This relative paucity of experience relates to concerns over the operative safety of the right-sided laparoscopic operation, principally the difficulties involved in obtaining the full length of right renal artery, and an adequate length of the short right renal vein. In a multicentre review of 97 right transperitoneal laparoscopic donor nephrectomies, Buell *et al.*[51] described the most common reasons for using the right kidney as multiple vessels on the left side (59%), small right kidney (8%) and right renal cyst(s) (5%). A 14% complication rate comprised 3 open conversions, 2 liver lacerations, 1 vena cava bleed, 2 recipient graft losses from renal vein thrombosis and 3 upper pole arterial injuries. Lind *et al.*[52] reported an historical review of 73 right and 28 left laparoscopic procedures, with no significant differences in any donor or recipient parameter, with the exception that right operations took less time. The Baltimore group report three post-transplant graft losses from 10 right donor kidneys in a series totalling 200 donor nephrectomies.[46] This high (30%) rate of thrombosis in right donor kidneys was presumed to be due to the short length of the right renal vein, and all occurred before introduction of the donor muscle splitting incision prior to excision to allow preservation of renal vein length (see above and Fig. 5).

Johnson *et al.*[53] described 15 right donor nephrectomies with hand-assisted laparoscopy; despite two cases of delayed graft function, graft function was equal to historic left sided grafts. Use of stapling devices on the renal vein leaves a line of staples on both the graft and patient side of the vessels. When staples are trimmed, approximately 5 mm of vessel length is lost. Additional length can be safely acquired by using a single Hem-o-lok® on the renal artery, a single Endo-TA® stapler (which has only one line of staples) on the renal vein, dividing the vessels with scissors and leaving the graft-side of the vessel unsecured.[54] Other techniques include the use of inter-aortocaval renal artery dissection to maximise the right renal artery length.[26,55] Mobilisation of the right lateral and posterior aspects of the vena cava through division of short lumbar veins and retraction of the cava to expose the right lateral aortic surface exposes the right aorto-renal junction and facilitates harvesting of maximum artery length (Plate XVI, p8).

This manoeuvre also allows the vein to be placed on slight traction, permitting division on the reno-caval junction. In 20 consecutive right-sided, hand-assisted procedures, this technique gave a mean renal vein length of 2.5 cm (compared to 2.7 cm by right open operation) and renal artery length of 3.6 cm (compared to 3.7 cm by right open operation).[26]

ECONOMIC CONSIDERATIONS

In two American studies, laparoscopic donation has been demonstrated to be marginally more expensive than open surgery ($10,310 versus $9850,[14] and $11,072 versus $10,840[56]), but quality of life for the donor was higher. Mackey and colleagues[57] estimated productivity loss was $4600 less in laparoscopic compared to open donors. Moreover, by potentially increasing organ donor rates, laparoscopic donor nephrectomy is likely to offer an overall cost saving by reducing the number of patients on dialysis.[14] For the hand-assisted technique, theatre costs are greater than with the open operation.[28] This is accounted for by the pneumosleeve and endovascular stapling devices, but is countered to some extent by a shorter hospital stay. Furthermore, loss of occupational income in the hand-assisted donors was 75% of that in the open donor group. With all these factors taken into consideration, there are no significant differences in the overall cost of the hand-assisted and open procedure.

TRAINING

Training issues in minimal access donor nephrectomy are likely to arise as patient demand increases. We have recently surveyed all renal transplant centres in the UK and Ireland, and whilst half of the units offer trainees the opportunity to undertake supervised training in open nephrectomy, only a small number of units perform laparoscopic donor nephrectomy, with consultants undertaking all of the work.[58] The wide spread use of animal laboratories for training may account for the greater prevalence of laparoscopic donation in the US; there is no scope for this kind of training in the UK. Indeed, studies in swine demonstrated the safety and efficacy of the laparoscopic procedure before its introduction in humans. The technical difficulties of transperitoneal laparoscopic donor nephrectomy confer a particularly steep learning curve, and the fact that lead-clinicians themselves need to learn the technique precludes, at least initially, the involvement of trainees. It may be that the hand-assisted technique has a place not just as an alternative, but also as a technical stepping-stone to the full laparoscopic technique.

Key point 6

- Laparoscopic donor nephrectomy is wide-spread in the US, but few centres in the UK offer the procedure. Training issues are likely to arise as demand for minimal access surgery increases.

DEVELOPMENT OF BLOOD GROUP-INCOMPATIBLE TRANSPLANT PROGRAMMES

Until recently, it was felt that ABO blood group compatibility was a prerequisite for successful transplantation because of the risk of hyperacute antibody-mediated graft rejection in non-compatible recipients and donors. A small proportion of otherwise suitable live donor/recipient pairs will be blood group incompatible. Such patients had not been transplanted but rather went onto, or remained on, the cadaveric transplant waiting list. Recently, the use of ABO-incompatible donor/recipient pairs has shown promise. This is particularly the case with A2 blood group donors (20% of blood group A Caucasians) transplanted into B or O recipients. A2 is expressed in a different form and at lower levels than the A1 subtype,[1,59] and A2 kidneys are less likely to undergo antibody-mediated rejection at a given level of anti-A antibody.[1] If the recipient's anti-A antibody titre is low, transplant can be performed without other interventions. If the titre is high, pretransplant recipient plasmapheresis to reduce antibody levels can result in safe transplantation. Alkhunazi *et al.*[60] reported 14 group O or B recipients of living or cadaveric A2 kidneys that received plasmapheresis and demonstrated a 1-year graft survival of 93%. The use of non-A2 donors (mainly A1 or B), has been also explored.[1,61] In this setting, antibody titres are high. As well as pretransplant plasmapheresis, recipients require splenectomy (at the time of transplant) and post-transplant monitoring of antibody titres. Winters *et al.*[62] reported their experience of 26 ABO-incompatible transplants at the Mayo Clinic. Conditioning consisted of plasma exchanges, intravenous immunoglobulin and splenectomy. Post-transplant immunosuppression comprised anti-T lymphocyte antibody, tacrolimus, mycophenolate mofetil, and prednisone. No hyperacute rejection occurred, and patient and graft survivals at last follow-up were 92 and 85%, respectively (mean follow-up 400 days). Antibody-mediated rejection occurred in 46% of recipients, but was reversed in 83% by plasma exchange and increased immunosuppression. The authors suggested that controlled clinical trials are needed to identify the optimum conditioning for ABO-incompatible renal transplants. Although the majority of the antibody-mediated rejections were reversible, there may be an element of irreversible damage caused by such episodes. Furthermore, the graft survival rates are slightly lower than that expected for ABO-compatible transplants.[63]

Tanabe *et al.*[61] described 141 ABO-incompatible living kidney transplants performed between 1989 and 2001. Plasmapheresis was used to remove anti-A and/or anti-B antibodies before transplantation and splenectomy was undertaken at the time of kidney transplantation. Patient survival rates were similar between groups. Acute rejection episodes occurred significantly more frequently among recipients of ABO-incompatible grafts (85 of 141, 60%) compared with ABO-compatible recipients (377 of 777, 49%). The 1-, 5- and 10-year graft survival rates among ABO-incompatible recipients were 82%, 76% and 56%, respectively. The graft survival rates among ABO-compatible recipients were 96%, 85%, and 67% at the same time points. There was a significant difference in the short-term graft survival rates between ABO-incompatible compatible renal transplants but no difference in long-term graft survival. With the introduction of newer immunosuppressants, graft survival since 1998 has markedly improved: the 5-year graft survival rate is now more than 90%, and is not significantly different from that of ABO-compatible cases. Almost all of the graft losses occur during the first year post-transplant. Thereafter, very few grafts are lost. Thus, the allograft seems to tolerate anti-ABO antibodies well over time (graft accommodation), despite recurrence of serum anti-blood group antibodies and the persistence of blood group antigens in the graft.[1]

Key point 7

- ABO incompatible transplantation is possible using A2 blood group donors, and B or O recipients. A1 donor into a B or O recipient requires recipient pre-conditioning with plasmapheresis (to remove anti-blood group antibodies) and splenectomy.

DEVELOPMENT OF DONOR EXCHANGE PROGRAMMES

Despite these encouraging data from ABO-incompatible kidneys, there remains an element of risk from early graft loss and severe antibody-mediated rejection. Although not yet utilised in the UK, other countries have developed donor exchange programmes as an alternative system. These enable simultaneous direct exchange between live donors (a paired exchange such that the two recipients are transplanted with ABO-compatible kidneys), or a live donor/deceased donor indirect exchange.[64] These arrangements yield an additional donor source for patients awaiting a deceased donor kidney. Every paired exchange transplant removes two patients from the waiting list and thereby increases access to deceased donor kidneys for the remaining candidates on the list.[64]

DIRECT EXCHANGE

With direct live donor exchange relative inequalities are still possible. For example one donor may be older than the other,[1] but as the exchange is direct, there is no negative impact on the cadaveric waiting list, apart from allowing two recipients the possibility of not entering the list, thus reducing pressures.

INDIRECT EXCHANGE

If an intended recipient has a potential but ABO-incompatible live donor, the donor can donate to a patient at the top of the cadaveric waiting list. The recipient originally paired with the live donor assumes a priority position on the cadaveric waiting list, but still remains behind 0 HLA-mismatched and sensitised donors, and children. The potential inequality is the swap of a live donor kidney for a cadaveric one. Further, if the living donor's intended paired recipient is blood group O, they are placed ahead of other group O recipients who already wait longer than those with other blood groups do.

Key point 8

- In some countries, recipients with a potential but ABO-incompatible live donor can enter donor exchange programmes. Kidneys are swapped between donor/recipient pairs so that each receives a compatible kidney, or a kidney is donated in exchange for a priority position on the waiting list.

CONCLUSIONS

Live kidney donation is assuming an increasingly prominent role in renal transplant programmes in response to the persistent rise in the number of patients requiring definitive treatment for end-stage renal failure. Minimally invasive donor nephrectomy was introduced to reduce the donor disincentives associated with the traditional open operation. A number of concerns have surrounded the introduction of this technique, but with attention to certain points of technique, graft outcomes equivalent to the open operation are achieved. Many potential donor/recipient pairs are blood-group incompatible, which has precluded transplantation in the past. New approaches to circumvent the blood group barrier include organ exchange programmes and ABO incompatible transplantation, possible with preconditioning of the donor using plasmapheresis and splenectomy where appropriate. The risk of antibody-mediated rejection is high, and it is still not clear from the literature whether graft survival is equivalent to ABO-compatible transplantation.

Key points for clinical practice

- Greater numbers of transplants are being performed from live renal donors because the supply of cadaveric organs is increasingly unable to meet demand.
- Spiral CT renal angiography is now the imaging modality of choice before live renal donation. It allows delineation of vascular anatomy and excludes gross donor renal pathology.

Key points for clinical practice (continued)

- Traditional open donor nephrectomy requires a large incision, with associated potential for postoperative complications. Laparoscopic donor nephrectomy is a relatively new technique that may reduce some of the disincentives for live donors.
- The most common minimal access technique is a classical transperitoneal laparoscopic operation. The hand-assisted laparoscopic and retroperitoneal approaches may have advantages in certain settings.
- Concerns over allograft damage during minimal access donation do not seem to be founded, as long as certain operative principles are adhered to.
- Laparoscopic donor nephrectomy is wide-spread in the US, but few centres in the UK offer the procedure. Training issues are likely to arise as demand for minimal access surgery increases.
- ABO incompatible transplantation is possible using A2 blood group donors, and B or O recipients. A1 donor into a B or O recipient requires recipient pre-conditioning with plasmapheresis (to remove anti-blood group antibodies) and splenectomy.
- In some countries, recipients with a potential but ABO-incompatible live donor can enter donor exchange programmes. Kidneys are swapped between donor/recipient pairs so that each receives a compatible kidney, or a kidney is donated in exchange for a priority position on the waiting list.

References

1. Stegall MD, Dean PG, Gloor JM. ABO-incompatible kidney transplantation. *Transplantation* 2004; **78**: 635–640.
2. Statistics and Audit Directorate UKT. More transplants – new lives. Transplant Activity in the UK 2003–2004. United Kingdom Transplant, 2004.
3. Ratner LE, Montgomery RA, Kavoussi LR. Laparoscopic live donor nephrectomy: the four year Johns Hopkins University experience. *Nephrol Dial Transplant* 1999; **14**: 2090–2093.
4. Rydberg J, Kopecky KK, Tann M *et al*. Evaluation of prospective renal donors for laparoscopic nephrectomy with multisection CT: the marriage of minimally invasive imaging with minimally invasive surgery. *Radiographics* 2001; **21**: S223–S236.
5. Riehle Jr RA, Steckler R, Naslund EB, Riggio R, Cheigh J, Stubenbord W. Selection criteria for the evaluation of living related renal donors. *J Urol* 1990; **144**: 845–848.
6. Derauf B, Goldberg ME. Angiographic assessment of potential renal transplant donors. *Radiol Clin North Am* 1987; **25**: 261.
7. Kaynan AM, Rozenblit AM, Figuera KI *et al*. Use of spiral computerized tomography in lieu of angiography for pre-operative assessment of living renal donors. *J Urol* 1999; **161**: 1769–1775.
8. Pozniak MA, Balison DJ, Lee FT, Tambeaux RH, Uehling DT, Moon TD. CT angiography of potential renal transplant donors. *Radiographics* 1998; **18**: 565–587.
9. Lewis GRR, Mulchay K, Brook NR, Veitch PS, Nicholson ML. A prospective study of the predictive power of spiral CT angiography in delineating renal vascular anatomy for live donor nephrectomy. *BJU Int* 2004; **94**: 1077–1081.

10. Shaffer D, Sahyoun AI, Madras PN, Monaco AP. Two hundred one consecutive living-donor nephrectomies. *Arch Surg* 1998; **133**: 426–431.
11. Ratner LE, Ciseck LJ, Moore RG *et al*. Laparoscopic live donor nephrectomy. *Transplantation* 1995; **60**: 1047–1049.
12. Brown SL, Biehl TR, Rawlins MC, Hefty TR. Laparoscopic live donor nephrectomy: a comparison with the conventional open approach. *J Urol* 2001; **165**: 766–769.
13. Shafizadeh S, McEvoy JR, Murray C *et al*. Laparoscopic donor nephrectomy: impact on an established renal transplant program. *Am Surg* 2000; **66**: 1132–1135.
14. Pace KT, Dyer SJ, Phan V *et al*. Laparoscopic v open donor nephrectomy: a cost-utility analysis of the initial experience at a tertiary-care center. *J Endourol* 2002; **16**: 495–508.
15. Ratner LE, Hiller J, Sroka M *et al*. Laparoscopic live donor nephrectomy removes disincentives to live donation. *Transplant Proc* 1997; **29**: 3402–3403.
16. Ratner LE, Montgomery RA, Maley WR *et al*. Laparoscopic live donor nephrectomy: the recipient. *Transplantation* 2000; **69**: 2319–2323.
17. Finelli FC, Gongora E, Sasaki TM, Light JA. A survey: the prevalence of laparoscopic donor nephrectomy at large U.S. transplant centers. *Transplantation* 2001; **71**: 1862–1864.
18. Statistics prepared by UK Transplant Support Service Authority (UKTSSA) from the National Transplant Database maintained on behalf of the UK transplant community. 1999.
19. Fabrizio MD, Ratner LE, Montgomery RA, Kavoussi LR. Laparoscopic live donor nephrectomy. *Urol Clin North Am* 1999; **26**: 247–256, xi.
20. Gill IS, Uzzo RG, Hobart MG *et al*. Laparoscopic retroperitoneal live donor right nephrectomy for purposes of allotransplantation and autotransplantation. *J Urol* 2000; **164**: 1500–1504.
21. Hemal AK, Singh I. Minimally invasive retroperitoneoscopic live donor nephrectomy: point of technique. *Surg Laparosc Endosc Percutan Tech* 2001; **11**: 341–343.
22. Wolf Jr JS, Tchetgen MB, Merion RM. Hand-assisted laparoscopic live donor nephrectomy. *Urology* 1998; **52**: 885–887.
23. Batler RA, Schoor RA, Gonzalez CM *et al*. Hand-assisted laparoscopic radical nephrectomy: the experience of the inexperienced. *J Endourol* 2001; **15**: 513–516.
24. Slakey DP, Hahn JC, Rogers E *et al*. Single-center analysis of living donor nephrectomy: hand-assisted laparoscopic, pure laparoscopic, and traditional open. *Prog Transplant* 2002; **12**: 206–211.
25. Fadden PT, Nakada SY. Hand-assisted laparoscopic renal surgery. *Urol Clin North Am* 2001; **28**: 167–176, xi.
26. Buell JF, Hanaway MJ, Woodle ES. Maximizing renal artery length in right laparoscopic donor nephrectomy by retrocaval exposure of the aortorenal junction. *Transplantation* 2003; **75**: 83–85.
27. Kercher K, Dahl D, Harland R *et al*. Hand-assisted laparoscopic donor nephrectomy minimizes warm ischemia. *Urology* 2001; **58**: 152–156.
28. Wolf Jr JS, Merion RM, Leichtman AB *et al*. Randomized controlled trial of hand-assisted laparoscopic versus open surgical live donor nephrectomy. *Transplantation* 2001; **72**: 284–290.
29. Yang SC, Rha KH, Kim YS *et al*. Retroperitoneoscopy-assisted living donor nephrectomy: 109 cases. *Transplant Proc* 2001; **33**: 1104–1105.
30. Hoznek A, Olsson LE, Salomon L *et al*. Retroperitoneal laparoscopic living-donor nephrectomy. Preliminary results. *Eur Urol* 2001; **40**: 614–618.
31. Lind MY, Ijzermans JN, Bonjer HJ. Open vs laparoscopic donor nephrectomy in renal transplantation. *Transplantation* 2002; **89**: 162–168.
32. Chow GK, Prieto M, Bohorquez HE, Stegall MD. Hand-assisted laparoscopic donor nephrectomy for morbidly obese patients. *Transplant Proc* 2002; **34**: 728.
33. Kavoussi LR. Laparoscopic donor nephrectomy. *Kidney Int* 2000; **57**: 2175–2186.
34. Dunn MD, McDougall EM. Renal physiology: laparoscopic considerations. *Urol Clin North Am* 2000; **27**: 609–614.
35. Rosin D, Brasesco O, Varela J *et al*. Low-pressure laparoscopy may ameliorate intracranial hypertension and renal hypoperfusion. *J Laparoendosc Adv Surg Tech A* 2002; **12**: 15–19.
36. Waller JR, Hiley AL, Mullin EJ *et al*. Living kidney donation: a comparison of laparoscopic and conventional open operations. *Postgrad Med J* 2002; **78**: 153–157.

3.2.98 - Jeffrey Braithwaite 85.
- P/R bleed.
- HB. 12.2.
- BP. Pulse - (N).

37. Hazebroek EJ, Cappel dVtN, Gommers D *et al*. Antidiuretic hormone release during laparoscopic donor nephrectomy. *Arch Surg* 2002; **137**: 600–604.
38. Nogueira JM, Cangro CB, Fink JC *et al*. A comparison of recipient renal outcomes with laparoscopic versus open live donor nephrectomy. *Transplantation* 1999; **67**: 722–728.
39. London ET, Ho HS, Neuhaus AM *et al*. Effect of intravascular volume expansion on renal function during prolonged CO_2 pneumoperitoneum. *Ann Surg* 2000; **231**: 195–201.
40. Ruiz-Deya G, Cheng S, Palmer E *et al*. Open donor, laparoscopic donor and hand assisted laparoscopic donor nephrectomy: a comparison of outcomes. *J Urol* 2001; **166**: 1270–1273.
41. Ibrahim S, Jacobs F, Zukin Y *et al*. Immunohistochemical manifestations of unilateral kidney ischemia. *Clin Transplant* 1996; **10**: 646–652.
42. Shoskes DA, Parfrey NA, Halloran PF. Increased major histocompatibility complex antigen expression in unilateral ischemic acute tubular necrosis in the mouse. *Transplantation* 1990; **49**: 201–207.
43. Kim FJ, Ratner LE, Kavoussi LR. Renal transplantation: laparoscopic live donor nephrectomy. *Urol Clin North Am* 2000; **27**: 777–785.
44. Stifelman MD, Hull D, Sosa RE *et al*. Hand assisted laparoscopic donor nephrectomy: a comparison with the open approach. *J Urol* 2001; **166**: 444–448.
45. Berends FJ, den Hoed PT, Bonjer HJ *et al*. Technical considerations and pitfalls in laparoscopic live donor nephrectomy. *Surg Endosc* 2002; **16**: 893–898.
46. Montgomery RA, Kavoussi LR, Su L *et al*. Improved recipient results after 5 years of performing laparoscopic donor nephrectomy. *Transplant Proc* 2001; **33**: 1108–1110.
47. Philosophe B, Kuo PC, Schweitzer EJ *et al*. Laparoscopic versus open donor nephrectomy: comparing ureteral complications in the recipients and improving the laparoscopic technique. *Transplantation* 1999; **68**: 497–502.
48. Jacobs SC, Cho E, Dunkin BJ *et al*. Laparoscopic live donor nephrectomy: the University of Maryland 3-year experience. *J Urol* 2000; **164**: 1494–1499.
49. Hsu TH, Su LM, Ratner LE *et al*. Impact of renal artery multiplicity on outcomes of renal donors and recipients in laparoscopic donor nephrectomy. *Urology* 2003; **61**: 323–327.
50. Goldfarb DA. Are concerns over right laparoscopic donor nephrectomy unwarranted? *J Urol* 2001; **166**: 2558–2559.
51. Buell JF, Edye M, Johnson M *et al*. Are concerns over right laparoscopic donor nephrectomy unwarranted? *Ann Surg* 2001; **233**: 645–651.
52. Lind MY, Hazebroek EJ, Hop WC *et al*. Right-sided laparoscopic live-donor nephrectomy: is reluctance still justified? *Transplantation* 2002; **74**: 1045–1048.
53. Johnson MW, Andreoni K, McCoy L *et al*. Technique of right laparoscopic donor nephrectomy: a single center experience. *Am J Transplant* 2001; **1**: 293–295.
54. Meng MV, Freise CE, Kang SM *et al*. Techniques to optimize vascular control during laparoscopic donor nephrectomy. *Urology* 2003; **61**: 93–97.
55. Chow GK, Chan DY, Ratner LE, Kavoussi LR. Interaortocaval renal artery dissection for right laparoscopic donor nephrectomy. *Transplantation* 2001; **72**: 1458–1460.
56. Buell JF, Hanaway MJ, Potter SR *et al*. Hand-assisted laparoscopic living-donor nephrectomy as an alternative to traditional laparoscopic living-donor nephrectomy. *Am J Transplant* 2002; **2**: 983–988.
57. Mackey TJ, Flowers JL, Bartlett ST *et al*. Cost comparison of laparoscopic versus open donor nephrectomy analysing provider charges and productivity loss. *J Urol* 1997; **157**: 156.
58. Brook NR, Nicholson ML. An audit over 2 years' practice of open and laparoscopic live-donor nephrectomy at renal transplant centres in the UK and Ireland. *BJU Int* 2004; **93**: 1027–1031.
59. Nelson PW, Landreneau MD, Luger AM *et al*. Ten-year experience in transplantation of A2 kidneys into B and O recipients. *Transplantation* 1998; **65**: 256.
60. Nelson PW, Landreneau MD, Luger AM *et al*. Renal transplantation across the ABO barrier using A2 kidneys. *Transplantation* 1999; **67**: 1319.
61. Tanabe K, Tokumoto T, Ishida H *et al*. ABO-incompatible renal transplantation at Tokyo Women's Medical University. *Clin Transplant* 2003: 175–181.
62. Winters JL, Gloor JM, Pineda AA *et al*. Plasma exchange conditioning for ABO-incompatible renal transplantation. *J Clin Apheresis* 2004; **19**: 79–85.

63. Tarantino A. Why should we implement living donation in renal transplantation? *Clin Nephrol* 2000; **53**: 55–63.
64. Delmonico FL, Morrissey PE, Lipkowitz GS *et al*. Donor kidney exchanges. *Am J Transplant* 2004; **4**: 1628–1634.

Plate XV Laparoscopic view at right donor nephrectomy.

Plate XVI Laparoscopic view of the inter-aortocaval dissection, demonstrating the right renal artery. The vena cava is displaced anteriorly. Adventitia is being dissected from the artery with hook diathermy.

Jonathan Winehouse Irving Taylor

15

Recent randomised control trials in general surgery

Rapidly evolving technology and a greater scientific understanding of disease process are paving the way for major technological and management advancements in surgery. Surgical dogma as well as new treatment modalities should ideally be validated scientifically using well-designed randomised control trials. We have selected a number of randomised controlled trials in general surgery from the past year.

INGUINAL HERNIA

INGUINAL HERNIA REPAIR

Inguinal hernia repair is the most frequently performed operation in general surgery. Following the introduction of the Bassini repair in the late 19th century, the methods for inguinal hernia repair remained little changed for over a century until 1984 when the Lichtenstein Hernia Institute introduced open 'tension-free' hernioplasty using synthetic mesh.[1] This was followed in 1991 by laparoscopic mesh hernioplasty initially in the form of a transabdominal preperitoneal repair (TAPP) and later, in 1992, with a totally extraperitoneal repair (TEP) which potentially reduced the likelihood of intraperitoneal complications and adhesions.[2] A systematic review of relevant randomised controlled trials recently compared open with minimal access laparoscopic mesh techniques.[3] No difference in recurrence was observed

Jonathan Winehouse MSc FRCS
Lecturer and Honorary Registrar in Surgery, Royal Free and University College Medical School, Charles Bell House, 67–73 Riding House Street, London W1W 7EJ, UK (for correspondence)
E-mail: JWinehouse@aol.com

Irving Taylor MD ChM FRCS FMedSci FRCPS(Glas)Hon
Vice-Dean and Director of Clinical Studies, Royal Free and University College Medical School, Charles Bell House, 67–73 Riding House Street, London W1W 7EJ, UK

between laparoscopic and open mesh methods of hernia repair. Length of hospital stay also did not differ between groups. However, the data suggested less persisting pain and numbness following laparoscopic repair and an earlier return to daily activities equivalent to a mean of 7 days. Operation times were longer for the laparoscopic group. As anticipated, there appeared to be an increased risk of serious complications in respect of visceral (especially bladder) and vascular injuries with TAPP repair,[2–4] although some authors in their personal series have not reported similar findings.[5] However, Neumayer *et al.*[6] recently suggested that laparoscopic hernia repair carries a higher complication rate than open mesh repair with more common recurrences in the laparoscopic group (87 of 862 patients [10.1%]) than in the open group (41 of 834 patients [4.9%]; odds ratio, 2.2; 95% confidence interval, 1.5–3.2). Rates of recurrence after repair of recurrent hernias were similar (10.0% and 14.1%, respectively).

In 2001, the National Institute for Clinical Excellence (NICE) recommended that open mesh should be the preferred surgical procedure for the repair of primary inguinal hernias and that laparoscopic hernia repair using TEP should only be considered for bilateral or recurrent hernias.[7]

Key point 1

- Open Lichtenstein mesh repair and laparoscopic hernia repair carry similar low recurrence rates.

Key point 2

- Laparoscopic hernia repair compared to open repair reduces the time to resume normal daily activities.

Key point 3

- Totally extraperitoneal laparoscopic inguinal hernia repair (TEP) potentially reduces the likelihood of intraperitoneal complications and adhesions when compared to transabdominal preperitoneal inguinal hernia repair (TAPP).

Key point 4

- NICE currently recommends that open mesh should be the preferred surgical procedure for the repair of primary inguinal hernias and that laparoscopic hernia repair using TEP should only be considered for bilateral or recurrent hernias.

ANTIBIOTIC PROPHYLAXIS

ANTIBIOTIC PROPHYLAXIS IN INGUINAL HERNIA REPAIR

Seven randomised clinical trials where prophylaxis was compared to control groups having either hernioplasty or herniorraphy were identified. Using pooled and subgroup meta-analysis, there was no clear evidence that routine administration of antibiotic prophylaxis for elective inguinal hernia repair reduced infection rates.[8]

ANTIBIOTIC PROPHYLAXIS IN APPENDICECTOMY

The age-old question of whether prophylactic antibiotics reduce wound and intra-abdominal sepsis following appendicectomy appears to have been answered in this systematic review of 45 relevant randomised controlled and controlled clinical trials.[9] A total of 10,000 patients were included in this study and the authors concluded that antibiotic prophylaxis is superior to placebo in the prevention of wound and intra-abdominal sepsis following emergency appendicectomy and that the potential benefits appeared to be independent of the extent of the appendicitis or the timing of peri-operative antibiotic prophylaxis.[9]

> **Key point 5**
>
> - Antibiotic prophylaxis reduces the risk of wound and intra-abdominal sepsis following emergency appendicectomy.

COLORECTAL SURGERY

MECHANICAL BOWEL PREPARATION

Pre-operative mechanical bowel preparation has been considered an effective remedy against postoperative anastomotic leak in elective colorectal surgery. To date, this belief has not been scientifically tested. In a systematic review of six randomised control trials where patients were randomly assigned to mechanical bowel preparation versus no preparation, no difference in leak rate was found between either group both for low anterior resections and for large bowel anastomosis overall. Complication rates were also similar.[10]

PROPHYLACTIC HEPATIC ARTERIAL CHEMOTHERAPY IN COLON CANCER

The liver is the most frequent site of recurrence following curative resection in advanced colon cancer with 83% of patients developing one or more liver metastasis.[11,12] Taylor *et al.*[13] reported that infusion of 5-fluorouracil (5-FU) into the portal vein in the peri-operative period resulted in significant reduction of postoperative liver metastasis in patients undergoing colonic resection for colon cancer.[14,15] In a recent randomised control trial of prophylactic hepatic arterial infusion (HAI) chemotherapy for the prevention of liver metastasis in patients with colon cancer,[16] 316 patients with pre-operative stage II and stage III colon cancer (TMN Classification 1997) received either surgery alone or a continuous 3-week course of 5-FU via HAI on an intention-to-treat basis. Results for stage II disease were equivocal; however, for stage III colon cancer there was a significant reduction in disease ($P = 0.0009$) and liver metastasis-free ($P = 0.0002$) and overall survival ($P = 0.002$). However, beyond 3 weeks, adjuvant chemotherapy was not dictated by the study and, therefore, the results need to be interpreted with some caution.

STAPLED (CIRCULAR) HAEMORROIDECTOMY

Despite initial excitement at the introduction of stapled (circular) haemorroidectomy, results do not appear to bear out enthusiasm for this new procedure. In a randomised controlled trial evaluating surgical and functional outcome of day-case stapled (circular) versus diathermy haemorroidectomy,[17] no difference was observed between groups for postoperative morbidity and time to return to work. Other studies[18–21] and current NICE guidelines[22] have suggested that time to return to work is more favourable for stapled (circular) haemorroidectomy but the authors of this paper advise caution in the interpretation of their results given their small trial numbers (n = 60).[17] Postoperative pain was significantly lower in the stapled (circular) versus diathermy group (median 1.88, range 0.1–4.8 versus 4.3, range 1.4–6.2 95 per cent CI difference medians, 1.15–3.85, P = 0.0002, Mann-Whitney U-test); however, 7 of the 30 patients assigned to the stapled (circular) haemorroidectomy group compared to one patient in the diathermy group necessitated further operative treatment within one year. In a further paper that considered minimum long-term follow-up at 33 months, overall satisfaction, continence and quality of life appeared to be equally effective with both techniques;[23] however, other authors have reported significant long-term morbidity of stapled (circular) haemorroidectomy.[24]

Key point 6

- It is currently unclear whether stapled (circular) haemorroidectomy carries any benefit over standard diathermy haemorroidectomy.

MULTIMODAL OPTIMISATION OF SURGICAL CARE

In this study, 25 patients undergoing elective colectomies were randomised to receive either multimodal or standard peri-operative surgical care. Both groups were similar for age and POSSUM (Physiological and Operative Severity Score for the enUmeration of Mortality and Morbidity). Optimisation significantly reduced hospital stay (3 versus 7 days; P = 0.02) and improve a patient's physiological and physical function.[25]

MODULATION OF PHYSIOLOGICAL RESPONSE BY EARLY BURN EXCISION

Two study groups (n = 35) of severely (full-thickness) burned children were randomised to either early skin burn excision (< 24 h; n = 20) versus conservative management and delayed skin burn excision (> 6 days; n = 15). Acute-phase and anabolic hormone levels were measured. Early burn wound excision abrogated hyper metabolic and hormonal responses in paediatric patients.[26]

BREAST SURGERY

BREAST-CONSERVING SURGERY WITH OR WITHOUT RADIOTHERAPY

A pooled analysis of published randomised clinical trials compared radiotherapy versus no radiotherapy after breast-conserving surgery. The outcomes studied were ipsilateral breast tumour recurrence and patient death from any cause. Fifteen trials with a pooled total of 9422 patients were available for analysis. The relative risk of ipsilateral breast tumour recurrence after breast-conserving surgery, comparing patients treated with no radiotherapy or radiotherapy, was 3.00 (95% CI = 2.65–3.40). Mortality data were available from 13 trials with a pooled total of 8206 patients. The relative risk of mortality was 1.086 (95% CI = 1.003–1.175), corresponding to an estimated 8.6% (95% CI = 0.3–17.5%) relative excess mortality if radiotherapy was omitted. The authors conclude that omission of radiotherapy was associated with a large increase in risk of ipsilateral breast tumour recurrence and with a small increase in the risk of patient mortality.[27]

Key point 7

- Adjuvant radiotherapy reduces the risk of breast recurrence following breast-conserving surgery.

SENTINEL LYMPH NODE BIOPSY

There is a vast amount of evidence in support of sentinel lymph node biopsy as an accurate predictor of lymph node status.[28–31] In a recent randomised control trial,[32] the efficacy and safety of sentinel-node biopsy was tested. A total of 516 patients with primary breast cancer in whom the tumour was ≤ 2 cm in diameter were randomised either to sentinel-node biopsy and total axillary dissection (the axillary-dissection group) or to sentinel-node biopsy followed by axillary dissection only if the sentinel node contained metastases (the sentinel-node group). A sentinel node was positive in 83 of the 257 patients in the axillary-dissection group (32.3%), and in 92 of the 259 patients in the sentinel-node group (35.5%). In the axillary-dissection group, the overall accuracy of the sentinel-node status was 96.9%, the sensitivity 91.2%, and the specificity 100%. There was less pain and better arm mobility in the patients who underwent sentinel-node biopsy only than in those who also underwent axillary dissection. Among the 167 patients who did not undergo axillary dissection, there were no cases of overt axillary metastasis during follow-up. The authors concluded that sentinel-node biopsy is a safe and accurate method of screening the axillary nodes for metastasis in women with a small breast cancer.

Key point 8

- Sentinel lymph node biopsy is an accurate (96.9%) predictor of axillary node status in small breast cancers and may be a very valuable diagnostic tool in patients in whom the value of axillary dissection is questionable. Longer-term studies are needed to demonstrate its safety and define its clinical role.

There was a reported false-negative group (n = 8) in the axillary dissection group (n = 257).[32] Although two of these patients had subcapsular micrometastasis, which is of doubtful clinical significance, one should be cautious to advise sentinel node biopsy as a substitute for the current gold standard axillary dissection outside of clinical trials on the basis of this and other papers.[28–31] However, in patients in whom the value of axillary dissection is questionable, sentinel lymph node biopsy maybe a very valuable diagnostic tool.

HEPATOBILIARY AND PANCREATIC SURGERY

ENTERAL VERSUS PARENTERAL NUTRITION FOR ACUTE PANCREATITIS

Surgical dogma has dictated that patients with acute pancreatitis remain nil-by-mouth in order to 'rest the pancreas' until the acute phase of their illness has subsided. However, acute pancreatitis creates a catabolic stress state that promotes nutritional deterioration. Total parenteral nutrition (TPN) provides exogenous nutrients and has become the mainstay of nutritional supportive treatment in patients with severe acute pancreatitis. It remains unclear whether patients with acute pancreatitis may actually benefit from early enteral nutrition (EN). This systematic review of randomised clinical trials in patients with acute pancreatitis compared the effects of TPN and EN on mortality, morbidity and length of hospital stay. Two trials with a total of 70 participants were included. The relative risk (RR) for death with EN versus TPN was 0.56 (95% CI, 0.05–5.62). RR for systemic infection with EN versus TPN was 0.61 (95% CI, 0.29–1.28). In one trial, RR for local septic complications and other local complications with EN versus TPN was 0.56 (95% CI, 0.12–2.68) and 0.16 (95% CI, 0.01–2.86), respectively. Mean length of hospital stay was reduced with EN (WMD –2.20, 95% CI, –3.62 to –0.78). Although there is a trend towards reduction in the adverse outcomes of acute pancreatitis after administration of EN, there was insufficient data to draw firm conclusions about the effectiveness and safety of EN versus TPN in acute pancreatitis.[33]

RESECTABLE PANCREATIC ADENOCARCINOMA

Randomised prospective trials have addressed various treatment approaches to pancreatic adenocarcinoma in order to try to improve the dismal prognosis associated with this disease. Surgical studies have demonstrated that morbidity and mortality are similar for pylorus-preserving (either as single[34] or double layer[35] end-to-side pancreatojejunostomy with duct stent) pancreato-duodenectomy and classic Whipple's[36] pancreaticoduodenectomy. Extended retroperitoneal lymphadenectomy can be performed with similar mortality but has increased morbidity compared with standard pancreaticoduodenectomy and does not prolong survival. Pancreatic-enteric anastomosis is associated with lower rates of pancreatic fistula and endocrine insufficiency than duct occlusion without anastomosis. However, a considerable source of morbidity and mortality is related to the integrity of the pancreatic-enteric anastomosis. Pancreatico-gastrostomy and pancreaticojejunostomy appear to be comparable techniques for pancreatic duct reconstruction. An end-to-side/duct –to-mucosa technique for pancreaticjejunal reconstruction can be performed safely with a lower rate of anastomotic dehiscence relative to that of the end-to-end/invaginating pancreaticojejunostomy.[37]

Intraperitoneal drainage after pancreatic resection is unwarranted and may contribute to intra-abdominal complications.[38] Routine use of prophylactic octreotide does not lower the rate of pancreatic fistula.[39] Chemoradiation after resection has failed to show a survival advantage over surgery alone.[40–45] Surgical resection remains the only potentially curative therapy for adenocarcinoma of the pancreas. There is still no clear indication as to a single preferable resection approach.[37]

Key point 9

- Pylorus-preserving pancreatoduodenectomy and classic Whipple's pancreaticoduodenectomy carry similar morbidity and mortality rates. There is still no clear indication as to a single preferable resection approach.

Key point 10

- Pancreatic-enteric anastomosis is associated with lower rates of pancreatic fistula and endocrine insufficiency than duct occlusion without anastomosis.

Key point 11

- Pancreaticogastrostomy and pancreaticojejunostomy appear to be comparable techniques for pancreatic duct reconstruction.

Key point 12

- Chemoradiation after resection of pancreatic carcinoma has failed to show a survival advantage over surgery alone.

UPPER GASTROINTESTINAL SURGERY

NEOADJUVANT CHEMORADIATION AND SURGERY VERSUS SURGERY ALONE FOR RESECTABLE OESOPHAGEAL CANCER

Oesophageal cancer carries a poor prognosis with surgery offering the only hope of a complete cure with long-term survival exceeding 20% in some series.[46–48] Micrometastatic disease not amenable to surgery is often present at initial presentation. Neoadjuvant chemoradiation with surgery may, therefore, improve survival; however, treatment morbidity remains a concern. In addition, chemoradiation may down-stage cancers that would otherwise not be amenable to surgery.[49,50]

A meta-analysis of randomised controlled trials (RCTs) compared the use of neoadjuvant chemoradiation and surgery with the use of surgery alone for oesophageal cancer.[51] Outcomes included survival, rate of complete (R0) resection, operative mortality, anastomotic leaks, and cancer recurrence. A random-effects model was used and the odds ratio (OR) was the principal measure of effect. A systematic quantitative review for outcomes unique to the neoadjuvant chemoradiation treatment group, such as pathological complete response has been carried out. Nine RCTs that included 1116 patients were selected with quality scores ranging from 1 to 3 (5-point Jadad scale). Odds ratio (95% CI; *P* value), expressed as chemoradiation and surgery versus surgery alone (treatment versus control; values < 1 favour the chemoradiation-surgery arm), was 0.79 (95% CI, 0.59–1.06; *P* = 0.12) for 1-year survival, 0.77 (95% CI, 0.56–1.05; *P* = 0.10) for 2-year survival, 0.66 (95% CI, 0.47–0.92; *P* = 0.016) for 3-year survival, 2.50 (95% CI, 1.05–5.96; *P* = 0.038) for rate of resection, 0.53 (95% CI, 0.33–0.84; *P* = 0.007) for rate of complete resection, 1.72 (95% CI, 0.96–3.07; *P* = 0.07) for operative mortality, 1.63 (95% CI, 0.99–2.68; *P* = 0.053) for all treatment mortality, 0.38 (95% CI, 0.23–0.63; *P* = 0.0002) for locoregional cancer recurrence, 0.88 (95% CI, 0.55–1.41; *P* = 0.60) for distant cancer recurrence, and 0.47 (95% CI, 0.16–1.45; *P* = 0.19) for all cancer recurrence. A complete pathological response to chemoradiation occurred in 21% of patients. The 3-year survival benefit was most pronounced when chemotherapy and radiotherapy were given concurrently (OR 0.45, 95% CI 0.26–0.79, *P* = 0.005) instead of sequentially (OR 0.82, 95% CI 0.54–1.25, *P* = 0.36). Compared with surgery alone, neoadjuvant chemoradiation and surgery improved 3-year survival and reduced locoregional cancer recurrence. Patients treated with surgery alone were more likely to undergo an oesophageal resection than those treated with chemoradiation and surgery (OR 2.50, 95% CI 1.05–5.96; *P* = 0.038); however, those patients having combination treatment had a higher rate of complete (R0) resection (OR 0.53, 95% CI 0.33–0.84; *P* = 0.007). There was no significant trend toward increased treatment mortality with neoadjuvant chemoradiation. Concurrent administration of neoadjuvant chemotherapy and radiotherapy was superior to sequential chemoradiation treatment scheduling.

Key point 13

- Compared with surgery alone, neoadjuvant chemoradiation and surgery improved 3-year survival and reduced local-regional cancer recurrence in oesophageal cancer.

Key point 14

- There was a higher rate of complete (R0) resection in patients undergoing neoadjuvant chemoradiation and surgery versus surgery alone in oesophageal cancer.

MELANOMA

EXCISION MARGIN IN HIGH-RISK MELANOMA

The necessary margin of excision for cutaneous melanoma with a depth of 2 mm or greater is unknown. A randomised clinical trial compared 1 cm and 3 cm margins in patients with melanomas over 2 mm in depth.[52] Of the 900 patients who were enrolled, 453 were randomly assigned to undergo surgery with a 1 cm margin of excision and 447 with a 3-cm margin of excision with a median follow-up of 60 months. A 1 cm margin of excision was associated with a significantly increased risk of locoregional recurrence. There were 168 locoregional recurrences (as first events) in the group with 1-cm margins of excision, as compared with 142 in the group with 3-cm margins (hazard ratio, 1.26; 95% CI, 1.00–1.59; $P = 0.05$). In all, 128 deaths were attributable to melanoma in the 1-cm margin group, as compared with 105 in the 3-cm margin group (hazard ratio, 1.24; 95% CI, 0.96–1.61; $P = 0.1$); overall survival was similar in the two groups (hazard ratio for death, 1.07; 95% CI, 0.85–1.36; $P = 0.6$). A 1-cm margin of excision for melanoma with a poor prognosis (as defined by a tumour thickness of at least 2 mm) is associated with a significantly greater risk of regional recurrence than is a 3-cm margin, but overall survival rates were similar in both groups.

Key point 15

- In patients with melanoma greater than 2 mm in depth, a 3-cm margin is recommended to avoid the risk of local recurrence.

Key points for clinical practice

- Open Lichtenstein mesh repair and laparoscopic hernia repair carry similar low recurrence rates.
- Laparoscopic hernia repair compared to open repair reduces the time to resume normal daily activities.
- Totally extraperitoneal laparoscopic inguinal hernia repair (TEP) potentially reduces the likelihood of intraperitoneal complications and adhesions when compared to transabdominal preperitoneal inguinal hernia repair (TAPP).
- NICE currently recommends that open mesh should be the preferred surgical procedure for the repair of primary inguinal hernias and that laparoscopic hernia repair using TEP should only be considered for bilateral or recurrent hernias.
- Antibiotic prophylaxis reduces the risk of wound and intra-abdominal sepsis following emergency appendicectomy.
- It is currently unclear whether stapled (circular) haemorroidectomy carries any benefit over standard diathermy haemorroidectomy.
- Adjuvant radiotherapy reduces the risk of breast recurrence following breast-conserving surgery.
- Sentinel lymph node biopsy is an accurate (96.9%) predictor of axillary node status in small breast cancers and may be a very valuable diagnostic tool in patients in whom the value of axillary dissection is questionable. Longer-term studies are needed to demonstrate its safety and define its clinical role.

Key points for clinical practice

- Pylorus-preserving pancreatoduodenectomy and classic Whipple's pancreaticoduodenectomy carry similar morbidity and mortality rates. There is still no clear indication as to a single preferable resection approach.
- Pancreatic-enteric anastomosis is associated with lower rates of pancreatic fistula and endocrine insufficiency than duct occlusion without anastomosis.
- Pancreaticogastrostomy and pancreaticojejunostomy appear to be comparable techniques for pancreatic duct reconstruction.
- Chemoradiation after resection of pancreatic carcinoma has failed to show a survival advantage over surgery alone.
- Compared with surgery alone, neoadjuvant chemoradiation and surgery improved 3-year survival and reduced local-regional cancer recurrence in oesophageal cancer.
- There was a higher rate of complete (R0) resection in patients undergoing neoadjuvant chemoradiation and surgery versus surgery alone in oesophageal cancer.
- In patients with melanoma greater than 2 mm in depth, a 3-cm margin is recommended to avoid the risk of local recurrence.

References

1. Lichtenstein IL, Shulman AG, Amid PK, Montllor MM. The tension-free hernioplasty. *Am J Surg* 1989; **157**: 188–193.
2. Felix EL, Michas CA, Gonzalez Jr MH. Laparoscopic hernioplasty. TAPP vs TEP. *Surg Endosc* 1995; **9**: 984–989.
3. McCormack K, Scott NW, Go PM, Ross S, Grant AM. Laparoscopic techniques versus open techniques for inguinal hernia repair. *Cochrane Database System Rev* 2003(1): CD001785.
4. Collaboration EH. Laparoscopic compared with open methods of groin hernia repair: systematic review of randomized controlled trials. *Br J Surg* 2000; **87**: 860–867.
5. Douek M, Smith G, Oshowo A, Stoker DL, Wellwood JM. Prospective randomised controlled trial of laparoscopic versus open inguinal hernia mesh repair: five year follow up. *BMJ* 2003; **326**: 1012–1013.
6. Neumayer L, Giobbie-Hurder A, Jonasson O *et al*. Open mesh versus laparoscopic mesh repair of inguinal hernia. *N Engl J Med* 2004; **350**: 1819–1827.
7. NICE. *Guidance on the use of laparoscopic surgery for inguinal hernia*. London: National Institution for Clinical Excellence, 2001.
8. Sanchez-Manuel FJ, Seco-Gil JL. Antibiotic prophylaxis for hernia repair. *Cochrane Database System Rev* 2003(2): CD003769.
9. Andersen BR, Kallehave FL, Andersen HK. Antibiotics versus placebo for prevention of postoperative infection after appendicectomy. *Cochrane Database System Rev* 2003(2): CD001439.
10. Guenaga KF, Matos D, Castro AA, Atallah AN, Wille-Jorgensen P. Mechanical bowel preparation for elective colorectal surgery. *Cochrane Database System Rev* 2003(2): CD001544.
11. Weiss LG, Torhorst J *et al*. Haematogenous metastatic patterns in colonic carcinoma: an analysis of 1541 necropsies. *J Pathol* 1986; **150**: 195–203.

12. Jemal A, Thomas A, Murray A, Thun M. Cancer statistics. *CA Cancer J Clin* 2002; **52**: 23–47.
13. Taylor I, Machin D, Mullee D, Trotter G, Cooke T, West C. A randomised control trial of adjuvant portal vein cytotoxic perfusion in colorectal cancer. *Br J Surg* 1985; **72**: 359–363.
14. Wolmark N, Rockette H, Wickerham DL *et al*. Adjuvant therapy of Dukes' A, B, and C adenocarcinoma of the colon with portal-vein fluorouracil hepatic infusion: preliminary results of National Surgical Adjuvant Breast and Bowel Project Protocol C-02. *J Clin Oncol* 1990; **8**: 1466–1475.
15. Beart Jr RW, Moertel CG, Wieand HS *et al*. Adjuvant therapy for resectable colorectal carcinoma with fluorouracil administered by portal vein infusion. A study of the Mayo Clinic and the North Central Cancer Treatment Group. *Arch Surg* 1990; **125**: 897–901.
16. Sadahiro S, Suzuki T, Ishikawa K *et al*. Prophylactic hepatic arterial infusion chemotherapy for the prevention of liver metastasis in patients with colon carcinoma: a randomized control trial. *Cancer* 2004; **100**: 590–597.
17. Kairaluoma M, Nuorva K, Kellokumpu I. Day-case stapled (circular) vs. diathermy hemorrhoidectomy: a randomized, controlled trial evaluating surgical and functional outcome. *Dis Colon Rectum* 2003; **46**: 93–99.
18. Rowsell M, Bello M, Hemingway DM. Circumferential mucosectomy (stapled haemorrhoidectomy) versus conventional haemorrhoidectomy: randomised controlled trial. *Lancet* 2000; **355**: 779–781.
19. Ho YH, Cheong WK, Tsang C *et al*. Stapled hemorrhoidectomy – cost and effectiveness. Randomized, controlled trial including incontinence scoring, anorectal manometry, and endoanal ultrasound assessments at up to three months. *Dis Colon Rectum* 2000; **43**: 1666–1675.
20. Shalaby R, Desoky A. Randomized clinical trial of stapled versus Milligan-Morgan haemorrhoidectomy. *Br J Surg* 2001; **88**: 1049–1053.
21. Ganio E, Altomare DF, Gabrielli F, Milito G, Canuti S. Prospective randomized multicentre trial comparing stapled with open haemorrhoidectomy. *Br J Surg* 2001; **88**: 669–674.
22. NICE. *Circular stapled haemorroidectomy*. London: National Institute for Clinical Excellence, 2003.
23. Smyth EF, Baker RP, Wilken BJ, Hartley JE, White TJ, Monson JR. Stapled versus excision haemorrhoidectomy: long-term follow up of a randomised controlled trial. *Lancet* 2003; **361**: 1437–1438.
24. Rowsell M, Bello M, Hemingway DM. Pain after stapled haemorrhoidectomy. *Lancet* 2000; **356**: 2188; author reply 2190.
25. Anderson AD, McNaught CE, MacFie J, Tring I, Barker P, Mitchell CJ. Randomized clinical trial of multimodal optimization and standard perioperative surgical care. *Br J Surg* 2003; **90**: 1497–1504.
26. Barret JP, Herndon DN. Modulation of inflammatory and catabolic responses in severely burned children by early burn wound excision in the first 24 hours. *Arch Surg* 2003; **138**: 127–132.
27. Vinh-Hung V, Verschraegen C. Breast-conserving surgery with or without radiotherapy: pooled-analysis for risks of ipsilateral breast tumor recurrence and mortality. *J Natl Cancer Inst* 2004; **96**): 115–121.
28. Keshtgar MR, Ell PJ. Clinical role of sentinel-lymph-node biopsy in breast cancer. *Lancet Oncol* 2002; **3**: 105–110.
29. Giuliano AE, Kirgan DM, Guenther JM, Morton DL. Lymphatic mapping and sentinel lymphadenectomy for breast cancer. *Ann Surg* 1994; **220**: 391–398; discussion 398–401.
30. Krag D, Weaver D, Ashikaga T *et al*. The sentinel node in breast cancer – a multicenter validation study. *N Engl J Med* 1998; **339**: 941–946.
31. Veronesi U, Paganelli G, Galimberti V *et al*. Sentinel-node biopsy to avoid axillary dissection in breast cancer with clinically negative lymph-nodes. *Lancet* 1997; **349**: 1864–1867.
32. Veronesi U, Paganelli G, Viale G *et al*. A randomized comparison of sentinel-node biopsy with routine axillary dissection in breast cancer. *N Engl J Med* 2003; **349**: 546–553.
33. Al-Omran M, Groof A, Wilke D. Enteral versus parenteral nutrition for acute pancreatitis. *Cochrane Database System Rev* 2003(1): CD002837.

34. Lin PW, Lin YJ. Prospective randomized comparison between pylorus-preserving and standard pancreaticoduodenectomy. *Br J Surg* 1999; **86**: 603–607.
35. Seiler CA, Wagner M, Schaller B, Sadowski C, Kulli C, Buchler MW. [Pylorus preserving or classical Whipple operation in tumors. Initial clinical results of a prospective randomized study]. *Swiss Surg* 2000; **6**: 275–282.
36. Whipple A. Present-day surgery of the pancreas. *N Engl J Med* 1942; **226**: 515–518.
37. Stojadinovic A, Brooks A, Hoos A, Jaques DP, Conlon KC, Brennan MF. An evidence-based approach to the surgical management of resectable pancreatic adenocarcinoma. *J Am Coll Surg* 2003; **196**: 954–964.
38. Conlon KC, Labow D, Leung D *et al.* Prospective randomized clinical trial of the value of intraperitoneal drainage after pancreatic resection. *Ann Surg* 2001; **234**: 487–493; discussion 493–494.
39. Li-Ling J, Irving M. Somatostatin and octreotide in the prevention of postoperative pancreatic complications and the treatment of enterocutaneous pancreatic fistulas: a systematic review of randomized controlled trials. *Br J Surg* 2001; **88**: 190–199.
40. Kalser MH, Ellenberg SS. Pancreatic cancer. Adjuvant combined radiation and chemotherapy following curative resection. *Arch Surg* 1985; **120**: 899–903.
41. Gastrointestinal Tumor Study Group. Further evidence of effective adjuvant combined radiation and chemotherapy following curative resection of pancreatic cancer. *Cancer* 1987; **59**: 2006–2010.
42. Bakkevold KE, Arnesjo B, Dahl O, Kambestad B. Adjuvant combination chemotherapy (AMF) following radical resection of carcinoma of the pancreas and papilla of Vater – results of a controlled, prospective, randomised multicentre study. *Eur J Cancer* 1993; **29A**: 698–703.
43. Klinkenbijl JH, Jeekel J, Sahmoud T *et al.* Adjuvant radiotherapy and 5-fluorouracil after curative resection of cancer of the pancreas and periampullary region: phase III trial of the EORTC gastrointestinal tract cancer cooperative group. *Ann Surg* 1999; **230**: 776–782; discussion 782–784.
44. Neoptolemos JP, Dunn JA, Stocken DD *et al.* Adjuvant chemoradiotherapy and chemotherapy in resectable pancreatic cancer: a randomised controlled trial. *Lancet* 2001; **358**: 1576–1585.
45. Neoptolemos JP, Stocken DD, Dunn JA *et al.* Influence of resection margins on survival for patients with pancreatic cancer treated by adjuvant chemoradiation and/or chemotherapy in the ESPAC-1 randomized controlled trial. *Ann Surg* 2001; **234**: 758–768.
46. Nigro JJ, DeMeester SR, Hagen JA *et al.* Node status in transmural esophageal adenocarcinoma and outcome after en bloc esophagectomy. *J Thorac Cardiovasc Surg* 1999; **117**: 960–968.
47. Lerut T, Coosemans W, De Leyn P, Decker G, Deneffe G, Van Raemdonck D. Is there a role for radical esophagectomy? *Eur J Cardiothorac Surg* 1999; **16 (Suppl 1)**: S44–S47.
48. Ando N, Ozawa S, Kitagawa Y, Shinozawa Y, Kitajima M. Improvement in the results of surgical treatment of advanced squamous esophageal carcinoma during 15 consecutive years. *Ann Surg* 2000; **232**: 225–232.
49. Lehnert T. Multimodal therapy for squamous carcinoma of the oesophagus. *Br J Surg* 1999; **86**: 727–739.
50. Geh JI, Crellin AM, Glynne-Jones R. Preoperative (neoadjuvant) chemoradiotherapy in oesophageal cancer. *Br J Surg* 2001; **88**: 338–356.
51. Urschel JD, Vasan H. A meta-analysis of randomized controlled trials that compared neoadjuvant chemoradiation and surgery to surgery alone for resectable esophageal cancer. *Am J Surg* 2003; **185**: 538–543.
52. Thomas JM, Newton-Bishop J, A'Hern R *et al.* Excision margins in high-risk malignant melanoma. *N Engl J Med* 2004; **350**: 757–766.

Index